Rose Prince is a freelance food journali[...] appears regularly in the *Daily Telegraph*, [...] *Independent on Sunday* and the *Spectator*. She has contributed to the *Food Programme*, *Woman's Hour* and *You & Yours* on BBC Radio 4. In 1999 she co-produced *In the Footsteps of Elizabeth David*, a two-hour film for Channel 4 presented by Chris Patten. *The New English Kitchen* is her first book. She lives in London with her husband, the journalist Dominic Prince, and their two children.

From the reviews of *The New English Kitchen*:

'If I am to be a good cook, by which I also mean a thinking cook, then it must mean more than making stock, saving my Parmesan rinds for soup and recycling my organic milk cartons. It may mean sometimes having to rethink the way I shop as well. With *The New English Kitchen* I have a blueprint with which to go forward.'
NIGEL SLATER, *Observer*

'A subtly transformative work.'
BEE WILSON, *TLS*

'A revolutionary new book. Prince has travelled around Britain and investigated food origins, learning from farmers, growers and specialist retailers. The insights she has gleaned are illuminating and often wittily expressed.'
JOANNA BLYTHMAN, *Ecologist*

'This is a notable first book from a respected journalist, a breath of fresh air, exuding good sense and full of unpretentious, desirably do-able recipes.'
PHILIPPA DAVENPORT, *Financial Times* Books of the Year

'A cookbook with a difference. I instantly warmed to its readability, fierce intelligence and admirable sense of economy. Practical, thoughtful and down-to-earth, this is a cookbook that prefers morals to morels.'
CHRIS HIRST, *Independent*

'No one bears Mrs Beeton's mantle better.'
The Economist

'This is a book for the stomach, from the heart. It passes the basic test that distinguishes a serious cookery book from a mass-production one. Pick it up just after you have had a very good lunch and you will immediately feel hungry again. Her prose takes on a shy songbird's lyricism.'

BRUCE ANDERSON, *Spectator*

'This is a gently riveting read that needs little embellishment. The chapters on bread, meat and fish are fascinating and the tone throughout authoritative and intimate.' *Daily Telegraph*

'Impassioned, principled and packed with practical and inspiring recipes. It is the antithesis of some extravagant big-name cookery books.' *Independent*

'The freshness is in her connections between sourcing, buying properly and knowing where the ingredients come from, and common-sense, delicious recipes.' *Mail on Sunday*

'An exceptional new cookbook.' *Sunday Telegraph*

'Rose Prince is a cook after my own heart, and her first book is one to put on the shelf.' *Country Life*

'Her information is accurate and deftly communicated; her recipes are inventive and homely.' *Daily Mail*

'She takes seriously the provenance of food, how it has been reared, grown, caught or harvested. One feature is the outmoded but crucial element of thrift. Prince recognises that if you pay a king's ransom for your organic chicken, then you want to make it go as far as possible. To add to its merit, the book is finely produced, with measurements in imperial as well as metric.' *The Tablet*

'This is a timely book with a practical and economical approach to sourcing and cooking top-quality, locally produced food.'

London *Evening Standard*

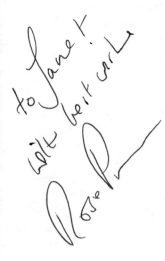

the new english kitchen

changing the way you shop, cook and eat

rose prince

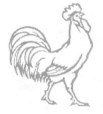

photography by
giacomo bretzel

FOURTH ESTATE • *London*

to dominic

First published in Great Britain in 2005 by
Fourth Estate
An imprint of HarperCollins*Publishers*
77–85 Fulham Palace Road
London W6 8JB
www.4thestate.co.uk

This edition first published in Great Britain in 2006
by Fourth Estate

1

A catalogue record for this book is
available from the British Library

ISBN-13 978-0-00-715659-7
ISBN-10 0-00-715659-6

Printed in Great Britain by Clays Ltd, St Ives plc

contents

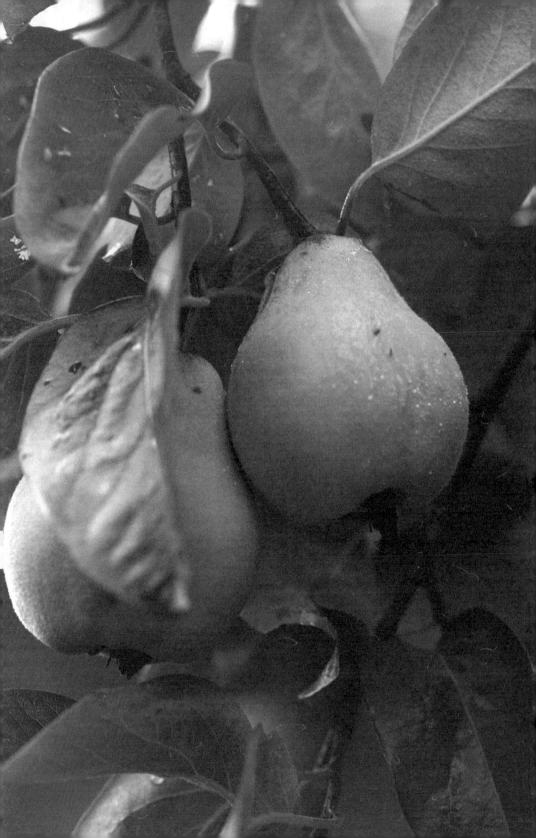

introduction

When you eat a langoustine, it gives you a present of its shell. Take that shell, toast it in a pan with some others, then boil in water – and you have a broth. That broth becomes one to pour over rice noodles with spices . . . You bought something good for a meal and it gave you two things good.

This simple idea not only enables you to eat well – twice – but is also a solution to the contemporary kitchen dilemma: how to make better-quality food something everyone can eat every day. This is possible not only through clever recycling – making, say, roast chicken leftovers into stock and so bringing to the table a second dish of risotto plus a third of smooth vegetable soup – but also by finding economical ways of buying the best, such as buying direct from farms using home delivery, or scouting vegetable stalls for good deals on seasonally abundant vegetables.

The New English Kitchen was born of a furious determination to connect the paths of two parallel stories. The first is a happy tale of lovely food, made using good recipes created by television chefs. It has been hard to ignore the cookery boom in all its guises. Up front, the message is all-embracing: *consume*, and choose what you want; it is all there in the lifestyle pages of the weekend supplements for the taking, cooking and eating.

The second story is unsettling. Looking regularly at the daily papers, it is clear that there is something wrong: the food chain is in crisis. Resources have buckled under consumer and retailer pressure to produce cheap food. Unpleasant stories emerge about food-related diseases in livestock and humans; UK farming faces financial ruin, the global market unfair, food is adulterated with chemicals and a growing number of children so unhealthy due to overeating fatty, sugary food that their parents may well outlive them. Rarely does a week pass without headlines reporting more trouble in the food industry.

Flick back to the recipe feature in the magazine – and to be quite frank you could be on another planet. Enjoy! Chargrill some more tiger prawns – to hell with the devastating effect warm-water prawn farming has had on the mangrove forests! Teriyaki another chicken breast – never mind where it comes from!

But beyond the headlines, there is a fledgling army of farmers, food producers, campaigners and food writers who are giving food and cookery back their integrity. More vital still is the consumer who wants to buy the best in order to eat well every day. This book is for you. It will help your good intentions into practical reality, proving that sustained good eating *need not* use up all your money and time.

The New English Kitchen's philosophy could equally be applied in Scotland, Wales, Ireland, the United States of America, Australia and Canada. It already exists in many European countries where the culture of home cooking has not faltered over the generations in the way that it has here. Focusing on English food was not an attempt to narrow the style but to broaden it, taking on the incredible variety of foods available in this province. True English food has always gone far beyond the Mrs Beeton concept of plain food economically produced. The national cuisine may be fossilised in people's minds as pies, roasts and nursery puddings, but there is now no reason why it could not include the rice noodle dishes of Southeast Asia or the delicious food of the Mediterranean. This is after all a country with a five-hundred-year-old history of food piracy: borrowing ideas from other shores, importing their raw materials and learning to cultivate them in our own soil, or rear new animal species on our pastures.

Then there is the impact of the last 50 years' food writing tradition. Without the great, inspirational books of those very English writers, Constance Spry, Elizabeth David and Jane Grigson, the good food renaissance would have been snail-pace slow. Multiculturalism and affordable worldwide travel have conspired to make English food in the 21st century more interesting still. So among the recipes in *The New English Kitchen* you will find pilaffs and soufflés, noodle soups and pasta dishes. They have every right to be considered as English as beef and Dover sole. There is one proviso: as far as possible, all the recipes must make use of UK-grown ingredients.

UK specialist and artisan food producers face a tough future, and in England the situation is uniquely difficult. I work in London but escape to a rented cottage in the West Country whenever possible. Bridging both worlds, urban and rural, has been insightful; essential to both my research and to the formation of the New English Kitchen concept. The English rural vote is small – and it affects the future of the food produced in the countryside. Small-scale farmers have often described as plain hostile the attitude of our authorities towards them. Enterprise is threatened constantly by both overseas competition and the crippling cost of the regulatory regime imposed on the food industry. Loyalty to the best that the country can produce will go a long way to help protect artisan food from extinction. Inside every shopper's wallet is power, no matter how large or small the amount.

There is much to take in. The commitment needed means a little sacrifice and asks that you take on more responsibility. My book won't solve every problem; indeed, confronting some of the information on its pages will add to your troubles and concern. Much of the methodology is easy to carry out but no, it won't make life easier. It will make it very different, though, because the idea is to empower you. A new enjoyment will creep into each day, infecting everyone in your home, literally engraving good aromas on to minds. *The New English Kitchen* is my own kitchen; these are my experiences with food, grasped at ground level through my work and in my home – now it's over to you.

acknowledgements

Very special thanks are due to Louise Haines at Fourth Estate for her truly extraordinary commitment and patience with this book. Also for the hard work put in by Catherine Blyth, Jane Middleton, Julian Humphries, Terence Caven, Silvia Crompton and Nicholas Pearson. Rosemary Scoular and Sophie Laurimore gave perfect guidance. Thanks, too, to Giacomo Bretzel for his beautiful photography.

This book has taken two years to write, but it would never have been possible without help from certain individuals during my career in food journalism. I am especially grateful to Nigel Slater; his friendship and advice were precious to me throughout. Also Sheila Dillon, Rosie Boycott, Chris Blackhurst, Roy Ackerman, Mark Halliley, Chris Patten, Catherine Pepinster, Michael Pilgrim, Georgie Brewster, Philip Beresford, Kim Fletcher, Carinthia West, Michelle Lavery, Carolyn Hart, Rachel Simhon, Gillian Carter, Maria Trkulja, Sophia Beddow, Dariel Garnett, Nicholas Faith, Fiammetta Rocco, Boris Johnson and Anne Sindall. Nicky Roche was the one who told me to stop talking about my ideas and to put them in a book instead, and the journalist Jonathan Cooper, sadly no longer with us, talked me through many tough moments, for which I will always be grateful.

Time and again, the following people helped with my research: Nicky Beresford, Joanna Blythman, Peter and Hen Greig, Matthew Stevens, Michael Stoate, John Sansom, Bob Dove, Martin and Vanessa Lam, Jeremy Lee, Michael Hart, Mark Newman, Aldo Zilli, Caroline Woofenden, Brendan May, Randolph Hodgson, Gregg Wallace, Barbara Garnsworthy, Teddy Bourke, Charles Nodder, Jeff Wheeler, Marlene Belbin, June Head, Paul Robinson, Caroline Cranbrook, David Willoughby de Brook, Bob Salmon, Alan Dangour, David Hammerson, Julia Moore and Jon Bullock.

Affectionate thanks to those in my family who kept up the encouragement far beyond their remit, especially Laura Jeffreys, Samantha and Samuel Clark, Carinthia and Teddy Clarke and Joyce Prince. Thanks to my mother, Sarah Clarke, whose cooking has always been an inspiration, and to my late father, Mark Jeffreys, for his confidence in me. My lovely children, Jack and Lara, have been so patient – never have the words 'nearly finished' been so untruly told, so often.

And above all my gratitude to Dominic, who started it all.

part one

the chapters that follow feature

foods that are especially suitable

to roll into several meals. bread,

stock, store vegetables, grains

and pulses, poultry, meat and

game are flexible enough to

adapt for many uses.

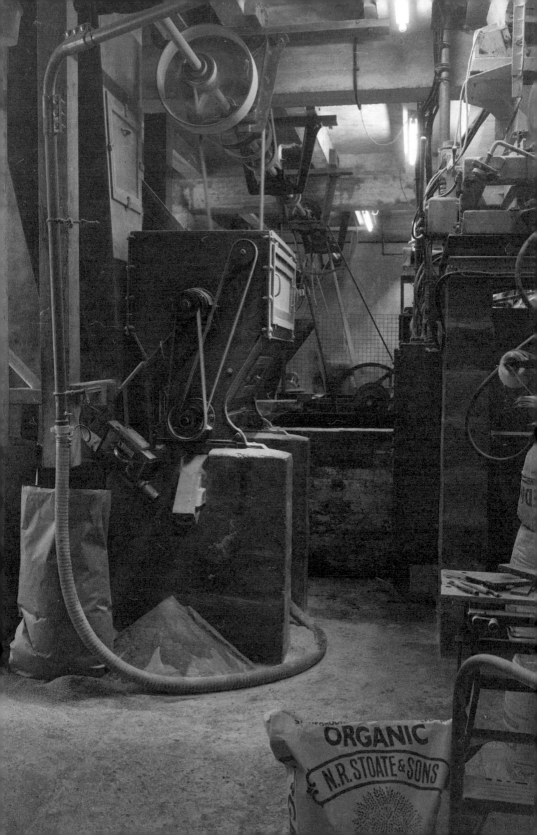

1

bread and flour

Bread can pull off a feat that few cooked foods are capable of: as it matures, it develops new and interesting uses. In other words, it ages gracefully. Once past its sandwich era, older bread fits easily into simple recipes: it lies beneath radiant vegetable broths, turns up in a bread, red wine and onion soup, blends smoothly into a clove-infused sauce, and can be sweetly saturated by a creamy, eggy custard with spices and fruit. There's always toast, too, an edible plate for favourite things. The bread that can do all this is not sliced and wrapped, sometimes costing little more than a first-class stamp, but made in the slower tradition. This bread has real integrity but it costs a bit more – which is why it is worth knowing how to use it as it ages.

The life of a good loaf of bread could unfold in the following way. On day one, it is as fresh as can be, the interior deliciously elastic and the crust crisp as an eggshell. A day or two later the crumb begins to dry, the crust to soften, and it's good for toast. Toast brushed with flavoured oil, then topped with salad leaves and soft fresh cheese; toast with creamy scrambled egg and marinated fish; or, best of all, toast spread with real beef dripping from yesterday's roast. Next day, put a slice of the now drying bread into a bowl and ladle over some vegetable broth. Or, if you are having a supper party, you might use the bread to make a toffee pudding or a fruit charlotte. By the end of the week, anything left from the loaf can be made into breadcrumbs. Eat them spiked with lemon zest beside roast poultry or game; mix them with garlic, herbs and olive oil for stuffing vegetables; or store them in the freezer for bread sauce. By now, I think it would be safe to say your loaf has earned its keep. You bought it to make a sandwich and it has contributed to at least four meals.

The economics of bread have an interesting pattern. A loaf of sliced, wrapped bread costs about 50 pence – although supermarket price wars have seen it drop down to 20 pence as a 'loss leader'. Better-grade, high-street-baked sliced white costs about £1. Handmade traditional bread is twice that, at around £2, but a loaf made at home with best-quality flour costs about 50 pence – again.

This leaves two choices: buy better, more expensive bread and learn how to reap more from it – as the recipes in this chapter will show – or bake bread at home and spend no more than usual. Obviously there's yet more to gain from baking your own bread and letting it earn its keep as it ages. I look at it this way: the time investment made when baking bread at home rewards you financially, leaving you more money to spend on other things. Having said that, it occurs to me that it is in fact quicker to make good bread than to go off and seek it out. Bread machines have made it easier still for busy people. But, putting the economics to one side, you can take real satisfaction in the fact that the bread you make in your own home will be the best. Unadulterated, wholesome bread is something of an endangered species nowadays . . .

the currency of bread

If the essence of this book is to know the value of food and make the most of it, then bread is the currency. Bread is money. It is slang for money and when you're on the breadline you have run out money. Two bestselling books that differ in their account of the value of bread wryly tickle. In *Angela's Ashes*, by Frank McCourt (Flamingo, 1996), a poverty-stricken boy glimpses through a Limerick window a piece of bread spread with jam. His mouth-watering description of it is enough to prove that even at a young age he knows the value of bread. The other book, *Dr Atkins' New Diet Revolution* (Vermilion, 1999), advises avoiding bread – or carbohydrates. Dr Atkins says that mixing carbs with protein, or meat, makes us obese – and so bread must be banished. It goes without saying that Dr Atkins' book is not a bestseller in the developing world. It walks off the shelves in Britain and America, however, because most of these countries' inhabitants are rich enough not to need bread.

the giant bread machine

'All our bakers are master bakers,' the factory manager told me. At that moment a master baker, dressed in regulation cover-up clothing, pushed a button and the bread production line swung into action.

Real master bakers are trained to use their hands to judge the texture of the dough, feeling its elasticity and warmth. They learn their trade in high-street bakeries or medium-sized bread wholesalers, where the bread is made at night. After leaving school, I worked as a shop assistant in a traditional bakery for nearly two years. The baker arrived at one in the morning to start the baking and clocked off at 8 a.m., half an hour after we turned the door sign to read 'open'. The hardship of beginning work at 7 a.m. was tempered by that gorgeous smell of bread emerging from the oven. As I walked to the bakery in the dark early morning, the aroma grew gradually more powerful until I was close enough to see a spectre of steam puffing out of the basement. The baker, Steve, who had spent time 'inside' after a fight, controlled his aggression with an interest in martial arts. But he also loved to bake. He liked the science and enjoyed using his skill – judging the readiness of the dough at every stage, shaping it by hand, and baking it in a century-old brick oven. He even liked to be up at night working while everyone else slept. His hours were strictly controlled by his trade union, in spite of his lonely job. Any slight alteration to the weekly timetable was subject to intense negotiation: well-muscled Steve versus a skinny shop manager, hell bent on not provoking the baker to lose his temper.

In the Midlands factory I visited many years later, the bakers use their hands only to push buttons during their eight-hour shift. This bread is made via the Chorleywood Process, the revolutionary high-speed mechanical baking system invented in 1961. The factory never rests, baking around the clock. It takes just one and three-quarter hours for a loaf to make its journey along the production line, helped by extra yeast and water and high-speed mixers. It is necessary to add flour 'improvers', usually in the form of soya flour, to ensure that the bread will literally rise to the occasion in such an artificially short space of time. Enzyme processing aids, softening agents, sugars, fats and preservatives are also sometimes added. These ingredients combine to speed up the natural breadmaking process, resulting in a soft, sweetish loaf with a long shelf life, which fits neatly into the modern maxim that shopping should happen just once a week.

And where do you, the consumer, fit in? The bread factories would say that all this is done for your benefit. This is the bread you want, and indeed for many, soft, sweet bread is easy to like; children in particular are swiftly seduced.

The high-tech mechanisation of bread comes at the cost of its integrity, however. Compare factory-produced bread to Italian dried durum wheat pasta, most of which is now made speedily in giant factories. The mixing is done high in their ceilings, the dough passes through giant tubes, is pressed through the various dies that make the shapes and then travels into vast drying machines that imitate the Neapolitan sun and sea breezes. But it still contains just flour and water. Pasta is perfect for mechanisation – the food itself never loses its integrity. Bread, on the other hand, needs a whole lot of help by way of additives if it is to survive the Chorleywood palaver.

bread in society

When I criticised sliced and wrapped bread in a newspaper for the first time, it provoked a reaction from the industry that both surprised and annoyed me. Their letters of complaint did not exactly defend their process; instead, they justified it by saying that it 'allowed everyone to eat cheap white bread'. This polemic takes us back over 140 years, when refined white bread had status. The upper classes ate white bread, the poor could afford only the rough, wholegrain type. Flour was ground between stones and then painstakingly sifted to remove the wheatgerm, leaving the flour pure and white – an expensive process.

Then roller mills were invented and suddenly white flour was cheaper to produce. The china rollers removed the brown (good) bits in the flour efficiently. This flour was the forerunner of our modern sliced and wrapped bread. It did indeed give cheap white bread to the poor, but I find it sickening that the modern industry is still arguing that this is the point of high-speed mechanisation. I believe that what it is really saying is: 'You're poor, so you get bread with additives, too much yeast, and no flavour; its integral goodness has been milled out, artificial vitamins have been added to replace it – but you can lump it because you are eating white bread, you lucky people.'

Food snobbery is alive and well, sadly. And highly divisive. There is still one form of nutrition for one group in society and one for another. What can you say in a country that still has two different words for the meal eaten in the middle of the day?

Mechanised breadmaking is no longer about feeding everyone white bread; it is about profit. It is about producing more for less, faster – and to hell with breadmaking tradition. But breadmaking, just like winemaking or rearing a beef steer naturally, is a slow process that yields results that are worth the wait. The recipes in this chapter help to solve the problem of how to afford good bread. They show that bread can be made inexpensively and retain its integrity, and they also show how to use every last crumb. This is bread for all.

how to recognise good bread

There has been a definite surge of interest in handmade or craft bread. This is bread made in the traditional way with two fermentations, during which time it builds true flavour. Good flour is essential. Bread made from stoneground flour retains wheatgerm, even if the 'brown' has been sifted out. Some bakers are interested again in good flour, in the slower baking process and also in traditional ovens – there are now commercial bakeries with domed brick ovens, offering all kinds of loaves made from a wide variety of grains.

When you buy bread, take a good look at it. The crust should not be too thick but its outer veneer should be brittle and crisp. The shape should be as the baker intended – bread that has been hurried will have a lopsided appearance where the interior has risen too fast, breaking through the crust. Smell the bread, too. The aroma of new baking should cling to a fresh loaf. Once it begins to fade, your bread is ready to use for toast or in recipes.

Feel the bread. The interior crumb should have elasticity, tearing when pulled rather than breaking. Despite its bubbly appearance, it should feel heavy for its size. Compare the weight of a piece of factory-produced sliced bread to a similar-sized slice of bread made with stoneground flour at traditional speed. Dry, crumbly bread has either been incorrectly made or is no longer fresh.

Finally, when you taste the bread, you should be able to detect the flavour of the grain. Even in white bread, if the flour is stoneground the flavour will be enhanced by traces of the oils that remain in it, and which are diminished in ordinary, roller-milled flour. Good bread will also taste ripe, indicating that it has been given a good long time to rise. This is most pronounced in sourdough bread, which undergoes a lengthy fermentation.

✳ Craft bakeries – Independent small bakers making bread using traditional techniques are still few in number but well worth seeking out. Don't forget that bread freezes very well, so a journey to buy good bread is a worthwhile mission. Keep an eye on the food media – magazines, weekend newspapers, local press – for new bakery businesses starting up and give them a try.

✳ High-street bakery chains – Home to the ubiquitous jam doughnut and bizarrely decorated buns and biscuits, the chains on the high street vary immensely but I have bought excellent bread from some of these shops. They can be a source of good everyday bread sold in whole loaves that can be sliced and bagged the moment you buy – a preferable alternative to ready sliced and wrapped.

✳ Farmers' markets and other specialist food markets – Worth visiting for good bakery stalls.

✳ Urban local shops and delis – Many corner shops now sell French-style baguettes and loaves 'baked on the premises'. The dough is made elsewhere, though, and the lack of labelling leaves you wondering how. But these Continental loaves often contain an element of authentic sourness, and I'd choose them over sliced and wrapped any day.

✳ Food chains and smaller supermarket chains – Shops such as Marks & Spencer, Waitrose and some Spar stores have responded to the demand for craft-made breads. While never as good as true artisan-made bread, because they are produced in considerable quantities, there are some imaginatively made loaves with plenty of flavour and a good crust.

✳ Supermarkets – The vast majority of bread sold in the Big Four supermarket chains (Asda, Morrison, Sainsbury's and Tesco) is sliced and wrapped but again they are making inroads to supplying traditional-style bread and flour and need your encouragement. Your questions and demands concerning bread and flour will be heard. Vote, as always, for good food with the power that your own money holds. Choosing craft bread over sliced and wrapped will send messages to the industry that it has no choice but to absorb.

organic bread and good flour

Many new craft bakers use organic flours milled with wheat that has been grown naturally. Organic grain farmers are permitted to use a very few fertilisers and pesticides that are deemed safe, but this is often criticised by the conventional food industry. However, it is undeniable that traditionally made bread using organic flour tastes wonderful. The technique is partly responsible for the flavour, but with organic flour the species of wheat also has an impact.

Organic farmers tend to use traditional grain varieties that are slow to grow but are more resistant to pests and disease. Some claim that the good health of the soil has an impact on the flavour of food. This makes sense, but the organic sector would be the first to say that more research is needed into the flavour and vitality of organic food. Independent research needs Treasury money – something that has not exactly been forthcoming since the popularity of organic food has quadrupled in recent times.

All craft bakers are interested in the flour they use because flour is bread's personality, its character. A craft baker will seek out good-quality flour, which may or may not be organic, for the greater good of the bread they bake. There is one simple way to find out – ask them. Good food producers love to talk about the food they make.

making bread at home

I make bread twice a week in a food mixer with an attached dough hook. Each batch of two loaves takes ten minutes to mix and knead.

Two hours later I shape it, and about an hour later the bread is baked. There is very little physical work – bread needs your presence more than anything else. People who go out to work will find breadmaking machines useful. Alternatively you can make the dough in a mixer, put it in the fridge for the day and shape and bake it when you get home.

hands versus machine

Making bread by hand is a real pleasure, but you will need to set aside a good 15 minutes to knead the dough. Food mixers make smooth, elastic dough. I have a KitchenAid but have also used a Kenwood mixer in the past. Use mixers fitted with a dough hook on a low setting.

Busy people swear by their bread machines. They can do the whole job for you, or be set to stop when the dough is ready so it can be shaped and cooked in a conventional oven. Beware of the manufacturer's recipe books. Some of them include recipes that are simply aping the factory process, with too much yeast and milk powder so the bread will be big and soft. Use traditional recipes instead, using the quantities given in the manufacturer's recipe book as a guide, and you will be very pleased with what a bread machine can do.

✳ kitchen note ✳

Look for used Kenwood mixers in local papers and car boot sales – a heavy old one with a good motor will go on for years.

the cost of bread

At the time of writing, I buy flour in bulk and it costs me approximately 50 pence to make a loaf, plus negligible costs for yeast, oil and oven power. A loose calculation based on baking four good-quality loaves a week shows that I can save up to £312 a year on buying bread of comparable quality – money for treats.

buying flour

I used to be hopeless at making scones. When I worked at the bakery, we threw away more scones than we sold because they were always dry, weighty and crumbly. Twenty years later I nibbled a sample scone from a stall at a farmers' market. Light and chewy, without a hint of dryness, this was the scone we were never able to make in the bakery. The stall-holder, slightly taken aback by the passionate interrogation I inflicted on her, casually remarked, 'Oh, it's the flour.' She bought her flour from Cann Mills, a local water mill in Dorset. She did not know why it was so good, it just was.

I wanted to know more, so I visited the mill. The miller, Michael Stoate, took up the story of good wheat flour, the type most commonly used for making bread, scones and cakes. The modern milling industry rolls the grain to remove the bran, taking out the wheatgerm and the flour's natural oil as it does so. This also removes a vital source of vitamins, which means that they have to be added back to the flour artificially. The wheatgerm oil is very valuable to the pharmaceutical industry, which puts it into creams to go on the *outside* of our bodies – oh, the irony of it. What's more, commercial bakers need not mention that it is missing from the flour. About 70 per cent of the bread bought in the UK is made from roller-milled white flour. That is a scandalous amount of missing wheatgerm from what most of us presume is a wholefood.

Stoneground flour, whether white or brown, still contains the wheatgerm – the white flour is simply sifted to remove the bran. Michael Stoate uses millstones to grind all his flour, including the white flour that was used in those scones, with their delightful texture. Traditionally milled stoneground flour can be bought direct from mills, and in some cases delivered to your home (see the Shopping Guide). Look also in specialist independent food shops, farm shops or farmers' markets, and on the internet. Some supermarkets stock British flour from traditional mills, but do check the label carefully.

Store flour in a sealed bin to keep out pests, or buy it in smaller bulk bags of about 5 kilos that can be sealed between use.

Bread baked in tins or shaped into high rounds needs strong flour, made from 'hard' wheat species. These contain a greater amount of glutenin and gliadin, essential for the bread to rise well and form a nice, elastic crumb. In the past, hard wheat was grown mainly in North America for the British bread industry, but with selective breeding it has been adapted over the last few decades to grow well in British conditions. Do not confuse strong flour with hard durum wheat flour, or semolina, which is used specifically for pasta making.

Soft wheat flour, sold as plain flour, is suitable for cake and pastry making and can also be used for soda bread and scones.

other types of flour

While the gluten in wheat flour is vital for the standard bread recipe, a percentage of another type of cereal flour can be added for variety, such as rye, barley, buckwheat or oats. These cereals, however, contain little gluten, and yeast bread made with rye, barley or oat flour alone will be heavy, and does not keep well. Alternative types of flour, made from vegetables like chick peas or potato, are more useful in other forms of cookery. There are recipes using these flours on pages 43–5.

yeast

Fast-action, or easy-blend, yeast is now the most widely available type. It can be mixed straight into the flour, speeding up breadmaking by about half an hour. Conventional dried yeast, sold loose in tins, should be used in the same quantity but must be dissolved in warm water first. Compressed or fresh yeast is not always easy to find now. The best places to try are independent bakeries and some health-food shops. It should be dissolved in warm water or milk before adding it to the dry ingredients. If substituting fresh yeast for dried, you will need double the quantity stated in the recipe.

a little bread science

The breadmaking process is easier to understand once you know a little piece of molecular chemistry. Yeast gives dough its oomph, but it needs gluten to do so. Live yeast makes bubbles of carbon dioxide in the soft, elastic dough. The legend of the first yeast goes that a cook left a piece of dough near a vat of beer and some of the wild yeasts from the ale got into the dough. The cook noticed the bubbles in the bread – the rest is history.

When water comes into contact with flour, it swells the proteins in it. Kneading the dough by hand or machine allows these proteins to blend, changing the molecular structure and forming the all-important gluten.

You must choose if you want to add fat to your bread. Fat improves bread's keeping qualities and gives it a denser texture. It can, however, prevent the dough becoming soft and elastic if it is rubbed into the flour before the water is added, because this delays the essential formation of gluten. Gluten is to dough what steel frames are to skyscraper construction. Its strength allows large spaces of air to form and hold within the dough. The best way to get bread going quickly is to add fat after the water. I do this by oiling the bowl that holds the dough as it rises, then mixing it in before the bread is shaped.

It is fine to leave fat out of bread; it simply results in a lighter dough with large bubbles. If you make small quantities of bread frequently, or rolls, there is no real need to add fat.

Two things kill yeast: too much salt, and heat. Don't be too free with salt – follow the amount specified in recipes until you get to the stage where experience teaches you how much to add. And don't leave the dough to rise anywhere too hot, such as on a radiator or beside a fire. In fact, bread doesn't have to be left in a warm place to rise at all, and will even rise perfectly happily – though slowly – in the fridge. The important thing is that it should be in a draught-free place.

how to knead bread by hand

Take the dough, which will still be sticky, out of the bowl and place it on a floured work surface. Use both hands to pull and stretch the bread, folding it back on itself, pulling and stretching again, giving it a quarter turn each time. Persevere for several minutes – 15 is best. The process helps the gluten develop, making the dough silky, soft and elastic. Be robust when kneading – you can be as aggressive as you want, since it will speed up the process.

basic yeast bread

This recipe works well in a food mixer and can be used for the classic, rectangular tin loaf or for any other shape. Strong white flour, malted wheat, wholemeal or a mixture all work well.

Makes 2 small loaves

700g/1½lb flour

2 x 7g sachets of fast-action (easy-blend) yeast

1 heaped teaspoon fine salt or 2 teaspoons soft sea salt crystals

1 heaped teaspoon unrefined sugar

425ml/14fl oz water, at blood temperature

1 tablespoon vegetable or olive oil (optional – see page 14)

Put the flour in a large bowl with the yeast, salt and sugar and stir until combined. Make a well in the centre and add the warm water, stirring all the time until the ingredients form a sticky dough. Continue to knead the bread – by hand (see above) for 15 minutes, or for 5 minutes on the slow setting of a food mixer fitted with a dough hook. If the dough is too sticky, add more flour; if it is too dry, work in a little water.

The dough will become smooth and elastic as the gluten forms. When you have finished kneading it, put it into an oiled bowl (if you are using the oil), cover with a cloth and leave in a warm, draught-free spot for 1½–2 hours, until doubled in size (or leave for longer at cool room temperature, or overnight in the fridge).

Knock the air out of the dough, kneading the oil into it. Prepare two 480g/1lb loaf tins by brushing all over the inside surface with a little oil. Divide the dough in half, shape each piece into a fat sausage and put into a tin or make 2 rounds and place each in the centre of a baking sheet. Scatter flour on top, cut a slash lengthways down the centre with a sharp knife and leave to rise again, uncovered, for 20–30 minutes. Preheat the oven to 230°C/450°F/Gas Mark 8.

Bake the loaves for 30–40 minutes. They are ready when they come easily out of the tin and sound hollow when tapped on the base with a finger.

✳ kitchen notes ✳

✳ To improve the quality of the crust, put a roasting tin half filled with water in the oven as you preheat it and leave in during baking.

✳ If bread goes wrong, it could be the weather. Ambience affects bread: on humid days the dough needs slightly less water; when the weather is dry, it will need more.

✳ You can freeze bread at almost any stage of the preparation – before the dough has risen; after knocking it back, or after baking.

more adventures with dough

Once you are hooked on making bread at home, it is easy to adjust the recipe or substitute different flours and ingredients. I am not crazy about adding olives, Parmesan, sun-dried tomatoes or fried onions to bread – I'd rather eat those things another way – but working fresh herbs or aromatics into the dough does have a good effect. A few chopped rosemary leaves or sage make a nice savoury bread. Steeping some saffron threads in the warm liquid before you add it to the flour makes a beautiful saffron-scented loaf, delicious with dry-cured meats and fresh cheeses.

To make tea bread, set aside a piece of dough and roll it into a rectangle. Scatter over a little brown sugar and some chopped dried fruit (figs, raisins, prunes or apricots), then roll it up into a Swiss roll shape. Either brush it with beaten egg and bake whole, or cut it into slices to make Chelsea buns, lay these on a greased baking sheet, brush with egg and bake. Scatter some golden caster sugar on Chelsea buns when they come out of the oven.

Substituting milk for water in your dough will make a softer, sweeter tea bread.

sourdough bread

Sourdough bread is a treat to buy from a specialist baker and can be eaten fresh or used in recipes. I admit I often beg mine from my sister and brother-in-law, Sam and Sam Clark. With apologies to the late M. Poîlaine, creator of the famous sourdough loaf, *pain Poîlaine* (see the Shopping Guide), and, honestly, no sibling conspiracy, I believe their experiments at their restaurant, Moro, have resulted in the absolute best there is. A recipe for it is given in *Moro – The Cookbook* (Ebury, 2001).

Slow fermentation of the yeast in bread makes a sour dough. You can make your own yeast, beginning with a combination of flour and fruit juice and 'feeding' the bacteria, but there are simpler methods for home kitchens. Leaving the dough to rise overnight in the fridge, rather than giving it a quick rise in a warm place, produces a more sour dough. You can also knead into it a piece of dough left over from breadmaking a few days earlier (keep it in the fridge, wrapped in cling film; it will sour as it matures). When you make your bread, use only half the yeast specified in the recipe and work the older dough into the new. Allow your dough to rise in the fridge either overnight or during the day. Once baked, the bread will have a full, ripe, savoury taste and the scent of toasted nuts. It will have a strong, tactile crumb, and larger bubbles even if you have used fat. There is no doubt at all that the inner crumb of sourdough keeps its elasticity longer. Nor will the flavour diminish as it ages: old sourdough bread will be as good eaten fresh as it is in your cooking.

soda bread

If you don't have any yeast, or prefer not to eat it, soda bread is a wonderful quick standby and the best bread to eat, buttered, with smoked fish or pastrami. While yeast comes to life with the changing temperature and moisture in the dough, bicarbonate of soda reacts with sour milk or buttermilk, making bubbles that raise the dough and set when baked.

> 480g/1lb wholemeal flour (or a 50/50 mix of white and wholemeal flour for a paler loaf)
> 1 teaspoon fine oatmeal
> 1½ teaspoons fine salt
> 1½ teaspoons bicarbonate of soda
> 30g/1oz butter
> 500ml/16fl oz sour milk (see Kitchen Note overleaf) or buttermilk (or low-fat yoghurt)

Preheat the oven to 230°C/450°F/Gas Mark 8. In a large bowl, mix together the flour, oatmeal, salt and soda, then rub in the butter. Make a well in the centre and slowly add the liquid, mixing all the time. Work the flour in using your hand, until you have a soft but not sticky dough. Turn it out on to a board and shape lightly into a smooth round. Place on a greased baking sheet, scatter with a little extra flour and cut a deep cross on the top with a sharp knife. Bake for 30–35 minutes, turning down the heat to 200°C/400°F/Gas Mark 6 halfway through. The loaf is ready when the base sounds hollow when tapped with a finger. If the loaf is soggy underneath, bake it upside down for a further 5 minutes.

✳ kitchen notes ✳

✳ To sour milk, warm it slightly, add about a teaspoon of lemon juice and leave to stand for a few minutes.

✳ Soda bread makes good breadcrumbs but can be dry and rubbery when toasted, so it is best made frequently in small quantities.

savoury pan scones

Try to find stoneground white flour for these scones; it will give them a lovely chewiness. A really heavy-based frying pan or flat griddle is essential if you cook them on the hob, otherwise they'll burn.

The nicest way to eat pan scones is while they are still warm, halved and buttered.

Makes 8–10 scones

480g/1lb plain flour

1 teaspoon bicarbonate of soda

1 teaspoon cream of tartar

2 teaspoons salt

90g/3oz beef dripping (see page 185) or butter (or 6 tablespoons olive oil)

300ml/½ pint sour milk (see above), buttermilk or low-fat yoghurt

Sift all the dry ingredients into a bowl and rub in the fat. Make a well in the centre and stir in the milk, buttermilk or yoghurt to make a smooth dough.

With floured hands, quickly shape the dough into small rounds, 2cm/¾ inch thick. Heat a heavy-based frying pan or a flat griddle and cook the scones for 4 minutes on each side, until golden and slightly puffed.

Alternatively, bake them in an oven preheated to 230°C/450°F/Gas Mark 8 for 10 minutes.

※ kitchen note ※

You can play around with the flavour of scones, adding grated or chopped cheese (it's a good way to use cheese that is no longer presentable on the table). Try to use one of the many interesting British farmhouse hard cheeses. Crumbled pork crackling makes them wickedly delicious, too. Alternatively, try chopped spring onions, dried thyme or rosemary.

drop scones

I include these because they were one of the first things I ever made myself, and because my mother often made them for tea to eat with golden syrup and butter. The ingredients are pure store cupboard, so you won't have to rush out and buy biscuits on a Sunday when someone drops in for tea. The recipe is from a much-Sellotaped 1950s copy of *The Constance Spry Cookery Book* – one of my bibles.

Makes about 12

240g/8oz plain flour

½ teaspoon bicarbonate of soda

½ teaspoon cream of tartar

½ teaspoon baking powder

1 tablespoon golden caster sugar

a nut of butter

1 tablespoon golden syrup

about 300ml/½ pint milk

1 egg

Mix the dry ingredients in a bowl, then rub in the butter and add the syrup. Add half the milk, mixing well with a wooden spoon. Break in the egg and beat well, then add the remaining milk. The mixture should just drop from the spoon. Allow to stand for 10–15 minutes, not more.

Heat an oiled flat griddle or heavy-based frying pan. When it is moderately hot, drop in the mixture in spoonfuls and cook for 2–3 minutes, until small bubbles appear on the surface. Flip the drop scones over and cook for about 30 seconds to brown the other side. Wrap the scones in a tea towel to keep them warm while you cook the rest, then serve with butter, jam and syrup.

✳ kitchen note ✳

It won't be necessary to re-grease the pan as you cook each batch; the drop scones are all the better for being cooked without much oil at all.

flat breads

The earliest breads were unleavened – they did not contain yeast. They were rolled or pressed out and baked absolutely flat. The offspring of these ancient flat breads can still be found in the Middle East, where there are hundreds of versions, including breads no thicker than card but floppy enough to wrap around herbs and salty cheese, and slightly thicker, round flat breads, which are put to use as a jacket for kebabs. I remember when pitta bread was considered avant garde, but now flat breads in every guise can be bought from Middle Eastern and Asian shops; even supermarkets sell several versions of flat bread, or 'wraps' – a word that came from the United States. There are soft breads such as Indian naan and chapatis or Mexican tortillas, crisp breads like lavash to crumble into soups and salads, or flaky roti to parcel up West Indian curries.

Making flat breads at home is good economics: a batch of up to ten can be made from 360g of good flour, worth less than 50 pence, which comes in at approximately a third of the cost of ten tortilla wraps or pitta breads.

basic flat bread

I cannot even begin to give an authentic recipe for every kind of flat bread but the recipe below, adapted from Tom Jaine's *Making Bread at Home* (Weidenfeld & Nicolson, 1995), makes a good, crisp, flat bread that can be broken into soup or a leafy salad, or used to scoop food into your mouth. It uses yeast, but you could use a little dough left over from the previous baking instead for the same lightening effect.

The secret of all flat breads is to rest the dough in the fridge. This gives the gluten time to relax, so that you can roll or press the bread out very flat. It also sours the dough slightly, adding flavour.

Makes 8–10

360g/12oz unbleached strong white flour (or 240g/8oz flour and
180g/6oz stored dough from the last bread)
1 teaspoon salt
7g sachet of fast-action (easy-blend) yeast
240g/8oz low-fat yoghurt

Mix together all the dry ingredients, then stir in the yoghurt. Knead, in a machine or by hand (see pages 11 and 15), until the dough is smooth and elastic. Cover with cling film and store in the fridge for at least 4 hours, or overnight.

Preheat the oven to 230°C/450°F/Gas Mark 8. Divide the dough into balls the size of a large walnut. Roll out each one on a floured work surface until it is very thin. Place on an oiled baking sheet, allow to rest for 5–10 minutes then bake for 8–12 minutes, until the flat breads are crisp and light golden in places.

✳ kitchen note ✳

You can also make these breads from maize flour (polenta), chestnut flour or gram (chick pea) flour, using them to replace a third of the ordinary flour.

dry flat bread

Bought and home-made flat breads become stale quickly but they can still be worked into other meals. If they are still soft, tear them up, then toast until dry. Alternatively fry gently in olive oil. Store in jars ready for use in salads or soups.

bread salad

Cut or tear a dry or toasted flat bread into postage-stamp-sized pieces. Make a salad with the bread, Cos or romaine lettuce hearts, spinach or other leaves, herbs (parsley and dill), sliced tomatoes – the juice soaks nicely into the bread – and cucumber. Dress with just extra virgin olive or walnut oil and lemon juice, salt and pepper.

pizza margherita

San Gennaro is the patron saint of Naples, the birthplace of spaghetti and that other international fast food, pizza. It is also the name above the door of our local pizzeria in London. We are lucky. At San Gennaro they make pizza in the traditional way, with ingredients from Campania, the region around Naples that is famous for its wheat, tomatoes and buffalo mozzarella. The proprietor, Enzo, operates on Neapolitan hours – the door never opens before 5.30 p.m. and it closes in the small hours. I first walked into this south London pizzeria late one August night. A few people were sitting at the bar drinking small glasses of home-made limoncello. We could have been in Campania itself and that was before we ate the pizza.

Good pizza dough is almost flaky, the air barely held inside, and breaks easily. It has a slight sourness, a faint smoky flavour where it has been charred by the heat of the oven. The secret of this recipe was revealed to me after an evening spent deep in the basement of San Gennaro, watching José make the dough. He refrigerates it overnight, so that it can be stretched to incredible thinness the following day.

'Anyone can make good pizza,' says Enzo. 'You can be from Ecuador, Nigeria or London, but you need two things: authentic ingredients and "the knowledge".'

Makes 2

4 tablespoons olive oil

8 basil leaves

6 tablespoons Tomato Sauce (see page 358)

120g/4oz buffalo mozzarella, cut into 1cm/½ inch pieces

freshly ground black pepper

extra virgin olive oil, to serve

For the dough:

540g/1lb 2oz plain flour

½ teaspoon salt

7g sachet of fast-action (easy-blend) yeast

150ml/¼ pint milk, warmed to blood temperature

200ml/7fl oz water, warmed to blood temperature

2 tablespoons olive oil

Put the flour, salt and yeast in a mixing bowl and slowly add the milk and water, mixing until it forms a dough. Knead by hand (see page 15) or in a food mixer until the dough is smooth and elastic. Add a little more flour if the dough is too sticky. Pour the oil into a large, clean bowl, add the dough and turn to coat it in the oil. Cover and place in the fridge for a minimum of 8 hours and up to 24 hours (you can use it sooner, after 2 hours, but it will not be pliable).

Preheat the oven to its highest setting (a commercial pizza oven cooks pizza at 350°C). A preheated pizza stone or perforated pizza baking dish helps; use in place of a baking sheet.

If you have time, bring the dough to room temperature before you shape the pizzas. Take half the dough and use your fingers to press it into a circle. Then pick it up and 'open' it with your hands by holding the edges and turning it about 45 degrees at a time. The pizza base should measure 30cm/12 inches across. Place on a baking sheet (or on the preheated pizza stone – but work fast when adding the tomato and cheese). Repeat for the second pizza.

Stir the oil and basil into the tomato sauce, then smear the sauce on to each circle of dough and scatter the mozzarella on top. Bake until the outer edge bubbles and turns crisp and the mozzarella is melted but not browned. Shake over a little extra virgin oil and grind over some black pepper before you eat the pizza.

✳ kitchen note ✳

Liquidised canned Italian tomatoes or *passata* can be used in place of the tomato sauce, but the pizza must cook fast at a high temperature for the tomatoes to sweeten and the juice to evaporate.

other uses for pizza dough

✳ Try the Tuscan *Schiacciata con l'uva*, which is eaten during the grape harvest. Roll out the dough to a thin rectangle, sprinkle over a little Pernod or aniseed-flavoured alcohol, then fold it in three and roll again to about 5mm/¼ inch thick. Scatter over a few red grapes – red wine grapes, if available, because their thin skins make them good for cooking. Bake at your oven's highest setting until the dough is crisp, then serve sprinkled with a little sugar.

✳ To make garlic bread, infuse 2 chopped garlic in 4 tablespoons of olive oil for an hour or two, then shake it over the uncooked pizza bases. Cut a few slashes in the centre of each one and bake as for pizza. Shake a little extra virgin olive oil over the bread as it comes out of the oven.

✳ To make goat's cheese pasties, roll out the dough thinly and cut it into rounds with a tumbler. In the centre of each one, put a spoonful of mild, fresh goat's cheese and a little finely chopped dill or lightly cooked greens (such as chard or spinach, with all the water squeezed out). Brush the edges with water, fold over and pinch together to make little pasties. Bake until crisp and golden in an oven preheated to 230°C/450°F/Gas Mark 8.

making the most of stale bread

It is easy to glance around the kitchen and say, 'I have nothing in the house', but that is not strictly true if the end of a loaf is lurking in the bread bin. This section of the bread chapter is intended to change 'I have nothing . . .' to 'hmmm, well perhaps . . .', or even to, 'I have eggs, I have some herbs and I can make toast . . .' Then there are breadcrumbs, so quick to defrost after storage in the freezer, then fry in olive oil with a little garlic and parsley to serve with pasta, or use as a coating for meat that has been hammered thin (see page 33).

The art of making bread go further has become almost extinct – partly because of the preservatives in commercially baked bread, but also because it is the kind of hand-me-down information that disappeared when mothers stopped cooking and broke the chain of food lore. It is not that recipes using stale bread are old-fashioned – Tuscan bread soups are now championed by contemporary chefs as one of the most delicious things in the world. Their recipes invariably suggest using the ubiquitous ciabatta but it is fine to make use of that old loaf of everyday bread.

Good bread deteriorates faster than sliced and wrapped factory-baked loaves containing preservatives such as citric acid. They will not, however, develop a mould quickly, but gradually dry out during the week. My experience with factory-made breads is that they deteriorate suddenly approximately six days after they are bought, when an outbreak of mouldy spots appear and the whole lot must go in the bin.

Sourdough bread, on the other hand, has an extraordinary life. The crust will dry but no spots appear for up to two weeks. Because it costs more, I tend to scrape or cut any mould away and continue popping the bread under the grill, where it obediently becomes springy inside and crisp on the outside – edible again.

This is what a home-made loaf can give, assuming it yields 10 slices of bread. Half the loaf is eaten fresh over a day for breakfast, or in packed lunches; 4 slices of the drying remains are toasted and put in the bottom of four soup bowls, then a vegetable broth spooned over; the remainder is made into breadcrumbs. Half the breadcrumbs are used to coat some hammered chicken thigh meat and the other half fried with herbs and nuts beside a separate dish of roast pheasant or partridge. Fifty pence goes a long way with food.

toast

There's nothing new. The French have croûtons, Italians crostini – we have toast. Crostini sounds so neo-Italian, so latter-day peasant that it is easy to forget that it is simply toast. Putting things on toast is genius – ordinary, everyday items of food are greatly elevated by their toasted mattress of bread. Toast belongs to the British Isles, and it is one of those things that we do better than anyone else. Thick slices of toast with butter and marmalade, what better breakfast? Apart from perhaps boiled eggs and toast. Or scrambled eggs on toast.

My father was very fond of savouries. These were small dishes, often on toast, served after the main course. They are out of fashion now, outside the gentleman's club. His favourite was sardines on toast – and yes, they were from a can. We quaked with horror at the table, but out came the macho Worcestershire sauce: 'They must have Worcestershire sauce!' And he was right. They were very good after a liberal shaking.

sardines on toast

I tried them again the other day, with very little modification, and liked them all over again. It is the same story of good and bad food in

England. They do need good bread, good butter and good sardines. You can buy line-caught canned sardines from Spanish shops and delis. Ramon Bue is an excellent brand that has been around for ever – as long as Worcestershire sauce, in fact.

Serves 4

8 canned sardines
4 medium-thick slices of day-old bread
butter
Worcestershire sauce
chopped parsley

Pick over the sardines without damaging their silver skins. Where possible, remove the gritty spines or obvious bones. Toast the bread and spread it with butter while it is still hot. Lay fillets from 2 fish on top of each slice, skin-side up, and put under a hot grill for 2 minutes. Dress with Worcestershire sauce and sprinkle with parsley.

dripping toast

When well-hung beef is roasted, it produces a full-tasting dripping with a jelly beneath that can only be described as nectar. Hot toast or Melba Toast (see page 30), cut nicely into triangles, with a fifty-fifty mixture of dripping and jelly spread on top, finished by black pepper and maybe a watercress leaf, is a completely respectable thing to serve with drinks. It fed the poor for centuries, but was killed off by tasteless, poorly hung meat. It is not an everyday dish; a little dripping is good for you but too much is not. But on those occasions when you splash out on the best beef joints, make sure you collect the dripping to make Roast Potatoes (see page 73), pilaffs (see page 202) – and for toast.

more good things on toast

✳ Melted cheese – Try some of the new British and Irish cheeses as well as traditional farmhouse Cheddar and Double Gloucester. Lord of the Hundreds is used often in this book – a hard ewe's milk cheese that melts to a tart, white cream. Other good melting cheeses include Saval, Malvern and Coolea, plus the obvious European mountain cheeses, Gruyère, Cantal, Emmental and Tilsiter.

✳ Fresh, young goat's cheeses – Soft white goat's cheese can be crumbled on to toast, with herbs, salad leaves and olives, and dressed with a few drops of those piquant oils you can buy, infused with chilli or aromatic herbs.

✳ Cooled scrambled eggs (see page 389) – With added cream, scrambled duck or hen's eggs on toast make a truly elegant starter or supper dish. If you like, you can add very thin, crisp bacon, fresh herbs or smoked fish, such as eel or trout.

✳ Chicken livers and other offal (see pages 156 and 223) – Chopped and fried with butter, chopped capers, anchovy and a little white wine.

✳ Smoked fish – Organic smoked salmon or trout, mackerel or kippers, or perhaps the more unusual fish now being smoked by specialists, such as pollack and ling.

✳ Herring – Filleted and fried in butter, then placed on hot toast that has been spread with a mixture of butter and mustard. Finish with lots of fresh dill.

✳ North Atlantic or other cold-water prawns or Morecambe Bay grey shrimps (see page 317) – Dress with a few herbs and scatter a little cayenne pepper and ground mace over the top.

✳ Fried tomatoes – Go a step further and fry the day-old bread, then cover it with sweet fried tomatoes. Add a blob of crème fraîche or soured cream and a few basil leaves for something richer.

melba toast

Melba toast is made by splitting a piece of toast apart and baking it in the oven. It has a lovely old-fashioned feel to it and is wonderful with those smooth duck liver pâtés from delis, finished with a slice of pickled cucumber. Use it also as a base for semi-dried tomatoes (sold as sunblush) and dress with virgin olive oil, or break it up and throw it into leafy salads with herbs, spring onions, lemon juice and olive oil.

The renowned chef, Auguste Escoffier, named Melba toast after the prima donna, Dame Nellie Melba, in 1897. But in her book, *English Bread and Yeast Cookery* (Allen Lane, 1977), Elizabeth David found an earlier recipe written by the Scottish home cook, F. Marian McNeill, proving that Melba toast belongs as much in our own kitchens as it does in the grand dining rooms of old hotels.

Serves 4

4 thin slices of white or brown bread

Preheat the oven to 180°C/350°F/Gas Mark 4. Toast the bread on both sides, then cut off the crusts. Using a serrated knife, split the toasted bread apart into 2 sides; you will find it comes away easily. Cut each side into 2 triangles, place them on a baking sheet and bake in the oven until dry. They tend to curl up, looking lovely as you bring them to the table in a basket.

✳ kitchen note ✳

To make a rich toast that will not go soggy, brush each side of the Melba toast with melted butter before you put it in the oven. This will keep for a week in an airtight container.

breadcrumbs

Like chicken bones, prawn shells and vegetable peelings, breadcrumbs are a gift to the cook. They are essentially 'free'. The crusted end of a dry loaf or the cut-away crusts from Melba toast, once headed for the duck pond in the park, still form the basis of another meal. They can perform a variety of jobs, from making a filling winter pasta dish to becoming a summer salad, spiked with chilli and soaked with olive oil.

There are two ways to make breadcrumbs:

Simply put stale but soft bread into the food processor and whiz. These crumbs can be used for stuffings, bread sauce and meatballs, but if you want to dry them, put them on a baking sheet and place in a moderate oven until golden.

Or – dry out old bread slices and rolls in a moderate oven, then either whiz them in a food processor or put them in a strong, thick plastic bag and crush with a rolling pin.

✳ kitchen note ✳

Dried breadcrumbs can be stored in an airtight container, where they will keep for at least three weeks. Fresh ones must be stored in the freezer.

bread sauces for poultry and game

These absorb and flavour the juices of poultry beautifully. I prefer them to bread-based stuffings which can take ages to cook, drying out the birds as they do so.

fried breadcrumbs with lemon

The pine nuts can be left out altogether, or replaced with pecans (for turkey), walnuts (for duck) or shelled unsalted pistachios (for partridge or pheasant).

Serves 4

4 tablespoons olive oil
4 heaped tablespoons fresh or dried breadcrumbs
zest of 1 lemon

4 sprigs of parsley, chopped

2 tablespoons pine nuts

½ teaspoon crushed pink peppercorns

Heat the oil in a small pan, add all the remaining ingredients and fry gently until golden. Serve with roast turkey, wild duck, partridge or pheasant.

✳ kitchen note ✳

Middle Eastern shops are the best places to buy dried nuts of every variety (and dried fruit, for that matter). Large bags of pistachios and walnuts are always fresh and cost about half the price of those found in conventional groceries and supermarkets.

almond, sherry and clove sauce

An aromatic sauce with a crumb base.

Serves 4

4 tablespoons olive oil

4 garlic cloves, chopped

4 tablespoons fresh or dried breadcrumbs

4 tablespoons ground almonds

8 sprigs of parsley, finely chopped

½ teaspoon ground cloves

a pinch of ground cinnamon

1 glass of sherry

175ml/6fl oz chicken stock

salt and freshly ground black pepper

Heat the oil in a pan, add the garlic and cook until golden. Stir in the breadcrumbs, almonds, parsley, spices and some black pepper. Add the

sherry, bring to the boil and simmer for a minute. Then pour in the stock and simmer for a further minute. Season to taste with salt. Serve with rice, beside roasted poultry or game.

traditional bread sauce

Serves 6

600ml/1 pint whole milk

1 onion, peeled and halved, studded with 5 cloves

a pinch of grated nutmeg

about 10 tablespoons fresh breadcrumbs

1 tablespoon butter

salt and freshly ground black pepper

Put the milk in a pan and add the onion halves and nutmeg. Heat to boiling point, then turn off the heat and leave to stand for at least half an hour. Reheat, adding enough fresh breadcrumbs to form a thick sauce, then stir in the butter and season to taste. If the sauce becomes too thick, let it down with more milk.

breadcrumb coatings – suspicious minds

In Italy, difficult food is made appetising for children by coating it in breadcrumbs: veal, chicken or lamb is hammered until thin, then concealed in a crust (see page 441–2). It is a proven means of getting children used to the flavour of real meat and away from fast-food nugget culture. You can also use the technique for plaice, prawns, green vegetables such as courgettes – in fact anything that you may not normally get past their suspicious minds on the basis that it is not chips. Crumbed food can be fried in a shallow layer of olive or sunflower oil. Keep an eye on the temperature; the food should emerge from the pan golden, not mahogany.

You need three bowls:

* ✳ Bowl 1 – contains about 3 tablespoons of plain flour with a tiny pinch of salt. Dip the raw food in this first; it allows the egg to stick to the breadcrumbs and puff away from the meat.
* ✳ Bowl 2 – contains 1 beaten egg. This is the glue, which firms up when cooking and prevents the breadcrumbs falling off. Dip the floured food in the egg, coating it fully. Use your fingers, tongs or 2 forks.
* ✳ Bowl 3 – contains the breadcrumbs. For 4 pieces of chicken, fill to 2cm/¾ inch deep. Use fresh or dried breadcrumbs; you will discover your own preference. Dip the egg-coated meat into the breadcrumbs and roll it around until evenly coated.

✳ kitchen note ✳

Any food that has been crumbed will keep safely in the fridge for the usual time without spoiling. You can also freeze the crumb-coated food before you cook it.

breadcrumbs and garlic with pasta

If possible, use orecchiette pasta for this dish, because the little, saucer-like shapes catch the breadcrumbs so neatly.

Serves 4

400g/14oz broccoli, broken into florets

400g/14oz short durum wheat pasta

2 garlic cloves, crushed

4 tablespoons fresh or dried breadcrumbs

4 tablespoons olive oil

salt and freshly ground black pepper

freshly grated Parmesan cheese, to serve

Bring 2 pans of water to the boil and add salt. Cook the broccoli for 5 minutes and the pasta for whatever time is recommended on the packet (reputable Italian brands give very accurate cooking instructions). The idea is for both to be ready at the same time, so you can drain them in the same colander.

Just before you serve, fry the garlic and breadcrumbs in the oil until golden. Drain the pasta and broccoli and return them to the pasta pan. Stir in the breadcrumbs, season with salt and pepper and serve with grated Parmesan cheese.

✳ kitchen note ✳

Use steamed courgettes, shredded Savoy cabbage, spring greens, calabrese or string beans instead of the broccoli.

breadcrumb, garlic and parsley butter stuffing for shellfish

A treat for large mussels or clams on the half shell. The butter and crumbs make expensive shellfish go further because you can mop up the juices with crusty white bread. You can also serve scallops in the same way.

Serves 4

120g/4oz unsalted butter, left at room temperature overnight

6 sprigs of parsley, finely chopped

6 heaped tablespoons fresh breadcrumbs

2 garlic cloves, finely chopped

24 large mussels or 40 clams, cleaned (see page 305)

sea salt

Pound together the butter, parsley, breadcrumbs and garlic and work in a pinch of salt.

Put the mussels or clams in a large pan, then cover and place over a fairly high heat for 2–3 minutes, until they open. Allow to cool. Remove the top half of each shell, leaving the mussel or clam in the other half. Spread a little stuffing into each (½–1 teaspoonful, depending on the size of the shell). Arrange on ovenproof plates – individual ones are best – and place under a hot grill. If you do not have a grill, preheat the oven to 240°C/475°F/Gas Mark 9. Cook until the breadcrumbs are singed and the butter bubbling.

✳ kitchen note ✳

If you have any leftover steamed mussels, cockles or clams, you can fill them with the breadcrumb stuffing and store them in the freezer if there is no immediate use for them. Even a few make an unusually good snack to have with drinks. Grill or bake as above.

soaked bread

I love recipes with soaked bread. It's funny but I could never stomach puddings or any dish made with soaked grains but sopping wet bread is in a realm of its own. Why else would just about everyone love bread and butter pudding? Bread dishes usually look a total mess but no one minds. The following recipes are for both fresh and stale bread.

breadcrumb salad

Another bread salad, this time one that uses breadcrumbs from sourdough or ciabatta bread. It is lovely and soggy, with oil, peppers, tomatoes and herbs. You can tailor-make it to your taste. Some prefer to leave out the garlic so you can really taste the quality of the olive oil. Serve it for dinner and most will think they are being given a plate of cold porridge but will come round after the first mouthful.

Italians call this dish *panzanella*, and the restaurant of the same name in Northcote Road (a wonderful market street in Battersea) gave me its approximate method, which I reproduce here. The restaurant uses Puglian bread but any rustic-style sourdough bread will work.

Serves 4

½ day-old ciabatta or sourdough loaf

3 tablespoons extra virgin olive oil

1 tablespoon white wine vinegar

1 garlic clove, finely chopped (optional)

1 carrot, finely grated

6 sprigs of parsley, chopped

salt and freshly ground black pepper

To serve:

½ fresh red chilli, chopped, or a strip of sweet red pepper, chopped

halved cherry tomatoes

small black olives

Tear up the bread, put it in a food processor and whiz to rough crumbs. Put them in a bowl, cover with cold water and leave for 5 minutes. Pour the breadcrumbs into a sieve and, using a ladle, press down to squeeze out all the water. Return the breadcrumbs to the bowl. They won't look too appetising but once you add the oil and vinegar, have a taste. Add the other ingredients, stirring them in well. Season with salt and pepper to taste. Scatter the chopped chilli, halved cherry tomatoes and olives on top.

sourdough bread, wine and onion soup

This is much, much nicer than French onion soup. Instead of one large croûton with cheese in each bowl, the bread is layered, club-sandwich style, with the cheese and baked separately. The hot soup is then ladled over the top.

Serves 4

5 tablespoons olive oil

1.4kg/3lb pink or white onions, sliced

a large pinch of dried thyme

175 ml/6 fl oz red wine

1.2 litres/2 pints well-flavoured beef stock

4 large slices of sourdough bread

1 garlic clove, lightly crushed but left whole

4 heaped tablespoons grated hard cheese (see Kitchen

Note overleaf)

salt and freshly ground black pepper

Heat 3 tablespoons of the oil in a large pan and add the onions, thyme and some salt. Cook over a very, very low heat for about 45 minutes, until pale gold, soft and sweet tasting. Add the wine, deglazing or scraping any cooking bits from the base of the pan with a wooden spatula. Add the beef stock and bring to simmering point. Taste for seasoning and add salt if necessary. Grind over a little black pepper.

Preheat the oven to 190°C/375°F/Gas Mark 5. Rub each slice of bread with the garlic, brush with the remaining oil and cut into quarters. Place 4 pieces of bread in a baking dish. Spoon a dessertspoonful of the cooked onions on to each, followed by a teaspoon of grated cheese, then place another piece of bread on top and repeat, continuing until you have used up all the bread and have 4 multi-layered croûtons.

Bake them in the oven for about 15 minutes, until the tops are golden and bubbling.

Put a croûton in each serving bowl. Bring the soup back to boiling point if you have set it to one side. Ladle the onion broth over the croûtons and serve immediately.

✳ kitchen note ✳

I recommend using a hard sheep's milk, Pecorino-style cheese, such as Lord of the Hundreds or Somerset Rambler, for the croûtons. You could also use a traditional farmhouse Cheddar or other cow's milk cheese, hard or crumbly. See page 425 for information on cooking with British and Irish cheeses.

summer pudding

This moulded pudding made from dry white bread and a mixture of lightly stewed berries doesn't require an exact recipe. You will need enough fruit to fill the pudding basin you wish to use, plus a little over. You could use a traditional pudding basin, a soufflé dish or any shallow dish. I sometimes make summer pudding in large plastic containers for children's meals, serving helpings from them as and when needed. Raspberries, blackberries, tayberries, red and blackcurrants are all suitable for the filling – it's best to use a mixture, but the pectin-rich raspberries are pretty much essential. You can use strawberries, but they tend to disintegrate wastefully when cooked.

Simply stew the fruit gently until the juices run and add enough sugar to remove any sourness. Line the pudding basin with slices of day-old white bread, pour in the compote and cover with a 'lid' of sliced bread, then a saucer small enough to fit inside the basin. Put a weight on top – a can of tomatoes will do – and leave in the fridge overnight.

Push any leftover compote through a sieve to make a sauce. To turn the pudding out, run a blunt knife between the bread casing and the bowl. Invert a plate on top and turn the basin and plate over. If you have ever got water in your gumboots, you will know the noise a summer pudding makes when it unmoulds. Pour over the sauce to cover any white patches. Serve with crème fraîche.

❋ kitchen note ❋

Frozen English berries, organic or conventionally farmed, are a wonderful source of winter fruit and, unlike exotic fruits, they are free of air freight and fossil fuel issues. I use them to make summer puddings in winter for school packed lunches or simply to cheer everyone up. I find them in supermarkets but also in farm shops in big chest freezers.

toffee pudding

Constance Spry again, with a pudding whose flavour has only to be tasted to be loved. I have fed this to everyone and, despite its obvious fudgy stickiness and collapsed appearance, they all say how light it is. Recipe trickery at its best.

Serves 4

120g/4oz butter
120g/4oz demerara sugar
240g/8oz golden syrup
300ml/½ pint milk
4 thick slices of bread, crusts removed, cut into fingers
whipped cream, to serve

Heat the butter, sugar and golden syrup in a small pan and boil for 3 minutes. Remove from the heat and keep warm. In a separate pan, heat the milk to boiling point. Put the fingers of bread in a dish and pour over the milk. Lift them out, put them into 4 serving bowls and pour over the sauce – you can dip them in the sauce instead but you will have to work fast. Serve immediately, with whipped cream.

winter charlotte with rhubarb and raspberries

For charlottes, buttered day-old bread is placed on top of the fruit and the pudding is baked. Apples and berries make good charlottes, and it is even possible to make a savoury charlotte with chicory, apple and spices that have been slowly cooked until sweet.

Here is a baked winter version of summer pudding, filled with forced rhubarb and frozen raspberries.

Serves 6

about 8 slices of day-old white bread, crusts removed (reserve them for breadcrumbs, if you like – see page 30)

softened unsalted butter

ground cinnamon

700g/1½lb forced rhubarb, cut into 2cm/¾ inch lengths
(see page 336)

400g/14oz frozen raspberries

golden caster sugar

Preheat the oven to 200°C/400°F/Gas Mark 6. Butter the bread slices and sprinkle with a little cinnamon. Cut each slice into quarters, then into 8 small triangles.

Put the rhubarb and raspberries into a pan, cover and cook over a low heat until the rhubarb is just soft. Add enough sugar to sweeten to your taste, then pour into a shallow ovenproof dish. Arrange the triangles of bread on top, buttered-side up, working in a fish-scale pattern. Bake the charlotte for about half an hour, until the surface of the bread is golden brown. Remove from the oven and sprinkle caster sugar on top. Serve with fresh custard (see page 401) or thick double cream.

brioche and fig pudding

For the last 15 years it has been easy to buy French-style breads in almost every town. Purists will quibble at their quality, but they have the slight sourness, crust and tearable dough that make French breads so wonderful. Next to arrive has been brioche – and no, it's not as good as the artisan-style buttery bread whose fragrance pours out of pâtisseries across the Channel, but it's not bad either. Our local late-night shop always sells brioche loaves wrapped in plastic, which keep for a suspiciously long time. They are too claggy to eat fresh but make terrific emergency puddings.

Serves 4

10 slices of brioche

5 ready-to-eat dried figs, sliced

4 egg yolks

300ml/½ pint whole milk

125ml/4fl oz double cream

1 tablespoon golden caster sugar

½ teaspoon vanilla extract

a pinch of grated nutmeg

caster sugar for dusting

Preheat the oven to 190°C/375°F/Gas Mark 5. Toast the brioche slices in a dry frying pan over a medium heat; they burn very easily, so be careful. Cut the slices into triangles and arrange them in overlapping layers in an ovenproof dish, points/corners up. Slot a slice of fig between each one.

Whisk the egg yolks into the milk and add the cream, sugar and vanilla. Put in a saucepan and heat gently, stirring, but do not let it boil. As soon as it thickens slightly, pour it over the brioche and figs and scatter a pinch of nutmeg on to the surface. Bake the pudding for 20–30 minutes, until golden on top and just set. Dust with caster sugar and serve with cream.

alternative flours

Flour made from wheat is clearly the most versatile, and the keeping qualities gluten gives to bread are a real advantage, as the previous recipes show. But there are alternative flours made from vegetables and nuts that are well worth discovering. Finding a bag of gram flour in an Asian shop in Tooting Bec was the beginning of a new friendship with flour in savoury cooking for me, and my favourite recipe for orange cake would be no good without potato flour.

gram flour

Gram flour is milled from dried chick peas and is a light, gentle-flavoured flour with a smooth texture. It is used extensively in Indian cooking, in fritters or to coat vegetables for frying.

gram coating for poultry, game and fish

A practical way to season poultry and game or whole fish like sole and trout before you fry it. Quicker than breadcrumbing, it also absorbs the sometimes unpleasant fat on poultry skin that spits as it cooks.

> gram flour
> 1 teaspoon salt
> 2 teaspoons dried oregano
> freshly ground black pepper

Scatter gram flour on to a dinner plate in a layer 5mm/¼ inch deep. Mix in the salt and oregano and grind over some black pepper. Roll the meat or fish in the mixture and cook.

gram and cheddar shortbreads

Makes 12–16 (enough to serve 4 people with drinks)

90g/3oz gram flour, sifted

75g/2½oz very mature farmhouse Cheddar cheese, roughly grated

75g/2½oz chilled unsalted butter, cut into cubes

a large pinch of cayenne pepper

½ teaspoon sea salt

a pinch of freshly ground black pepper

1 tablespoon very cold water

Preheat the oven to 190°C/375°F/Gas Mark 5. Put the flour, cheese, butter, cayenne and seasoning into a food processor and whiz until the mixture has a breadcrumb consistency. Add the water and whiz again. As soon as the crumbs begin to form a dough, tip them on to a board and knead together until smooth. Work quickly; the mixture should not become greasy.

Shape the dough into a cylinder and cut it into 1cm thick slices. Put them 2cm/¾ inch apart on a baking sheet lined with baking parchment or greaseproof paper. Place in the fridge for 20 minutes, then bake for 15 minutes, until the shortbreads are slightly puffed, their edges lightly brown.

✳ kitchen note ✳

To decorate and add flavour, roll the cylinder of dough in chopped pistachio nuts, or scatter toasted black cumin seeds or flaked almonds on to the sliced biscuits before baking.

potato flour

In Italy, potato flour is added to sweet cakes with ground nuts, giving them an almost impossible lightness and delicious dry crumb. It is also used to coat pork before frying. Also known as *fécule*, potato flour is available from Italian stores and wholefood shops. It is very white, and squeaks when rubbed between your fingers.

almond and orange cake

Based on Anna del Conte's recipe in her book, *Secrets of an Italian Kitchen* (Bantam Press, 1989), this is a subtle cake to eat after a meal with a little crème fraîche.

150g/5oz blanched almonds, whole or flaked

3 eggs, separated

150g/5oz golden caster sugar

60g/2oz potato flour

1½ oranges

a pinch of salt

30g/1oz butter, softened

icing sugar for dusting

Preheat the oven to 160°C/325°F/Gas Mark 3. Chop the almonds in a food processor, or finely by hand, until they have a crumb-like texture. Whisk the egg yolks with the sugar until pale and creamy. Add the almonds and the potato flour. Grate the zest of the whole orange into the mixture, then add the juice of 1½ oranges.

In a separate bowl, whisk the egg whites with the salt until they form stiff peaks. Fold them into the orange and egg mixture. Butter a 20cm/8 inch round cake tin – use up all the butter; when it cooks it will be absorbed into the cake and form a delicious crust. Pour in the mixture and bake for 50 minutes, until the cake has shrunk from the side of the tin and feels springy when you press the surface with a finger. Unmould the cake and cool on a wire rack. Dust with icing sugar.

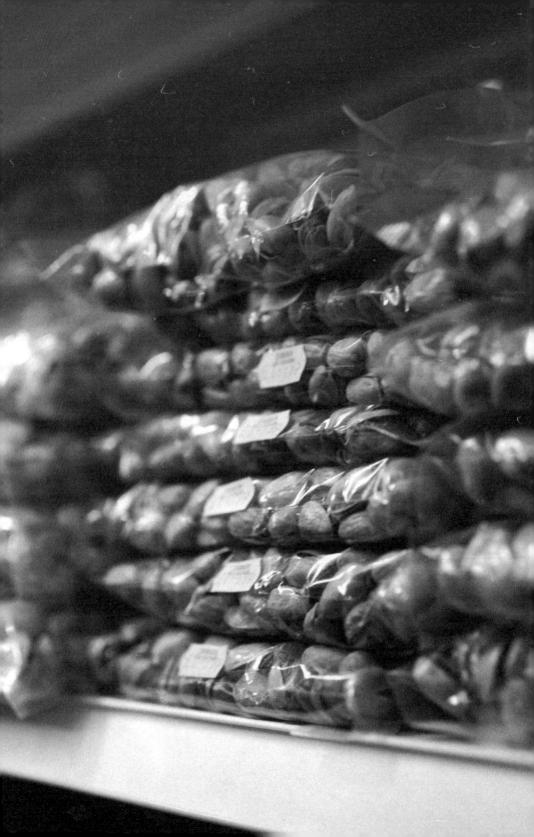

2
store

A good cook knows how to squirrel food away, storing it to save not just time but money, too. Squirrelling reduces the number of occasions when you hear yourself say, 'I haven't the time to cook.' It is also a comfort when you don't want to shop. It's not that taking an evening off cooking is a bad thing, but with the pressure upon everyone to work longer hours and spend more time on other pursuits, a night off cooking can turn into six nights. And unless you really hate cooking, it's not just the cost that is irksome but the sensation that you are 100 per cent reliant on others to choose the food you eat.

A good store of food not only means more home cooking and therefore more pleasure, it makes good economic sense, rewarding you with more money to spend on other things.

A few organisational skills are needed. Briefly imagine living on a boat. The bulk of what you eat must come from packets, cans, or sacks kept in the dark to prevent the contents rotting. Before the days of fridge freezers, the ship's cook must have been a man of talent, able not only to improvise with the few fresh ingredients available but – who knows? – perhaps also to prevent a crew going stir-crazy from meal tedium. Knowing how to use your stores is a good discipline. Even with the advantages of refrigerated storage, store food has changed little from centuries ago.

The miles of aisles devoted to bottled, canned, frozen and packet food are endless. Spoilt for choice, that's us – yet look again and there are very few things that anyone really needs. Cooking sauce? Try a little oil, spice and lemon. Flavoured rice? Add dried wild mushrooms to ordinary rice. Ready-made vegetable curry? Heat canned tomatoes, coconut milk and spices with canned chick peas.

Food manufacturers are always keen to show journalists their latest innovations. Warrens of laboratories are devoted to the imaginings of their development teams. In the name of convenience, they bottle and preserve our favourite foods and create some weird new ones. My heart sinks when I see all this effort in pursuit of the impossible. Fresh pesto tickles every sense; bottled is, well, all right. Home-made tomato sauce is sweet, light and delicate; commercially bottled tomato sauce is salty and acidic, bulked out with thickeners to make money for the manufacturer. None of these is essential. Lazy cooks could save themselves the bother of carrying it all home if only they would shake a little good olive oil on to cooked pasta, chop a bit of chilli and mash a little garlic. This is *olio d'aglio* – the sauce to make when you come in at midnight, desperate not just for food but for real cooking.

The contents of my store cupboard are minimal. Actually, that's not entirely true. The contents of my store cupboard are vast, but most of it is food bought that is never finished. No matter how clever the manufacturer, I don't want their poppy seed, tarragon and lemon salad dressing – I want my bottle of olive oil and a lemon, and a little soft crystal sea salt. The contents of my store cupboard *that I use* are minimal. That is the truth.

This is about the sum of it. I could potentially survive on the following but the children would complain:

dried foods

* Grains – Rice, couscous, bulgar, hulled durum wheat.
* Dried pulses – Green lentils, including Puy, and red lentils.

* Cans – Tomatoes, coconut milk, artichokes in brine; beans (cannellini, flageolet, butter beans) and chick peas; plus there's always a tin of dried Colman's mustard powder, ready to mix with water to eat beside Saturday breakfast chipolata sausages.
* Bottles – French mustard, capers and gherkins.
* Packets – Flours – strong white and wholemeal, plain and self raising plus some alternative flours like gram and potato flour; pasta – both long and short durum wheat pasta, and nests of noodles made with egg; sugar – unrefined caster and soft brown; spices, seeds (sesame and pumpkin), dried fruit (figs, prunes, sultanas), pine nuts and pistachios.
* Fruit and vegetables – Oranges and lemons, potatoes, garlic, shallots and onions.
* Finally, by the hob, there are two bottles of olive oil – standard and good – plus sesame oil, avocado oil (both good wok oils), soy sauce, red wine vinegar and rice vinegar.

the Fridge

* Fats – Butter, dripping, coconut cream and duck fat.
* Dry-cured meat – bacon, ham, salami and chorizo.
* Fresh herbs and salad leaves – wrapped in damp newspaper these keep a long time.

the Freezer

* Meat – A variety of cuts, plus sausages and chicken (see the chapters on meat and poultry).
* Stock – frozen in plastic bottles.
* Seafood – Atlantic prawns and squid.
* Bought pastry, breadcrumbs.
* Fruit and vegetables – red berries, plus oddities like stewed quince and rhubarb, peas and broad beans, and invaluable cooked tomato sauce.

The dried foods listed above are items that have, more or less, been in store cupboards for ever. The important thing is to put them into a modern context, making them fit the life you lead now. It isn't necessary to buy 50 different foods a week. Just a few will do, each put to more than one use. Look at what is fresh in the house, or what can be bought at the shop you pass on the way home. Can it be used with one of your store foods? The shop has spring onions, you have some eggs, frozen peas, and cooked rice left over from last night. A bowl of fried rice is yours, and very good it can be.

cooked store foods

There is a group of storable foods that, since they are already cooked, can be swiftly added to something else for an almost-instant meal. Leftover rice; tomatoes simmered until sweet with oil; mashed potato; braised lentils; meat sauce, and stock – these are the things that really do save time shopping and cooking, while simultaneously helping to provide the home cooking that everyone craves deep down.

food-safety rules

Modern food-safety advice can be the enemy of good home economics. It encourages wastefulness and, worse, it promotes the idea of microwaving chilled or frozen food in sealed containers. Talk of reheating food is viewed by the food-safety authorities as subversive stuff – dangerous talk perverting the nanny state's plan to make all food safe. But there's no hope of making all food safe. Not when 60 million humans are on the loose – eating dirt as babies, sharing dinners with family pets as toddlers. Who hasn't occasionally sampled the glory of a dropped 99 ice cream with its topping of earth and grass, or gallantly rescued a dusty boiled sweet from under the sofa? And in adulthood there are all sorts of opportunities to eat living food, as you begin to enjoy handmade cheeses, air-dried meat and reheated leftovers.

The thing to bear in mind is that the most dangerous thing about food is the person handling it. If you store and reheat food, use your common sense, and your senses. Keep cooked food in clean, sealed containers in the fridge and check it for signs of deterioration in terms of appearance and smell. Always make sure you reheat food thoroughly before use, and the risk to anyone who's had that dirt-eating, dropped-lolly childhood should be low.

rice

I recommend deliberately cooking more long grain or basmati rice than you need. Kept in a sealed container in the fridge, it yields almost-instant meals throughout the week: reheated into a pilaff with meat or vegetables; stir-fried with peas; or stirred into lemongrass-infused coconut milk. Short grain or risotto rice can be partly cooked, then stored to make into quick risottos; any leftover risotto can be rolled into balls, crumbed, fried and eaten with green salad.

rice economics

The value of rice – and all grains, beans and pulses, for that matter – lies in its ability to provide a cheap, meatless meal. Once you accept the principle that more must be paid for better meat, inexpensive foods such as rice become essential. A kilo of good-quality basmati rice should cost around £2.75, while Arborio rice will be about £4. They will yield 20 servings of 50g, each serving costing 14 pence and 20 pence respectively. The cost of added fat, vegetables, herbs and spices is minimal, so this is great food, economically and gastronomically.

buying rice

To make it easy, I buy just two types of rice: genuine long grain basmati from India or Pakistan, and Italian short grain rice, usually Arborio but I have also made short grain rice dishes with Carnaroli, Spanish paella rice and even 'pudding rice', which works magnificently in emergencies.

Basmati rice is grown in the foothills of the Himalayas, in both India and Pakistan. It is the rice I eat plain with curries and sometimes with fish, or make into pilaffs and re-fry in a pan. Good basmati lengthens to almost twice its size when cooked, so it is worth paying for the best. Choose genuine brands, labelled 'pure' basmati, rather than the cheaper, inferior hybrids, which do not lengthen in the same way.

Asian stores and some supermarket delivery services sell 5-kilo bags of pure basmati rice. They have nylon zips so they can be properly sealed to keep out bugs and mites, which is very important. A bag of this size costs approximately £10, bringing the price of one helping of best basmati rice down to 10 pence.

American long grain rice is the other choice. But, while it is cheaper and meatier, it does not have the elegant scent of basmati or its enjoyable texture in the mouth.

Short grain rice is used for risotto and rice puddings. It can absorb twice or more of its weight in liquid, and should retain a tiny opaque pearl of hardness in the centre when perfectly cooked. There are many brands, most of which perform their task well, but makers of specialist varieties from Italy or Spain will wax on about their superiority – which is, in my view, less obvious than it is with genuine basmati.

to cook basmati or long grain white rice

The following method should solve your rice troubles, but given time you will instinctively know when to turn off the heat, how long to leave the lid on, and so on. I like to wash and soak the rice first, as it shortens the cooking time by a few minutes and also helps to produce perfectly cooked, unbroken grains. However, you can omit this procedure if you prefer.

Serves 4–8, depending on appetite

480g/1lb long grain white rice
600ml/1 pint water

To wash the rice, place it in a saucepan, fill the pan with water, then swirl the rice around a bit to release the starch. Carefully pour most of the water away, leaving the rice in the pan. Repeat twice, then cover the rice with water again and leave to soak for a minimum of 15 minutes.

Drain the rice in a sieve, then return it to the pan and add the 600ml/1 pint of water. Bring to the boil, stirring once. Let the rice simmer, uncovered, for about 10 minutes, until all the water has been absorbed, then cover the pan with a well-fitting lid – put foil between the lid and the pan if it is loose. You do not want the vapour to escape. Turn the heat down very low and continue to cook for 5–7 minutes. Turn off the heat and leave the rice for a further 5 minutes, without removing the lid. Fork the rice to loosen the grains and it is ready to eat.

✳ kitchen note ✳

Regular rice cooks rely on their rice steamers, which not only cook perfect rice but keep it warm safely. The best are available from Asian shops.

how to store cooked rice

Cool the rice quickly in the pan with the lid slightly off, immersing the base of the pan in a bowl of very cold or iced water. When the rice is cold, transfer it immediately to a clean plastic container with a tight-fitting lid. It will keep in the fridge for about five days. Smell it and inspect for deterioration before use.

The following three recipes serve two and can be made in minutes – they make perfect TV dinners.

Fried rice

An enormous bowl of this, on the knee – a big cup of jasmine tea beside – makes an immaculate dinner on its own.

Serves 2

2 tablespoons vegetable oil

a few drops of sesame oil

2 helpings of cooked basmati rice (see page 53)

4 spring onions, chopped

1 egg, beaten

4 tablespoons frozen peas

Heat the oils in a non-stick frying pan or a well-seasoned wok, add the rice and stir-fry quickly over a high heat. Mix the spring onions with the beaten egg, push the rice to the edge of the pan and pour in the egg mixture. Turn the heat down to medium and cook, stirring, for a minute. Bring the rice back over the egg and stir thoroughly but with a light touch, flicking the egg through the rice. Once the egg has turned from transparent to pale yellow, stir in the peas, heat for a minute until they defrost and warm through, and eat.

cooked rice with coconut, lemongrass and galangal

Southeast Asian shops can be few and far between but passing one should mean popping in for tubs of real green, red and yellow curry paste, coconut cream and milk, huge bags of rice, galangal, fresh lime leaves and lemongrass. This rice meal takes the edge off the craving for a sour-hot curry, but without the need for a fresh supply of meat.

Serves 2

1 tablespoon oil

1 tablespoon green curry paste

1 red pepper, cut into 1cm/½ inch squares (optional)

2cm/¾ inch piece of lemongrass, outer layers removed, then very thinly sliced

2cm/¾ inch piece of fresh galangal, crushed, or fresh ginger

2 fresh or dried lime leaves

250ml/8fl oz canned coconut milk, or 4cm/1½ inches cut from a block of coconut cream and broken into 250ml/8fl oz water

2 helpings of cooked basmati rice (see page 53)

leaves from 4 sprigs of mint or basil

salt

Put the oil in a saucepan with the curry paste and heat through. Add the red pepper, if using, plus the lemongrass, galangal and lime leaves, followed by the coconut milk. Bring to the boil and simmer for 3 minutes. Add the rice and bring back to the boil, then stir in the herbs and season with salt to taste. Tip into bowls and eat with a spoon.

aubergine and pumpkin seed rice

When I want a warm and filling lunch that will not see me slump fast asleep over my desk mid afternoon, I heat a little cooked rice in a pan with some cooked vegetables, cumin and a few nuts or seeds. I eat it with plain yoghurt – there is usually some in the fridge – and a teaspoon of bought harissa, the hot pepper sauce of North Africa. The fresh ingredients in the following recipe could be replaced by tomatoes, shallots, spring greens, squash or pumpkin.

Serves 2

3 tablespoons olive oil

1 aubergine, diced

1 onion, chopped

2 celery sticks, chopped

1 tablespoon green pumpkin seeds

1 teaspoon ground cumin

2 tablespoons stock or water

2 helpings of cooked basmati rice (see page 53)

leaves from 2 sprigs of mint

salt and freshly ground black pepper

Heat the oil in a pan and add the aubergine, onion and celery. Cook, stirring, until the aubergine is soft, then add the pumpkin seeds, cumin and stock or water. Mix in the rice and reheat thoroughly. Add the mint and season to taste.

✳ kitchen notes ✳

✳ For a richer, sweeter dish, substitute sherry for the stock or water.
✳ A recipe for pilaff using cold cooked rice and leftover roast lamb can be found on page 202.

kedgeree

We made this for a big Christening party recently and agreed that kedgeree is hard-to-beat party food. The bare bones can be made in advance and assembled just before everyone arrives. It's also incredibly rich. A little fish goes a long way in kedgeree, which is an advantage with the high price of sustainable fish. For information on how to choose fish, see page 281.

Serves 8–12

480g/1lb smoked fish fillet – haddock, pollack or hot-smoked organic salmon (see the Shopping Guide)

1 onion, cut in half

6 cardamom pods, crushed

250ml/8fl oz creamy milk

90ml/3fl oz single cream

1 quantity of cooked basmati rice (see page 53)

180g/6oz cooked peeled North Atlantic prawns (optional)

1cm/½ inch piece of fresh ginger, grated

1 teaspoon cumin seeds, toasted and ground in a pestle and mortar

6 fennel seeds, toasted and ground as above

½ teaspoon ground turmeric

30g/1oz butter, melted

4 semi-soft boiled eggs (see page 380), peeled and quartered

8 sprigs of coriander, chopped

Put the fish in a pan with the onion and cardamom pods and pour over the milk and cream. Place over a medium heat and bring up to boiling point. Turn down to a simmer and cook for 5 minutes, or until the fish begins to firm up and flake apart (if you are using hot-smoked salmon, you will not need to cook it – just bring to the boil). Strain off the creamy milk and reserve.

Break the fish into large flakes, discarding any skin or bones, and mix lightly with the rice and prawns. Add the remaining spices, pour over the reserved creamy milk and the melted butter and mix quite thoroughly. Strew the eggs on top and scatter over the coriander.

rice, cucumber and dill salad

The herbs lend their aromas, the onion seed gives a sharp little kick and the cucumber cools down this salad. It will not spoil if you take it to work in a carton. It's also very good eaten outdoors, with barbecued sardines or lamb.

Serves 2

2 helpings of cooked basmati rice (see page 53)
4 tablespoons extra virgin olive oil
juice of ½ lemon
a pinch of sea salt
½ cucumber, cut in half lengthways, then peeled, deseeded and sliced
4 sprigs of dill, chopped
4 sprigs of chervil, if available, or flat-leaf parsley, torn into smaller sprigs
½ teaspoon black onion seeds (nigella)
freshly ground black pepper

Put the rice in a deep bowl, add the oil, lemon juice and salt and mix well. Add a little more oil if you want a wetter salad. Add the cucumber and dill and mix again. Strew the chervil leaves on top. Throw over the onion seeds and finish with a grind or two of black pepper.

short grain rice

There are various traditional risotto recipes in the Stock chapter (pages 130–32) but here is the store-method recipe.

store-method risotto

This technique is used in very busy Italian restaurants that want to be able to make a genuine risotto in 15, not 30, minutes. Although it is frowned upon by purists, it is very useful for anyone who works long hours.

  1 tablespoon butter

  1 onion, finely chopped

  300 g/10 oz short grain Italian rice, such as Arborio

  1 glass of white wine (optional)

  1–1.5 litres/1¾–2½ pints chicken, vegetable or beef stock

Melt the butter in a large pan, add the onion and cook until soft. Add the rice and cook, stirring (preferably with a wooden fork), for 1 minute. Stir in the glass of wine, if using. When it has been absorbed, begin to add the stock a ladleful at a time, stirring constantly over a medium heat. After 10–15 minutes, taste the rice – it should be half cooked, with a white, opaque centre. Strain it, reserving any cooking liquor. Cool the cooking liquor, add it to the remaining stock and store in the fridge, clearly marked. Spread the rice out on a plastic tray, no more than 2cm/¾ inch deep. Allow to cool, cover with cling film and store in the fridge. It will keep for 2–3 days.

  To finish the risotto, cut a piece of the rice from the tray – as much as you need – and put it in a pan. Cover with just enough of the cooking liquor to make it sloppy when stirred. Bring to the boil, then turn down the heat and cook gently for a few minutes, until the rice is tender but firm to the bite – *al dente*. Do not stir. The risotto should be cooked perfectly and ready for Parmesan or a grated hard ewe's milk cheese, plus any other ingredients (see the recipes on pages 130–32 for risotto inspiration).

Fried risotto cakes

Leftover risotto can be shaped into little cakes – a cube of mozzarella hidden inside – then dipped first in flour, then beaten egg, then dried breadcrumbs. Shallow-fry them in a little olive oil and eat as a lunch dish, with a lush green salad.

couscous, bulgar and other grains

This is my sister Sam's domain. She runs Moro, the Moorish-influenced London restaurant, with her husband, Sam, and they know more about grains and allied North African dishes than I can shake a stick at. But in the New English Kitchen, where your pricy piece of meat is reserved for special occasions, grains provide diversity – a lively change from rice. Use whole durum wheat (sometimes sold as pasta wheat or Ebly) in broths (see page 134) and salads, and use grains such as bulgar wheat (cracked whole wheat) and couscous (grains of semolina paste made from durum wheat) in salads with herbs. If you have the chance, buy your grains – along with wonderfully fresh nuts, juicy dried fruits and big bunches of herbs – from Middle Eastern shops. They usually do good bulk deals and take great pride in the quality of these essential goodies. Middle Eastern shops also sell a finer version of bulgar, the true grain to use in a tabbouleh salad with parsley, oil and lemon juice. Couscous is usually sold pre-cooked in the UK, and needs only moistening with water.

to make a store of couscous

To create a store of 6 helpings, put a 240g/8oz teacupful of couscous in a plastic container that will take twice that amount and pour over 200ml/7fl oz cold water and 3 tablespoons of olive oil, stirring. Stir in a large pinch of salt and leave the couscous to swell. After 15 minutes, test the grains to see if they are tender – add a little more water if they are still dry. Use a fork to loosen the grains, then cover the container and put it in the fridge, where it will keep for about 5 days.

Couscous can be eaten very simply with boiled purple sprouting broccoli (see page 339) or with the baked chick pea recipe on page 70. For a decorative, mighty feast, see the recipe below. Its flavour benefits from being made well in advance.

reheating couscous

There are two ways to do this. Put the couscous in an ovenproof dish with a large knob of butter, cover with foil and place in an oven pre-heated to 180°C/350°F/Gas Mark 4 for 20 minutes. Alternatively, melt some butter in a pan, add the couscous and stir over a low heat until warmed through.

a couscous feast

It must be 20 years since I first saw a bowl of hot couscous next to a grand platter of simmered meats and vegetables. It was in France, close to the Mediterranean coast, where merguez sausages, tabbouleh and harissa – a paste made with hot red peppers – could be bought in almost every grocery. Then it seemed so alien. Now couscous, like risotto and dal, has become neo-English; it has a second home and a new following. I like to cook it in a festive way, covering the table with all the component dishes: a large platter of braised lamb and poultry, plus steamed courgettes, carrots, runner beans and golden beetroot (when I can find it – the colour of red beetroot invades in an unpleasant way). There's a bowl filled with fresh parsley and mint leaves, another with toasted nuts and golden sultanas, a dish of harissa, and finally a large pan filled with the cooking juices from the meat, ready to ladle over everything. It's probably inauthentic, but it works.

Serves 8 generously (I am always happy to have leftovers from this for reheating later)

2 small, corn-fed chickens, jointed and skinned (ask the butcher to prepare them for you, with the lamb)
8 lamb shanks, trimmed of fat
10 sprigs of flat-leaf parsley, finely chopped
4 onions, finely chopped
about 2 litres/3½ pints water or chicken stock
120g/4oz butter
2 teaspoons ground coriander
8 spring carrots, trimmed of leaves, then halved lengthways
4 courgettes, cut lengthways into quarters
about 10 runner beans, cut on the diagonal into 2cm/¾ inch lengths
240g/8oz string beans
4 golden beetroot, scrubbed, cut into quarters, and boiled for 30 minutes
salt and freshly ground black pepper

To serve:
leaves from 8 sprigs of parsley
leaves from 8 sprigs of mint
4 tablespoons flaked almonds, toasted in a dry frying pan until golden
4 tablespoons sultanas or 4 dried figs, sliced

harissa sauce (available from Middle Eastern shops and
specialist shops)

480g/1lb couscous, cooked (see page 61)

Put the chickens in one saucepan and the lamb in your largest pan.
Throw half the parsley and half the onion into each pan. Grind about
half a teaspoon of black pepper into each, then cover with the water or
stock. Bring to the boil, skimming away any foam that rises to the
surface. Turn down to a simmer and cook for about 20 minutes, then
put half the butter and ground coriander into each pan. Let the chicken
simmer for another 20 minutes, then turn off the heat. Continue to cook
the lamb for 1½ hours; it should become very tender.

Put all the vegetables in a steamer, or simply put them on top of the
lamb, and cook, covered, for 10–12 minutes, until they are just tender.
Bring the chicken back to the boil (if there is no room for all the vegetables in the lamb pan, you could put the rest in with the chicken and cook
as for the lamb).

To serve, put the herbs, almonds and sultanas or figs into separate
bowls. Lift out the meat and arrange it on a large dish with the vegetables all around. Pour all the stock into a pan, then taste and season with
salt and pepper if necessary. Bring back to the boil. Spoon the heated
couscous on to each serving plate, followed by the meat and vegetables,
then some of the herbs, nuts and sultanas or figs. Ladle over the stock
to moisten, then offer the harissa to those who like a bit of heat in their
food.

to make a store of bulgar wheat

Put 240g/8oz bulgar in a pan, cover with water and add a good pinch
of salt. Bring to the boil and simmer for about 8 minutes, until tender.
Drain and either use immediately or cool quickly and put into a sealed
container. Store in the fridge for up to 5 days.

bulgar and parsley salad for barbecued meat

The salad to make during a parsley glut – you will need a lot of tender leaves.

Serves 2

2 tablespoons pine nuts

2 helpings of cooked bulgar wheat (see page 63)

4 tablespoons extra virgin olive oil

juice of ½ lemon

a pinch of sea salt

8 sprigs of parsley, very finely chopped

2 spring onions, finely chopped

freshly ground black pepper

Toast the pine nuts in a dry frying pan over a medium heat until golden. Add them to the bulgar wheat with all the other ingredients and stir well. Eat with flat breads (see page 22) or grilled meat.

lentils

With lentils you enter the realms of pulses, and the many braised dishes that can be made with them. These are foods that can form a meal in their own right, without meat, fish or eggs, because they contain proteins and fats, but you can also feast on them with those foods. Lentils that have been hulled and split, such as red lentils, are best for soft, sloppy dal-like dishes to eat with hot flat breads (see page 22), while whole lentils belong in stews and salads.

You can make a store of lentils – green ones are good because they will stay firm in a sealed container – eating them once with a big meal, then dipping into them for little dishes of curry, or in salads with semi-soft boiled eggs and herbs.

Puy lentils are the finest. They have blue-grey marbled skins and cost more than standard green lentils, which are over twice the size. Cooked, they have a shiny, almost caviar-like quality and pop pleasingly in your mouth. Both types are easy to overcook, becoming a dry, powdery hash, so keep an eye on them when they are on the go.

to cook puy lentils

Serves about 10

3 tablespoons vegetable oil

1 garlic clove, chopped

1 white onion, finely chopped

480g/1lb Puy lentils

½ teaspoon dried thyme

sea salt and freshly ground black pepper

Heat the oil in a saucepan and add the garlic, onion, lentils and thyme. Swish them around in the warm oil for a minute or two, then cover with water (or stock). Bring to the boil and simmer for about 30 minutes; when cooked, the lentils should be tender inside, with firm skins. Add more liquid during cooking if you need to.

Remove the pan from the heat and tip the lentils into a large, cold bowl – it is important to stop the cooking process and – if you are storing them – to cool them quickly before putting them in the fridge. Season with salt and pepper. When the lentils are completely cold, cover and place in the fridge, where they will keep for about 5 days.

✳ kitchen note ✳

Use a combination of red wine and water for a rich lentil stew to eat with beef or game.

lentils and eggs

Undeniably pretty to look at, this recipe has become a picnic lunch regular.

Serves 2

8 heaped tablespoons of cooked lentils (see page 65)
1 tablespoon olive oil
1 teaspoon red wine vinegar
3 sprigs of coriander, chopped
4 semi-soft-boiled eggs (see page 380), peeled and halved
lengthways
sea salt and freshly ground black pepper

Put the lentils in a bowl and add the oil, vinegar and three-quarters of the coriander. Season with salt and a few grinds of black pepper. Spoon on to a flat dish and arrange the eggs on top. Scatter the remaining coriander leaves over them.

✳ kitchen note ✳

You can use a few pinches of a good curry powder to devil up the eggs a bit.

spiced green lentils with buttered spinach

Scoop this rich, green stew up with strips of hot flat bread – either bought naans or bread made using the recipe on page 22.

Serves 4

2 tablespoons vegetable oil
1 white onion, chopped
1 tablespoon ground cumin
1 teaspoon ground coriander

1 teaspoon turmeric

½ teaspoon cayenne pepper

12 heaped tablespoons of cooked lentils (see page 65)

150ml/¼ pint water or stock

150g/5oz unsalted butter, melted

480g/1lb frozen spinach leaves, defrosted, the water squeezed out

salt

Heat the oil in a saucepan, add the onion and fry over a low heat until it turns the colour of fudge. Add the spices and heat through, then add the lentils and cook for 1 minute, stirring slowly. Add the water or stock and bring to the boil. Simmer for 5 minutes, then remove from the heat and season with salt.

Melt the butter in a large frying pan. When it foams, add the spinach and cook for 1 minute, until it wilts. Pour the spinach on top of the lentils, with the butter, and take it to the table without stirring.

braised red lentils with lime juice and fresh ewe's milk cheese

A meal in itself – soft hulled red lentils, citrus, lots of spice as for dal and lumps of fresh, lemony ewe's milk cheese – feta is best – added at the end. Serve in big bowls and abandon forks, giving everyone a big spoon instead. It can also be stored in the fridge for a few days and successfully reheated.

Serves 4–6

240g/8oz red lentils

1 onion, chopped

a pinch of ground turmeric

3 tablespoons vegetable oil

2 garlic cloves, chopped

2 hot green chillies, chopped

2cm/¾ inch piece of fresh ginger, peeled and finely chopped

juice of 1 lime

2 kaffir lime leaves, slightly torn

240g/8oz feta cheese, broken into lumps

Put the lentils in a pan with the onion and turmeric, cover with water (or stock) and bring to the boil. Simmer for 45 minutes, then strain.

Heat the oil in a large frying pan, add the garlic, chillies and ginger and cook over a medium heat until singed light brown, but not burnt. Stir in the lentils, lime juice and lime leaves, then bring to the boil and add the cheese. Take to the table when very hot – the cheese will soften as it heats through.

beans

Beans are the pasta of Spain and the Latin American countries where they come from, but they do not share pasta's convenience-food factor – unless bought in cans. Dried beans bought in the UK take a seeming age to cook and there is a reason for this. In countries where beans are really valued, they tend to be fresher even when dried, since they are taken from the new-season crops. Ageing beans, dry as can be and prob-ably years old, are sent to those who care less about them – to, er, places like Britain, where everyone happily consumes chicken breasts and tiger prawns for their protein fix. So we get the old beans – the ones that take ages to cook. No wonder everyone prefers pasta. Chick peas are the worst – I once waited seven hours for a pan to produce a batch soft enough to eat. The energy cost must have run to the price of a rib of beef. You *can* buy better beans (there are specialist varieties in Spanish groceries), and patience – or a pressure cooker – will deliver nice tender beans eventually. It's not that you have to do anything while they go through their eternal simmer, just that you have to be around – and most people would prefer to be doing something else.

It's because of this that I am a fan of canned beans. I buy my haricots, cannellini, flageolet and black-eyed beans in cans. They still go a long way – averaging 30 pence per helping – and are perfectly cooked and ready to use. They keep for ever and, apart from being damned heavy to carry back from the shop, are a practically perfect food.

windowsill bean sprouts

Not the oriental sprouts but mung bean sprouts, left on damp paper. This is a lovely, crunchy little sprout that gives its liveliness to open sandwiches made with cold meat and mustard. Children can be put in charge of production – the biology lesson alone is healthy stuff.

Use an old wooden or plastic seed tray with drainage holes and put it on something leak proof. Cover with four layers of kitchen roll and dampen with water. Scatter mung beans on top and leave to germinate, moistening the paper again if necessary. When the sprouts are about 2cm/¾ inch high, after about four days, they are ready to eat.

You can do the same with herb seeds, and slavishly follow the current fashion for pointless but fun infantile plantlings. Frankly, bigger leaves have far more oomph. But there's no harm in them, and buying big packs of coriander seeds will produce coriander babies in a matter of days, to chuck on to green salads, open sandwiches and shut ones.

butter beans marinated with shallots and watercress

To eat with cold meat, such as ham, pork, chicken or beef.

Serves 4

6 shallots, sliced

6 tablespoons olive oil

2 cans of butter beans, drained

the leaves from 2 bunches of watercress (the stalks can be
reserved for soup)

sea salt and freshly ground black pepper

In a saucepan, stew the shallots in the oil for about 2 minutes to remove their raw aroma. Add the beans, remove from the heat and leave to steep in the shallot-flavoured oil until cold. Season to taste and add the watercress, stirring the salad well.

This salad will keep in the fridge for a week – the watercress will wilt but it will still taste lovely. Again, this goes against standard food-safety advice but I check it, smell it, and look for any bubbles or bad signs.

✳ kitchen note ✳

Add canned tuna to this recipe (see page 82).

baked chick peas, peppers and potatoes with yoghurt sauce

Another one-pot standard to keep in the fridge for busy weeks when you don't want to cook. The yoghurt sauce will brighten it, and it's good alone or as a side-of-the-plate number.

Serves 6–8

3 teaspoons ground cumin

2 teaspoons ground coriander

1 teaspoon ground ginger

1 teaspoon freshly ground black pepper

½ teaspoon salt

4 tablespoons vegetable oil

2 onions, sliced

2 red peppers, cut into strips

1kg/2¼lb new potatoes, scrubbed and sliced

2 cans of chick peas, drained

20 cherry tomatoes, or 6 small tomatoes, halved

2 sprigs of thyme

600ml/1 pint chicken, vegetable or beef stock

1 tablespoon butter

For the yoghurt sauce:

8 tablespoons plain yoghurt

1 tablespoon olive oil

a pinch of salt

1 teaspoon black onion seeds (nigella)

Preheat the oven to 200°C/400°F/Gas Mark 6. Mix the spices, pepper and salt together in a small bowl – you will need them as you layer the dish.

Heat the oil in a large casserole and add the onions and red peppers. Cook them over a medium heat until they soften, then add a layer of sliced potatoes and season with the spice mixture. Add a layer of chick peas with half the tomatoes and a sprig of thyme, then season again. Repeat the layering process, finishing with a layer of potatoes and using all the spice mixture. Pour over the stock, dot the surface with the butter and bake for 1 hour, or until the potatoes are tender. Leave for half an hour before you eat, to let the flavours merge.

For the sauce, combine the yoghurt with the olive oil and salt in a bowl. Scatter the black onion seeds on top and serve with the baked chick peas.

potatoes

Buying sacks of British potatoes at the roadside, even in cities, is a great economy. They should be sold in paper sacks to keep the light away from them and prevent them turning green. I now keep a metal dustbin outdoors for potatoes but as long as you store them in a cool, dark place they should be fine.

Looking at the supermarket shelves, you would think that only two or three potato varieties grow in the UK. It's not that Maris Piper, King Edwards or Desiree are dull, simply that there are dozens of other varieties in danger of vanishing unless there is a demand for them – and we, the cooks, are missing out. Many of them are lovely, with colours ranging from white to yellow, and purple to a strange blue-black. Some are waxy, some are earthy and fibrous, some even taste of lemons or chestnuts. Seek out Kerrs Pink, Shetland Black, Wilja and Golden Wonder, as well as some interesting varieties of new potato (see the Shopping Guide). The types of potato grown in domestic gardens are more exciting still – these are the places where you will find old-fashioned varieties such as British Queen, Arran Pilot, Majestic, Suttons Foremost and the various Pentlands.

I would always choose British potatoes over imported but there is a window, between March and May, when supplies are low and the quality is frankly poor. I compromise by buying imports from Cyprus and Spain. I look out for organic when I can, as I do with British potatoes, for clear reasons:

organic potatoes

The season for organic potatoes in Britain is shorter than that for conventionally grown potatoes. The first organic new potatoes are dug in late April/early May and the first large, storable potatoes arrive in shops in September. The late arrival is due simply to the slower growth rate – conventional potatoes grow fast with the help of fertiliser and a lot of water. Using less water and allowing the potato to grow at a natural rate not only strengthens it, protecting it from disease, but it gives the potato more flavour. Here is an instance where there is no doubt at all that an organic food has more flavour than its conventional counterpart. Ordinary potatoes are routinely treated with anti-blight spray – their fast growth means weaker plants that need frequent treatment. They are also treated with sprout suppressants and insecticides after harvest. Organic farmers find that growing several types of potato throughout the season in soil that has been well nourished with manure will also help control disease, but they are allowed to spray with copper to prevent blight. Copper treatments are controversial, as residues remain in the soil, but still greatly preferable to the numerous chemical treatments used on conventional potato farms.

the price of potatoes

Potatoes are caught up in the supermarkets' price wars – sold at less than their value in order to attract customers. Some poorly flavoured varieties are sold for just a few pence per kilo. The real price of the best conventionally farmed potatoes should in fact be up there with the price of organic potatoes, odd as it may seem. This is around £1.40 per kilo. With a kilo of potatoes yielding about five helpings, that's 28 pence per helping – still a bargain for a high-quality food.

roast potatoes

Dripping or duck fat is ideal for making really crisp roast potatoes but you can get a good result with vegetable oil using the following method. I routinely sprinkle flour on to the potatoes after the par-boiling stage because it guarantees crispness, especially in summer when potatoes can be watery, but you can leave it out if you wish.

> 1 large, floury potato per person, plus a couple more for good measure
> a little flour for sprinkling
> dripping, duck fat or vegetable oil

About 1¼ hours before you are due to eat, peel the potatoes and cut them into a shape you like. I cut them lengthways into quarters for a sleek look. Put them in a large pan, cover with water and bring to the boil. Simmer for 5 minutes, then drain in a colander and leave them there to steam for a minute. Sprinkle with a light coating of flour and shake the potatoes around in the colander.

Heat some fat in a separate roasting tin or, if there is room, in the tin you are roasting your meat in. The fat should be about 5mm/¼ inch deep. When it is hot, lift out each potato from the colander and place at even intervals in the tin. Place in the oven and roast until tender and browned – you will probably have to take them out of the oven and turn them over once.

more roast winter vegetables

About half an hour before you serve the roast, slice 1 sweet potato, cut 3 medium parsnips into quarters lengthways and peel a small squash – any sort – and cut it into slices 1cm/½ inch thick. Add them to the tin with the roast, or the roast potatoes, if there is room. Or heat some fat in a separate tin and roast for 25 minutes.

leftover roast potatoes

The season for large potatoes that will keep through the winter begins in August. Cooking too many potatoes is a habit of mine, probably brought about by greed. Before I had children, we always had lots of roast potatoes left over, and I used to fry them until crisp and eat with peppery or bitter greens such as rocket, watercress or curly endive. They become yet more colourful with the addition of diced red chilli and dabs of black olive tapenade.

unused potato skins

Leftover potato peelings that are clean and unblemished can be shallow-fried, preferably in dripping or groundnut oil, until crisp. Serve with soured cream and a chilli sauce.

roast potato soup

You need only a few leftover roast potatoes – or parsnips if you routinely add them to your roasts – to make a heartening soup for very cold weather.

Serves 4

6 roast potatoes or parsnips, cut into cubes

1 large onion, chopped

600ml/1 pint milk

600ml/1 pint chicken or beef stock

salt and freshly ground black pepper

Put the potatoes or parsnips, onion, milk and stock in a pan and bring to the boil. Simmer for about 20 minutes, then cool slightly and liquidise until very smooth. Reheat gently, season to taste, and serve in large bowls, with maybe some chopped fried bacon to make more of a meal of it.

mashed potato

This is easily the most useful of all types of cooked potato and, like rice, it keeps well in the fridge in a sealed container. If it begins to discolour, I throw it away immediately. Milk adds lightness to mash – and scalding it accentuates the potato flavour.

Makes about 10 helpings

2kg/4½lb old potatoes, peeled
300ml/½ pint milk
60g/2oz butter
sea salt and freshly ground black pepper

Boil the potatoes in a large pan of salted water until soft (test by spearing a potato with a sharp knife and holding it just above the pan; if the potato falls off the knife after a second, it is ready – if it sticks, it is not). Drain in a colander and leave in the colander for 10 minutes to steam. The more liquid that leaves the potato, the better the mash. Some people put their (metal) colander of potatoes in a preheated oven for a few minutes, to be sure.

You can either mash the potatoes in the traditional way with a potato masher or purée them through a food mill (mouli-légumes). Then heat the milk to boiling point in a separate pan and beat it into the potato with the butter. Season to taste.

✳ kitchen note ✳

Peeling the potatoes before cooking is an old habit, and I know that boiling potatoes with the skin on works beautifully, too. Doing this means slipping off the potato skins when they are still hot. It's up to you.

potato cakes with watercress sauce

Makes 8

½ quantity of mashed potato
2 eggs, beaten

flour for coating

sunflower or groundnut oil for shallow-frying

For the sauce:

1 bunch of watercress, finely chopped

150ml/¼ pint crème fraîche

1 egg yolk

salt and freshly ground black pepper

Mix the mashed potato thoroughly with the eggs and return to the fridge to firm up. Form the mixture into little cakes, about 5cm/2 inches in diameter and 1cm/½ inch thick, and coat them in flour. Heat a thin layer of oil in a frying pan, add the potato cakes and shallow-fry over a medium heat for about 5 minutes on each side, until lightly browned.

Meanwhile, heat the watercress, crème-fraîche and egg yolk together in a small pan, whisking gently. Remove from the heat before it boils and season to taste. Serve the potato cakes with the sauce poured around the edge.

smoked trout potato cakes

Follow the above recipe, mixing 2 flaked fillets of hot-smoked trout into the mashed potato, together with 2 chopped hard-boiled eggs, if you like. These fishcakes are very good with the watercress sauce.

bubble and squeak

What more can be said about a classic leftovers hash? Except that I add egg yolks for richness, which is not authentic but very good. You can leave them out, if you prefer.

240g/8oz leftover cooked cabbage

½ quantity of mashed potato (see page 75)

2–4 leftover egg yolks

3 tablespoons dripping

Mix the cabbage, potato and egg yolks together. Heat the dripping in a large frying pan, add the potato mixture and fry over a medium-low heat on both sides, until it forms a crisp cake that is hot all the way through.

✳ kitchen note ✳

You can use the same method with all the brassica family, whether the much-maligned Brussels sprout or the ultra-chic Italian cavolo nero. You can also use cooked leeks, anything from the squash family, or sweetcorn – a hash is a hash.

salad potatoes

Salad potatoes are small with firm skins. They are available all year round, and while it is always the right move to buy British during our own new-potato season – from April to July – imported types can be fine when there are no home-grown to be had. Varieties omnipresent in supermarkets are Charlotte and Nicola but do seek out the rarer breeds, too. These include La Ratte, Pink Fir Apple, Belle de Fontenay, Duke of York and Kestrel (see the Shopping Guide). Organic salad potatoes are grown slowly, a factor that no doubt accounts for their deeper flavour. Cook more than you need and use them to help other meals happen. Don't confuse year-round salad potatoes with specialist seasonal types like the papery-skinned Jersey Royals, which begin to arrive in Britain as early as February, or their Cornish early equivalent.

potato salad

This is the best salad to eat with cold ham or beef. The sweeter the onions, the better it will taste. If you can find Breton or Roscoff onions – they are still sold in strings – so much the better. So-called banana shallots, which are in fact onions, make a good substitute.

Serves 4

1kg/2¼lb salad potatoes

1 teaspoon salt

6 shallots, or pink Roscoff onions if you can find them, sliced

Mayonnaise (see page 393)

Put the potatoes in a pan, cover with water and add the salt. Bring to the boil and cook until just tender – they should still be waxy in the centre when you cut them open. Drain and leave to cool, then slice thickly. Put them in a bowl and add the shallots and enough mayonnaise to coat. Mix well.

the freezer

Before you run screaming from the room, I am not about to make you cook for the freezer. I do freeze extra food, but not great bags of every type of vegetable and fruit, which only become soggy and tasteless when defrosted. I make a few shepherd's and fish pies, and braised meat stews and sauces to store in the freezer. Otherwise I prefer to cook from stored ingredients. However, there are foods that are ideal for freezing: peas, broad beans and spinach come to mind. Sweetcorn freezes well – so much better for the children than canned – as do all red berries apart from strawberries.

broad beans

Frozen broad beans have to be used in a certain way because one of their weakest points serves them very well in the freezer. The pale skin that surrounds the inner, podded bean toughens unpleasantly but in doing so protects the flesh of the bean from the ice crystals that make most frozen vegetables go soggy. Broad beans are inexpensive, so the method that follows is not as wasteful as it seems.

Defrost the beans in a colander and put them in a pan. Pour over boiling water and reheat to boiling point. Drain, splash with plenty of cold water and then pinch off the pale skin of each bean. It doesn't take long and you are left with beautiful bright green kernels, perfect to dress with oil and lemon juice and eat with dry-cured meat, hard-boiled eggs, soft goat's cheese, or even quite alone.

frozen peas

A terrific vegetable, and ingredient. It is true that frozen peas often taste better than fresh, unless you can be sure that your fresh supply has been picked within two or three days. This is because fresh peas deteriorate quickly, becoming hard and starchy. It is now possible to buy organic frozen peas and petits pois. I recommend them. not least because it is an inexpensive way to eat naturally produced food (see the Shopping Guide).

Blend frozen peas with stock for an almost-instant pea soup, stir them into rice dishes, or combine them with skinned broad beans (see above), spinach, olive oil and fresh mint for a simple salad that will put the colour green into your winter food.

pea soup with potatoes and bacon

Serves 4

1 litre/1¾ pints chicken, beef or vegetable stock

2 spring onions, chopped

480g/1lb frozen peas, defrosted

150ml/¼ pint single cream or whole milk

4 rashers of unsmoked back bacon, cut into thin slivers

8 salad potatoes, boiled in their skins until just tender then thickly sliced

leaves from 4 sprigs of dill

sea salt and white pepper

Heat the stock to boiling point and add the spring onions and peas. Bring back to the boil and simmer for 1 minute. Allow to cool for a few minutes, then liquidise with the cream or milk. Season to taste with salt and pepper.

Fry the bacon over a low heat until crisp, then add the potatoes and stir to warm them through. Serve the soup in deep bowls with a large spoonful of bacon and potatoes in each. Scatter the dill on top.

frozen spinach

Defrosted slowly, frozen spinach can be as good as fresh. All the water must be squeezed out, and the spinach cooked either with plenty of butter, or heated with good olive oil to make this quick vegetable dish.

spinach with pine nuts

Serves 2

2 tablespoons pine nuts

480g/1lb frozen whole-leaf spinach, defrosted and the water

squeezed out

2 tablespoons olive oil

1 tablespoon lemon juice

salt and freshly ground black pepper

Dry-toast the pine nuts in a frying pan until lightly browned, then set them aside in a bowl. Warm the spinach through in a pan and add the oil. Transfer to a dish, season with salt and freshly ground black pepper and scatter the pine nuts on top. Finish with the lemon juice.

canned food

Canning is ideal for certain foods, a good and pure way to store them without preservatives. It can even improve them in some cases – skipjack tuna being an example.

skipjack tuna

I could never understand why anyone would want to eat a lot of seared fresh tuna. Half the time it is dry and tasteless and, when buying it, it can be hard to tell how long it has been out of the water. What's more, at the current rate of consumption, blue and yellow fin tuna will soon go the way of the dodo. Blue fin – the type favoured by the Japanese for top-quality sushi – is at an all-time low, while yellow fin is in serious decline. The only tuna not listed as endangered is skipjack. The standard of canned skipjack tuna varies from dubious and disgusting small flakes that look like factory-floor sweepings in unidentifiable oil, to tender fillets that, when packed in the tin, look like the cross section of an old tree trunk. This tuna is far superior and has a light texture, because it does not absorb too much oil. The unique double-cooking technique – before canning and then again when the sealed cans are heated to preserve the contents – seems to improve and tenderise the flesh. It can then simply be softly flaked into a salad or sandwich, or made into a delicately flavoured fish cake.

choosing tuna

Trawling for any fish using nets puts other wild species at risk of getting caught up in the gear, but the risk is greater to these lovely mammals when netting tuna. Check labelling on cans to be sure it contains 'dolphin friendly' tuna, looking for mention of monitoring by the EII (Earth Island Institute). The 'dolphin safe' motto you may find on cans from North and South American tuna fisheries is not, according to marine conservationists, so closely monitored. In coming years, the EII hope to develop a logo to make it easier for shoppers.

Catching tuna by pole and line is the only truly sustainable means. Not all 'line-caught' tuna is sustainable. Ask for hand-lined, troll-caught tuna; or tuna caught on long lines that are 'seabird friendly'. It is currently very difficult to tell what fishing method was used for catching skipjack tuna. This is because it is a commodity – like coffee or tea – traded on a world exchange. It's a system of trading that undermines efforts to conserve the tuna numbers. If well-managed fisheries are not rewarded, why bother? In the coming years the Marine Stewardship Council hope to certify the pole and line tuna fisheries as sustainable – watch out for their logo on tins and jars.

You can also find handline-caught albacore – a pale, delicate-fleshed relative often dubbed 'white tuna', and found mostly around the coast of Spain, Portugal and France (see the Shopping Guide).

Always buy tuna packed in either olive or sunflower oil, draining it away before you use the fish.

tuna cakes

Lovely, delicate cakes to eat for supper – tuna-loving children will adore them. Serve with a green sauce (see page 91).

Serves 4

3 tablespoons butter

3 tablespoons plain flour

300ml/½ pint milk

180g/6oz canned tuna, drained

2 shallots, finely chopped

juice of ½ lemon

2 tablespoons freshly grated Parmesan cheese

dried breadcrumbs (see page 30)

sunflower oil for shallow-frying

salt and white pepper

Melt the butter in a small pan and add the flour. Cook gently for a minute, then remove from the heat. Gradually stir in the milk, then cook, stirring, until the sauce thickens and finally boils. Remove from the heat, add the tuna, stirring to break up the flakes, then add the shallots, lemon juice and Parmesan. Season with a little white pepper and the barest pinch of salt. Refrigerate the mixture until very cold, then roll it into a cylinder shape, about 4cm/1½ inches in diameter. Cut it into pastilles 2.5cm/1 inch thick and roll each one in dried breadcrumbs. Shallow-fry the tuna cakes in sunflower oil for 3–4 minutes on each side, then drain on kitchen paper.

tuna salad with skinless tomatoes

I mix preserved tuna with lots of herbs, lemon juice, and virgin olive oil if necessary, then add black pepper and a few capers and eat it with tomatoes. The secret, by the way, of great tomato salads is skinning them. Note to the 'time sceptics': it takes 3 minutes to skin 4 tomatoes. This is how to do it: nick the skin of ripe tomatoes with a knife, submerge the tomatoes in boiling water for a minute, then drain and push the skins off. They have a wonderful way of homogenising the dish, absorbing the olive oil and the flavour of the herbs and allowing the tuna to stick to them.

✳ kitchen note ✳

Add drained, canned cannellini or haricot beans to make a more substantial plateful.

other uses for tuna

✳ Flake tuna over a pea and broad bean salad dressed with olive oil.
✳ Tuna can be added to semi-soft-boiled eggs and lettuce hearts (see page 384).
✳ Tuna is always good with Mayonnaise (see page 393). For an interesting sauce to eat with cold veal or chicken, blend 150g/5oz tuna with 2 anchovy fillets and 150ml/¼ pint mayonnaise, then stir in 1 tablespoon chopped capers. This is a take on the dish Italians love – *vitello tonnato*.

canned anchovies

The best-quality anchovies have a sleek, carefully handled appearance, and come from artisan fisheries. Spanish groceries are a good source of the best, which come packed in olive oil (see the Shopping Guide).

anchovy butter

Melt this butter over green beans, haricots or even a dish of hot new potatoes. If you like anchovies, make a pot and keep it, covered, in the fridge.

Serves 6

150g/5oz unsalted butter

60g/2oz canned anchovies

4 sprigs of parsley, chopped

freshly ground black pepper

Soften the butter in a bowl with a wooden spoon. Drain the oil from the anchovies and pat them with a paper towel to remove any extra. Chop finely, add to the butter with the parsley and mix thoroughly. Season with black pepper and mix again; it will temper any saltiness.

canned tomatoes

Buy canned tomatoes from Italian specialist food shops, choosing authentic brands from the south of Italy. They will be genuinely sun ripened, and canned at source. The tomatoes should have a rich dark red appearance and a thick juice. It does not matter whether you buy whole, quartered or chopped tomatoes, but if you use whole ones for the following sauce, chop them roughly using a pair of kitchen scissors while they are still in the opened can.

canned tomato sauce

Since beginning to make my own Tomato Sauce (see page 358), I have used canned tomatoes less, but was once shown a clever technique for an instant sweet sauce that has rescued a meal or two.

This sauce has been very useful in emergencies for pizza or pasta. It is rather thick because the hot oil instantly caramelises the tomatoes, but it has a character of its own. The technique was shown to me by Carla Tomasi, a wonderful cook from Rome.

3 tablespoons olive oil

1 can of chopped tomatoes

8 basil leaves

salt and freshly ground black pepper

You need a heavy frying pan with a lid to make this sauce safely and successfully. Have the canned tomatoes open and ready.

Put the oil in the frying pan and heat to smoking point. Working quickly, pour in the tomatoes and slam on the lid, otherwise the sauce will spit. When the sound of sizzling has died down, remove the lid and add the basil. Season with salt and pepper.

✳ kitchen note ✳

Substitute *passata* for tinned tomatoes for a very smooth sauce.

tomato juice

The strained juice from canned tomatoes makes a wonderful Bloody Mary. For every 90ml/3fl oz juice, add a dash of Lea & Perrins, a pinch of celery salt, a shot of vodka, half a shot of sherry and as much Tabasco as you like – start with 2 drops. Shake in a cocktail shaker with ice.

canned artichokes

A secret store-cupboard weapon. Canned artichokes come in brine, cost very little and taste bland – until you get to work with your olive oil, herbs, garlic and lemon juice. Eat them on toast, with chopped hard-boiled eggs or soft, fresh cheese.

bottled and canned sweet peppers

Much less fuss than roasting peppers yourself, bottled peppers in oil should be an ideal store-cupboard food but the majority of them are sour from undercooking and, worse, still have leathery skins attached. Go in search of Navarrico, a Spanish brand (see the Shopping Guide). The outlay for a can seems high until you realise that it contains over 20 genuine Spanish, sun-ripened, wood-roasted peppers in olive oil. They have so much flavour you need add only a few to a paella, or use a few at a time in Roasted Pepper Mimosa (see page 386).

cured meats

Bacon is the most obvious example of British cured meat, with hams following closely behind. There's a lot of dry-cured bacon about, but virtually no culture of dry-cured ham such as prosciutto at all. Every other European country has its dry-cured *saucissons* and *salami*; its *charcuteries* and *salumerie* – where are ours? The answer, as explained to me by a successful English butcher, is very interesting: 'We are happy to make sausages and bacon; they're quick to make and we sell them fast. But why would we want to put money on a shelf for six months?' Because you would reap more from it if you waited – there's a real passion for this stuff and we are importing tonnes of it.

The analogy brings Tabasco to mind. Its Louisiana originator, Henry McIlhenny, made the first batch, then forgot about it for a year. When he came back to it, the sauce had fermented slightly and developed a mellow, mature flavour, though it still had the heat of red chilli. It has been made in the same way ever since. Long maturation gives Tabasco its subtle taste. Pity the poor Caribbean sauce makers. They make superb hot sauces but, try as they might, they cannot make a similar sauce or a similar sum of money because they cannot afford the time for maturation. It's an attitude to aged food shared by most British meat curers. We are slowly but surely reviving genuine mature Cheddar and making better wine. But, with few exceptions, British butchers will never see the point of the great starter plate of thinly sliced, dry-cured meats and sausages, with a little pile of vinegary cornichons beside.

Cured meats such as chorizo, bacon and ham hocks are very useful in the New English Kitchen. They can be served as instant meals or used to flavour stews. Take advantage of British-based charcuterie makers (see the Shopping Guide) – your spending power will see others jump on to the bandwagon.

herbs

Herbs give so much to cooking. They lift and freshen dishes and, when matched to the right foods, they turn the flavour volume up – by this I mean they sing, not shout. Herb oil half stirred into a potato soup invades it with its flavours; the same beside grilled or roast meat, or spooned over boiled meats and offal, will make the grey-brown of the dish evaporate and give it a new vitality.

herbs and english cookery

Herbs have always belonged in English cooking. There is a general idea that the English are a nation of rehabilitated mistresses of the bland, rescued by Elizabeth David's *Book of Mediterranean Food* in 1952. Wrong – David herself was perfectly aware of that, as her later books testified. If you believe some of what is said about English cooking, we are masters of roasting joints but otherwise stole everything from the French and Italians. Many people believe the first statement and are subsequently shamed into accepting the second. But this is not an argument about cookery – who made custard first, the English or the French – it is about the real tools: ingredients.

Visit a house that still has its eighteenth-century gardens and you will see a herb or knot garden. Fresh herbs once had a vital place not only in the kitchen but also in the medicine chest. They were used in early recipes for salads along with edible flowers, and in sauces, soups and stuffings. Cooking with them was considered an art. I blame the puritanism that invaded the kitchens of this country in the nineteenth century for the disappearance of fragrant green leaves from our cookery – the twisted concept that exotically flavoured food is vulgar, suspect and bad for the gut. In the southern Mediterranean, aromatics are used to bridge the gap between humble, locally grown ingredients and elegant cuisine, creating an egalitarian cookery available to people on every income level. The prime example is the addition of basil leaves to a plate of sliced tomatoes, refining and cultivating the salad.

Now to those silly plastic packs of herbs that hang on hooks in supermarkets. Hopelessly, guiltily smitten is how I feel about them. They make wonderful food possible, yet I know they should be in big, generous bunches or, better still, in pots on my windowsill. I do grow a few herbs in pots but what I really want is a knot garden because I use a lot of them.

If you can, buy herbs in bulk from Middle Eastern shops. Many of them are grown in the Middle East and arrive here impeccably fresh. Wrap them in damp newspaper and then in a plastic carrier bag – they will keep for at least a week. They are ten times cheaper than the triangular, plastic containers sold in supermarkets and it is well worth lobbying the supermarket you use for larger bunches of a wide variety of herbs. Insist!

✳ kitchen note ✳

My sister Laura, unlike me, has only to glance at a plant and it seems to do whatever she wants. She takes home from the supermarket a potted herb such as basil or coriander. These are usually immature and soft, being 30 or so plants crammed very close together, which is why they do not grow, and drink like camels at a watering hole. She pulls them apart at the root, replants them in compost, three to a pot, and keeps them on a windowsill that gets the sun. Two weeks later, she has ten healthy pots of basil, all from one pot. If you have the time, this is well worth it; the supermarket has done the tricky part for you, you reap the reward.

green sauce

This is a standard to eat with poached, roast or grilled meat, poultry and fish. You can also stir it into mayonnaise or salad dressing. Make a small jar to store in the fridge; it will keep for 2 weeks.

Serves 4–6

5 sprigs each of tarragon, basil, chervil and parsley

about 10 chives

1 heaped teaspoon capers, rinsed, the liquid squeezed out

olive oil

salt

Chop all the herbs and the capers very finely and put them in a jar. Barely cover with olive oil and stir. Taste and add salt to bring out the flavours of the sauce.

herb oils

Herb oils can be used, a few drops at a time, to flavour salads, cooked vegetables and pasta. A pestle and mortar is the best tool to get the right effect. Parsley, basil, dill, oregano and chives are all suitable.

Roughly chop 4 sprigs of either herb, or the equivalent of chives, and put them in a pestle and mortar. Add a few drops of olive oil and begin to work it into the herbs, grinding with the pestle and mortar. Add more until you have a smooth, green oil. Season with a little salt to taste.

✳ kitchen note ✳

Oil blended with fresh or dried smoked chillies makes a good addition to a noodle soup.

herb, oil and breadcrumb 'stuffing'

This can be spooned on to halved tomatoes, cylinders of courgette or thick aubergine slices before baking them in the oven. You can also fry it and serve it beside game or poultry with the gravy.

> 4 tablespoons breadcrumbs, fresh or dried (see page 30)
>
> 2 sprigs of basil or oregano, chopped
>
> 1 garlic clove, crushed with a little salt
>
> 3 tablespoons olive oil

Preheat the oven to 220°C/425°F/Gas Mark 7. Mix together all the ingredients until they are well blended and have the texture of wet sand. Spoon on to the vegetables and transfer them to an oiled baking dish. Cook for half an hour or until the vegetables are soft. Eat them on their own, or beside meat or fish.

year-round salad vegetables

lettuce

While I am grateful for those herbs in their little plastic packs, bags of washed infant lettuce leaves are expensive and taste suspiciously of chlorine. Washing salad in a strong solution of chlorine and water to kill the bugs that cause food poisoning seems to wash away the flavour, too. It can also make the leaves smell downright manky once they have sat on the shelf for a time. This is not to say that all small leaf salad is bad. You can buy fresh leaves, loosely packed, all year round – some from British farmers. Rocket, mizuna, ruby chard, sorrel, purslane, dandelion and pak choi have a beautiful fresh taste and can be bought from specialist grocers and farmers' markets. At £10 per kilo, however, it hurts. The popularity of fresh wild rocket makes it easier to obtain, and slightly cheaper.

Whole Cos or romaine lettuces, on the other hand, are inexpensive, keep for ages and have a good mineral flavour. A salad made with torn romaine lettuce and herbs will be as good as any so-called gourmet leaf mixture. Use the inner leaves for salads and the outer leaves for stock or for creamy lettuce soups (see page 129).

Store whole lettuces and salad leaves as you would herbs. They will keep for a week wrapped in slightly damp newspaper in a plastic bag. Limp lettuce can be revived by separating the leaves and putting them in a ceramic bowl. Cover with a dampened tea towel and leave in or out of the fridge.

cucumber

The standard supermarket cucumber is a watery creature but you can boost its flavour with a simple method. Peel the cucumber, halve it lengthways and scoop out the seeds. Slice thinly, then place in a colander in the sink and throw a little salt over it. Leave for an hour, during which time the water will seep out of the cucumber flesh. Pat dry with a towel, which will absorb the water and excess salt.

Cucumbers store well in the lower drawers of the fridge.

cucumber sandwiches

Butter very fresh white bread and sandwich a few layers of cucumber, prepared as above and seasoned with freshly ground black pepper, between 2 slices.

cucumber salad with mustard

Serves 4

1 cucumber, prepared as on page 93

6 tablespoons olive oil

2 tablespoons red wine vinegar

2 tablespoons Dijon mustard

2 teaspoons golden caster sugar

½ teaspoon soft crystal sea salt

2 tablespoons water

4 sprigs of dill, chopped

10 chives, chopped

freshly ground black pepper

Combine the cucumber with all the remaining ingredients, scattering the herbs on top. Serve with Fried Sole (see page 298).

spiced braised cucumber

An easy, instant curry to eat with flat bread (see page 22).

Serves 2

1 tablespoon butter or ghee

1 onion, chopped

1 green chilli, chopped

1 tablespoon mild curry paste

½ can of coconut milk

4 tablespoons water

1 cucumber, peeled, halved, deseeded and cut into slices

1cm/½ inch thick

1 teaspoon black onion seeds (nigella)

4 sprigs of coriander, chopped

Melt the fat in a pan, add the onion and cook until soft. Stir in the chilli and curry paste and cook for 1 minute, then add the coconut milk and water. Finally add the cucumber slices, bring to a simmer and cook for 5 minutes. Finish with the black onion seeds and coriander.

pickled cucumber

½ cucumber, peeled, prepared as on page 93

1 teaspoon golden caster sugar

2 tablespoons white wine vinegar

a pinch of salt

2.5cm/1 inch piece of fresh ginger, grated

3 small green chillies, chopped

Combine the cucumber with all the remaining ingredients. It's good served with curries or boiled ham.

avocado

When an avocado is perfectly ripe, its oil-rich flesh is almost a sauce, a kind of green mayonnaise that goes so well with crustaceans – yes, it's a refugee from the avocado-and-prawn generation talking – but also matches red chilli, lime and fresh coriander. Avocados are imported into the UK from South Africa, the Caribbean and Mexico. The dark, knobbly-skinned variety, the Hass avocado, has more flavour but some prefer the gentle taste of the smooth, soft-skinned type. Both are available all year round and are as welcome to me as bananas and oranges – fruit that I cannot do without.

avocado mash with coriander and curry oil

Treat this as a starter. It looks dazzling with the yellow oil, particularly if decorated with a few sprouting beans or pea shoots. Smooth-skinned avocados are ripe if the skin gives a little when pressed at the round end; knobbly avocados are ripe when the skin turns from green to a dark greeny-black.

Serves 4

2 teaspoons Madras curry powder

6 tablespoons avocado oil (see the Shopping Guide)

2 ripe avocados

2 tablespoons yoghurt

juice of 1 lime

4 sprigs of coriander, including their roots, well washed

2 shallots, finely chopped

salt

Stir the curry powder into the oil and leave to infuse for 30 minutes. Strain through a fine sieve and reserve.

Peel and stone the avocados, then mash the flesh until almost smooth. Beat in the yoghurt and lime juice. Tear the leaves from the coriander stalks and roots and set to one side. Chop the stalks and roots finely and stir them into the avocado mixture. Season with salt.

To serve, spoon the avocado mash into a neat mound on each starter plate, then scatter over the shallots and coriander leaves. Zigzag the curry oil over the top and eat with toasted flat bread.

✳ kitchen note ✳

If the curry powder does not contain turmeric, add 1 teaspoon to colour the oil a zingy yellow.

watercress

Watercress now grows all year round, and stores well in the fridge. It relies on a supply of clean water to grow and only several days of hard frost will dry up the supply. Most British watercress comes from an admirable co-operative of farms in the south of England, particularly Hampshire and Dorset. Choose this type in preference to French imported – there is no excuse for shops to sell this. Watercress is very underrated, and so English.

The nutritional qualities of watercress were once valued so highly that it was known as poor man's meat. I use watercress frequently in this book as a replacement for the ubiquitously trendy rocket. Its peppery leaf goes with dozens of dishes, and finds a place in sauces and salads, too. Grumble if you are sold sealed bags of watercress that smell of rank water when opened; it means it has been hanging around a bit.

Watercress has the winning attribute of being slow to change colour from bright green to dull olive when cooked, unlike spinach or herb leaves. For that reason, as well as its powerful, clean flavours, I use it in dumplings and soups and in the simple sauce below.

watercress oil

1 bunch of watercress

6 tablespoons olive oil

a pinch of sea salt

Cut off and discard the lower 5cm/2 inches of the watercress stalks. Either whiz the watercress with the oil and salt in a food processor or pound using a pestle and mortar until you have a smooth sauce.

Use in the same way as Herb Oils (see page 91). Good with roast beef, or zigzagged over toast spread with fresh cheeses or smoked fish.

watercress sandwiches

Children once took watercress sandwiches to school, in place of real meat. They are, in fact, very good and, cut small, are nice to eat with drinks before dinner.

Spread slices of good brown or white bread with farmhouse butter, then sandwich with watercress, the lower stalks cut away.

year-round fruit

Oranges and bananas, mangoes and papayas – I cannot do without them, and rely on a supply to cheer up fruit bowls when the English apples and pears have all been eaten, the berry season is over and soft orchard fruits are a memory in a pickle jar to eat with cold Monday leftover meat. I have travelled to Tobago twice and eaten so-called exotic fruits in their home – ripened in the sun and not in the hold of a ship – and was cheered to find that although they tasted better, it was only marginally so.

These fruits are made for travel. They ripen without sunlight in the dark, in our cold shops and quickly on our radiators. The gentle fingers that pack them in boxes in the Caribbean and Africa do so knowing how easily bananas bruise. I once asked a banana trader in London's Nine Elms wholesale market why Caribbean bananas are small and curled and South American bananas long and straight. It was a conversation that has always stayed with me. 'Ah, that is because there is less investment in the banana plantations of the Caribbean,' he said, 'and the bananas are picked before they grow to their full size.' It was 1999 and we were talking about the World Trade Organisation's decision to apply levies on certain European 'luxury' goods to the US, in retaliation for European loyalty to the Caribbean banana market over the largely American-owned plantations in South America/Costa Rica. 'The Caribbean bananas,' the trader continued, 'are picked early because the farmers cannot afford to leave them on the trees even for another week. To me,' he added, 'they always look like small, hungry hands.'

This is an analogy of a worldwide problem for food producers. Lack of investment is the enemy of small food production. Along with coffee, tea, chocolate and dried fruits, Fairtrade bananas are now in most supermarkets. They are still small and curled but I am watching with hope.

fresh mango chutney

This chutney can be made in half an hour or less. Eat with sausages or hot ham.

150ml/¼ pint white wine vinegar

3 cardamom pods

120g/4oz golden granulated sugar

1 red chilli, deseeded and chopped

3 mangoes, peeled, stoned and cut into 1cm/½ inch cubes

1 tablespoon black onion seeds (nigella)

Put the vinegar and cardamoms in a small saucepan and add the sugar. Heat slowly, allowing the sugar to dissolve before the mixture boils. Simmer until the mixture has reduced in volume by about one-third and then remove from the heat. Add the chilli and stir. Pour the mixture over the mangoes and throw the onion seeds on top. You can eat it immediately or store it in the fridge for up to a week.

plantains

If you have never visited an Afro-Caribbean market, you are in for an experience. At Brixton Market in London, you will see some of the most demanding shoppers in action. African and West Indian women, and men, shout at market traders to push prices down and go for bulk deals. They pick up everything, squeeze it and smell it; they are terrific buyers of fresh vegetables and understand their true value.

Plantains are large, banana-like fruits that are eaten cooked. On my trip to Tobago, I ate them sautéed in butter or ghee for breakfast and they were wonderful. Their skins must be completely black before you cook them or they will have no flavour. Eat them with baked chicken legs and Corn Fritters (see page 357).

fried plantain

Serves 2

1 plantain, peeled and cut slightly on the diagonal into slices
1cm/½ inch thick
ghee or butter mixed with vegetable oil
1 lime

Shallow-fry the plantain slices in the fat until golden on both sides and tender when prodded with a fork. Squeeze a little lime juice over them and serve.

pomegranates

Pomegranates are in Middle Eastern shops all year round, although they are particularly plump and fresh in late summer to autumn. They do keep a long time, though – I bought some for Christmas once and they were still there in April, albeit a little shrivelled, but the pips inside were red and juicy. Pomegranates appear frequently in Iranian cooking. I tend to buy them because I like the look of them, and then use only a few in a pilaff or a salad with oranges and spinach. What to do with the rest? What the Iranians do, of course. Make a pomegranate syrup to eat with roast poultry or game.

pomegranate syrup

I am ever grateful to the exhaustive research of Claudia Roden for this recipe. This is an adaptation of her version.

> 4 pomegranates
>
> juice of 2 lemons
>
> 1 tablespoon golden caster sugar
>
> 150ml/¼ pint water
>
> a pinch each of salt and pepper

Cut the pomegranates in half and dig out the seeds. Put them in a food processor and blend for a few seconds – enough to break the skin that surrounds the seeds. Transfer the pulp to a sieve placed over a bowl and squeeze out the remaining juice by rubbing it through with a wooden spoon. Four pomegranates should yield about 300ml/½ pint.

Put the pomegranate juice in a pan with the lemon juice, sugar, water, salt and pepper. Heat slowly and bring to the boil. Turn down to a simmer and cook until the mixture has reduced by about a third. Add more lemon juice if it is too sweet. Pour into a jar and store in the fridge.

✳ kitchen notes ✳

✳ To eat pomegranate syrup with poultry or game, pour it over browned chicken, mallard or pheasant, then cover and simmer for 1–1½ hours, until the meat is tender. Thin the sauce with water if you wish.

✳ Throw fresh pomegranate seeds over the pilaff on page 202 – substituting pheasant or other game for lamb will be even nicer.

dried fruit

Dried fruit has gone though a renaissance and you can now buy wonderful, freshly dried soft pineapple, plums, figs, cherries and cranberries.

I cook them with ordinary dried figs, adding them sliced to stock when braising partridge or pheasant. I make trifle with them too, having discovered by accident when short of fresh berries that they make a much more interesting pudding that is nice for Christmas meals.

winter trifle

Serves 8

480g/1lb dried fruit, such as figs, cherries, pineapples, plums and peaches, roughly chopped
2 glasses of marsala
2 glasses of freshly squeezed orange juice
6 sponge fingers, spread with any jam or Quince Cheese (see page 367)
1 quantity of Lemon Syllabub (see page 104)
dried rose petals and unsalted slivers of pistachio (optional – both available from Middle Eastern shops) or flaked almonds
double cream, to serve

Soak the fruit in the marsala and orange juice for about 1 hour. Put the sponge fingers in the nicest glass bowl you own and pour over the fruit and liquid. Spread the syllabub on top and chill for at least 1 hour. Scatter the petals and nuts on top, then put the trifle on the table with a small jug of cream.

dried fruit meringues

Based on an Australian recipe, this is basically a meringue with chopped fruit and nuts folded in. You can make it into a pavlova-style cake with a layer of cream and fresh figs, which go well with the dried fruit inside, or make small, macaroon-style cakes to put on the table with cheese and coffee after a big dinner.

Serves 6–8

4 egg whites

270g/9oz golden icing sugar, sifted

90g/3oz dried apricots

90g/3oz dates

90g/3oz pecan nuts or green pistachios

Preheat the oven to 150°C/300°F/Gas Mark 2 and line 2 baking sheets with baking parchment.

Put the egg whites and icing sugar in a large bowl and beat with an electric whisk until stiff peaks of white foam are formed. This will take about 9 minutes, so a tabletop food mixer is best, although you can use a handheld mixer.

Chop the dried fruit and nuts finely in a food processor, but do not allow them to become a paste. Fold them into the meringue. Drop dessert-spoonfuls of the mixture on to the baking parchment, 5cm/2 inches apart. You should fit approximately 9 on each sheet. Bake for 30 minutes, until very pale brown and slightly cracked. Allow the meringues to cool on the trays, then lift them off the baking parchment.

lemon and orange zest

Lemons and oranges should be washed or scrubbed before you use the zest, as they are sprayed with a protective covering, unless they are labelled unwaxed. In honesty, I do not always do this, and hope not to suffer as a result of my laziness.

A strip of orange zest in a beef stew, or a few parings of lemon in the cavity of a chicken, is all that is needed to brighten the flavour. You can also dry citrus peel by hanging strips of it on a mini 'washing line' in a warm cupboard – 48 hours should do it. It can be stored indefinitely and added to stews and sauces.

pasta with lemon

Keep the Parmesan away from this. It is delightful alone, clean flavoured and comforting, too. You could serve it as a side dish with grilled sardines.

Serves 4

zest and juice of 2 lemons
175ml/6fl oz best quality, extra virgin olive oil
400g/14oz dried egg linguine
15g/½oz butter
salt and freshly ground black pepper

Add the zest and juice to the oil and leave to infuse for 2 hours.

Simmer the pasta in a large pan of boiling salted water until it is cooked to the bite – there should still be a tiny opaque dot at its heart when bitten or cut crossways. Drain, leaving 1 tablespoon of the cooking liquor in the pan, then add the oil mixture and toss it into the pasta over a low heat. Season with salt and pepper and eat.

lemon syllabub

Syllabub is whipped cream thickened with lemon juice and white wine that has been infused with lemon zest. In spite of its double cream content, it forms a light, lemony mousse that makes a suitable end for any meal, from roasts to curries. Once made, it can be poured into individual pots and kept in the fridge for a few hours, making it an ideal pudding if you want to avoid too much last-minute cooking.

Serves 4

zest and juice of 1 lemon
125ml/4fl oz white wine or sherry

a pinch of grated nutmeg

90g/3oz golden caster sugar

300ml/½ pint double cream

borage or heartsease flowers, or dried Moroccan rose petals, to decorate (optional)

Mix together the lemon zest, juice, white wine or sherry, and nutmeg and leave to infuse for at least 1 hour. Stir in the sugar and then pour in the cream. Whisk together for a minute or two, until the cream thickens. Spoon into small tumblers or old-fashioned teacups. Decorate with an edible flower from the garden, such as borage or heartsease, and chill.

✳ kitchen note ✳

Substitute a different alcohol for the wine. Dry Somerset cider, or a combination of cider and apple brandy (Calvados), is good with a little apple purée in the bottom of the cup; tawny or white port makes a festive, perhaps Christmassy, syllabub – decorate with sultanas that have been soaked in the port beforehand. End a Burns Night dinner with a syllabub made with whisky, served with buttery shortbread.

caramelised oranges

Peel and slice 6 oranges and put them in a dish. Put 2cm/¾ inch golden granulated sugar into a small, heavy-based saucepan and cover with just enough water to soak it. Bring to the boil slowly, then cook at a fast boil until the contents darken to the colour of maple syrup. Before the caramel becomes too dark, pour it over the oranges. Decorate them with borage flowers, if it grows near you.

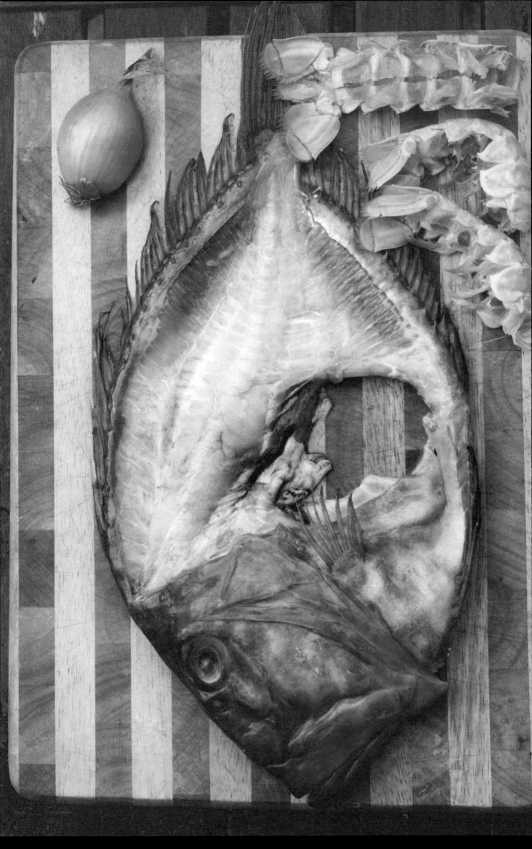

3
stock

The natural ingredients in home-made stocks transform the flavour of a dish. In a soup it brings to the fore the taste of the vegetable, reducing the need to 'cover' it with salt before you eat. A risotto is enveloped with the goodness in the stock, a stew thoroughly heartened. But there is more goodness to stock – of the non-sensual type:

✳ Stock costs almost nothing, and makes valuable items like meat and fish go just that bit further for you economically, rolling on to an extra meal.

✳ Stock makes use of things you might otherwise throw away, recycling the remains of a roast, some mushroom stalks or vegetable peelings – even the shells of prawns.

✳ A store of good stock saves shopping time – it is a meal half made. It easily links the foods stored in your fridge or cupboard: a few ladlefuls put together with a can of white beans, maybe some broken pasta and windowsill herbs, can make a cheerful soup you'd be happy to serve to others.

✳ Making stock does not take up your time. While the simmering water around those bones and peelings extracts their flavour, cooks need do nothing at all.

the economics of stock

As I have said, there is a wider argument for making stock than the glories of its taste; one that demands a complete readjustment in the approach to good home economics. As successive disasters related to intensive food production have unfolded over the last ten years, it has become glaringly obvious that if we want uncontaminated raw food, we will inevitably have to pay more. But if you keep the roast free-range chicken carcass, ask for extra bones from naturally reared beef, or reserve those organic mushroom peelings, you will get twice, even three times, as much from costlier food. Now that a naturally reared chicken costs at least twice as much as a broiler-house bird, it is necessary to extract every bit of its worth. It becomes, I promise, very hard to sling away a chicken bone when you know it still has value in its marrow.

Making stock also solves the 'what shall I cook next?' problem. Many cooks, inspired by television cookery programmes or recipes in the press, admit they love the idea of cooking everything with fresh ingredients, but complain that this means too much shopping, overfilled fridges, and too many dishes that must be begun from scratch. A store of stock tells, even dictates, what to do next – it is one half of a risotto or pilaff; one half of a lamb braise or fish stew and at least one half of any soup. If there is a supply of stock in the fridge, there's no tough decision – the meal you have just made rolls neatly into the next one, be it half a day or half a week later, because stock keeps so well.

A last word of encouragement: making stock in the home creates an atmosphere. You walk in the door to an aroma that tells you there's good food in this place. The atmosphere never really leaves. When the pot is on the go, the welcome scent buckles knees – but even when it has been stored away in plastic bottles and containers there hangs a message in the air: we love food enough to make stock.

bought stock (stock cubes, stock powder and ready-made fresh stock)

There is no knowing where the meat in standard stock cubes comes from. It could have been imported, you have no idea what the animals were fed on or to what standard of welfare they were reared (there is more detail about these issues in the chapters on poultry and meat). It must be said that there is little meat in stock cubes – but there will be a whole lot of other things.

To make up for their lack of flavour, most conventional, non-organic stock cubes contain flavour enhancers, whose main purpose is to conceal the fact that they contain so little meat (or fish or vegetables, depending on the type of stock cube). These additives include hydrolysed vegetable protein (HVP) and monosodium glutamate (E621) – both of which have associated health risks. HVP is a highly processed food, not permitted in manufactured baby foods. To make it, vegetable proteins are treated with hydrochloric acid, converting them into amino acids. Food scientists discovered that the flavour of these acids can imitate meat when they are added to stock cubes or powder, and manufacturers of some of the best-known brands have been merrily doing so ever since. HVP is added to vegetable stocks, too, so they taste of meat. Hmm – is this what vegetarians really want? It is also used in the manufacture of other seasonings, particularly soy sauce. The vegetable proteins in HVP are various: soya beans, wheat, cottonseed, peanuts and corn are used but this essential information is not supplied on stock- cube labels. HVP has been found to contain small quantities of the carcinogen, chloropropanol, sometimes called 3 MCPD. These levels have not been assessed as dangerous, but it is still wise to buy natural stock and naturally fermented soy sauce (see the Shopping Guide).

Monosodium glutamate (MSG) is celebrated by manufacturers as a seasoning that brings out the natural flavours of food without adding its own, but it is associated with risk as an allergen and, controversially, as a cause of hyperactivity in children.

Contacting the Food Standards Agency department responsible for advice to consumers about these two types of additive produced a reply, *after five weeks*. Their response was not user friendly:

'MSG (E621) is permitted at a maximum level of 10g/kg either singularly or in combination with Glutamic Acid (E620), Monopotassium Glutamate (E622), Calcium Diglutamate (E623), Monoammonium Glutamate (E624) and Magnesium Diglutamate (E625). It is also allowed in condiments and seasonings at *quantum satis* levels (i.e. in accordance with good manufacturing practice).' FSA 09.03.04.

Enlightened? Reassured? I wasn't. The only reason these chemicals end up in food is because the manufacturers are not using enough real food to give their products real flavour. Real food is expensive; chemical additives cheap. Manufacturers profit from the low proportion of real meat, fish or vegetables in their stock.

Stock powder is widely held to be an improvement on stock cubes – perhaps it's the hippy-style package designs on some tubs – but if you read the label, there is little difference between them. And all are heavily over-salted. This goes for organic stock cubes and powder, too, although Soil Association standards do not allow the use of HVP or MSG. The meat used in organic stock should have been organically reared – a guarantee of good animal welfare standards and natural feed. Examine the label for evidence of this; the word 'organic' should appear in brackets after meat in the ingredients list.

For emergencies, buy freshly made stock in plastic tubs – it is sold refrigerated – and choose organic; labels reveal very little about the quality of the meat used in conventional freshly made stock (see the Shopping Guide). This is an extravagant way to go about it, though – you will soon be hesitating before tipping those roasted bones into the bin.

Canned consommé is not a good substitute for stock. Ideally consommé should be made only from beef or chicken and vegetables but manufacturers happily tip in bouillon powder and salt with extra gelatine to give the broth the gelatinous texture it would have had if it had been made properly in the first place.

Try this test. Once you have made your first-ever batch of home-made stock, reserve a cupful. Make a second cup of stock using a stock cube and taste them both, looking for the separate flavours of real ingredients and artificial ones. It's a good exercise for the palate – in future you will have a heightened ability to identify stock-cube-based gravy or risotto in restaurants and, 'fraid to say, other people's houses.

meat stocks

bones

It is very easy, as a shopper in the new century, to hide away from awkward issues about food. Almost no one in the West hunter-gathers, so there's no need to confront or take responsibility for the way in which our food is produced. However, there are concerns about bones that every meat lover should be aware of, and which now seriously threaten the producers of naturally reared meat.

The best meat comes from artisan producers and butchers. The word 'artisan' means 'made with skill', and in the traditional sense this means made by hand. Artisan butchers tend to seek out meat from live-stock that have been fed a natural diet, reared without stress in small herds and killed locally. They then carefully hang and artfully cut the meat, which will, inevitably, taste good and cook beautifully. These artisan meat retailers, which may include butcher's shops, farm shops and home delivery companies (see the Shopping Guide), have thrived since the food scares of the 1990s. BSE has, in effect, been good for them and good for their customers. No matter how hard the super-markets try – and some have made great efforts, albeit with marginal amounts of the meat they sell – supermarket meat will always lack the quality of that sold by the artisan butcher. This is because supermarkets don't have access to the relatively small number of prime animals, and even when they get good meat they are unlikely to hang it properly.

BSE has, however, been bad for the bone business. The food scares triggered a raft of new and sometimes draconian regulations affecting everyone in the meat industry, including a rule specifying that bones and other 'waste' material must be collected for safe disposal in rendering plants. The cost of this collection falls to the butcher – a tax, in other words. So the artisan meat companies that have enjoyed an increase in their sales of good-quality, traceable meat since BSE are now seeing their survival threatened by the cost of the new regulatory regime. The authorities are dismissive of their pleas to keep the administrative expenses low. The regulators are hostile to paperwork-heavy small businesses, and artisan producers suspect they would happily see them go out of business.

the real waste

'Indeed, it has been said, and not altogether facetiously, that the only industry in which some part of the cow is not used is concrete production.' *BSE Inquiry: The Report* (Volume 6, Chapter 4)

In 1996 Devon farmer and artisan butcher, Peter Greig, was being paid for his bones – or, put another way, the surplus bones and fat from his butchery were collected and he received a cheque from the Prosper de Mulder Group, a company that was given state subsidies to collect waste. Guess where this waste went? It was rendered – quite literally melted into meat and bonemeal (MBM) – and fed back to cattle. Further waste material was made into tallow, a grease once used for candles but more recently added to human food, pet food and pharmaceuticals. A table put together in the report following the BSE enquiry listed the many uses of cattle waste: they included buttons, glue, racquet strings and musical instruments, dye and paint, fire extinguisher foam, toothpaste, chewing gum, door handles, felt, ankle support dressings, glycerine, collagen, leather and surgical implants.

All in all, if you value animals, it's terrific to know that a steer can be not only your Sunday roast but also the button on your coat – or it could have been. Everything changed after 1996, the year the possible link between BSE and its human form, CJD, was established. All British beef waste must now be destroyed in giant furnaces – leather is about the only by-product it is still easy to obtain. And the odd horn button.

At the end of all of this, Peter Greig now finds himself having to pay the Prosper de Mulder Group – same people, eight years on – an average of £6,000 per year to take away his waste (all animal waste, not just cattle). It was less after the BSE crisis but, as the subsidies have gradually been picked off by Brussels, the waste collectors have put the price up. The cost of collection has even risen above inflation, year on year. Why, I suggested to Greig, doesn't he get someone else to take it away for less? Because Prosper de Mulder has the monopoly on the practice, he said, at least in the Southwest.

the more bones the better

Because he'd like very much to reduce the amount of bones he has collected, the butcher will be your instant friend if you ask for extra bones for stock, or take those attached to the piece of meat you buy even if you do not need them for a particular dish. You are reducing his burden.

Stock making can become a habit, almost addictive. Whenever you roast something, add some bones to the roasting tin and they will brown with the meat, ready to be put in the stock pan later. The more bones you use for stock, the richer and more flavourful it will be.

Asking for bones for soups and stock will surprise supermarket managers or employees on the meat counters, but keep asking even if you get a negative response, because word will filter back to their buyers, whose job is to please *you*.

Bones should be given to you for free, but you may be charged a nominal sum by a butcher whose marrow bones are in high demand. Ask your butcher to saw the bones into manageable chunks to fit your saucepans.

time to make stock

I don't want to be precise about making stock; it is easy, yet there is an art to it. The recipe below for stock can be used with bones from all types of meat. You can be versatile about adding other flavours in the form of alcohol, vegetables or herbs, but it is necessary to understand how to extract the most taste from the stockpot.

Stock does not take long to make in terms of hard work – putting all the ingredients into the pan and straining it when done is about as strenuous as it gets. The period of simmering that each type needs varies from 1–3 hours. You can be in, doing whatever you like, or out shopping. Some people make stock in a slow cooker, overnight or while they are at work. It requires a different method, so I have written a recipe for Slow-cooker Stock (see page 119). Making stock arguably saves time because it means you have less shopping to do, plus a convenient store of a vital ingredient in soups, rice and pasta dishes.

making stock from raw bones

If you roast meat off the bone, ask the butcher to give you the bones wrapped separately, then roast them beside or under the meat. The meat for a forerib of beef, for example, will sit neatly on its cradle of rib bones; this has the dual benefit of preventing the meat drying out while browning the bones for stock.

If you buy raw bones on their own, rub them with a little vegetable oil and roast them at 200°C/400°F/Gas Mark 6 until browned – when the bones brown, it creates molecules of flavour. You can also brown meat and vegetables in a heavy-based pan over a high heat. Allow the 'bits' to stick to the bottom of the pan; they will add colour and flavour, too.

meat stock (beef, veal, lamb, pork and ham)

Real stock is easy to make – not with artificial flavour enhancers or loads of salt but by simmering meat, fish or vegetables in a pot until their flavour, aroma and colour have been extracted into the water.

Makes about 1.5 litres/2½ pints

1kg/2¼lb bones taken from either:

marrow or rib bones from beef or veal (British milk-fed veal only – see page 415)

½ leg of baked or roasted ham

roast loin, shoulder or leg of pork

or any part of lamb

Plus vegetables, chosen from:

2 onions, peeled and halved

3 celery sticks, roughly chopped

4 carrots, cut in half

1 fennel bulb, or its outer layers

2 leeks, cut in half

Plus herbs (optional):

1 bay leaf

a pinch of dried thyme

4 sprigs of parsley

Put all the ingredients in a large pan, cover with 1.75 litres/3 pints of water and bring to the boil. A little foam will rise, from the fat combined with the heated water – skim it off if you wish. Otherwise it will boil back into the stock, which is harmless, but it makes for a cloudier broth.

When the stock boils, turn it down to a slow simmer and cook for 2 hours (for pork, ham and lamb) or 3 hours (for beef and veal). Turn off the heat and cool slightly. Strain the stock through a large sieve or colander and chuck away the bones, vegetables etc. Leave the stock to cool completely, then refrigerate. It should set to a jelly. If there is any hardened fat on the surface after chilling, you can lift it off if you wish but I often leave it there as a hygienic seal.

❋ kitchen note ❋

Adding wine to stock deepens and enriches the flavour and sweetens it slightly. Use dregs of red or white wine when making meat stock, or white wine for poultry or fish stock.

concentrated stock

After straining, you can reduce stock to concentrate its flavour. Pour the stock into a clean pan and simmer until reduced by the desired amount. The longer you let it simmer, the more intense the flavour will become. It is possible to boil it down to just 300ml/½ pint and reconstitute it later with water. This is a good method for anyone with little storage space.

storing stock

Cool the stock quickly, then store it in either the fridge or the freezer. I store stock in everything from double polythene freezer bags to Tupperware boxes and plastic water bottles – you can just snip the narrow neck off with kitchen scissors and cut the bottle open when you want to use the stock, in order to defrost it.

I have found that fresh stock will keep in the fridge for 1–2 weeks, left undisturbed in the coldest area. Always smell stock before you use it. If it smells of anything other than the ingredients in it, or sour and lemony, throw it away. Make sure all stored stock comes to the boil before use or in the recipe, and simmers for a minute or more. Frozen stock keeps for at least 3 months and can be melted in a pan over a low heat.

clarifying stock

This method will produce very clear stock. It's a job for the perfectionist but fun to try just for the magic of it.

To make about 1 litre/1¾ pints of clarified stock, place approximately 1.5 litres/2½ pints of well-flavoured stock in a pan over the heat and bring it to the boil. Whisk 3 egg whites until foamy, then add them to the stock. Keep whisking – the egg whites will harden and form a crust on the surface of the stock. Leave to simmer on a very low bubble for about 45 minutes. The egg whites will absorb the bits, leaving a clear liquid. To strain, ladle a little of the stock at a time into a muslin-lined sieve set over a bowl.

Use clarified stock for clear soups, adding sherry or brandy, thinly sliced vegetables or cooked haricot beans.

✳ kitchen note ✳

Save egg whites from making Mayonnaise (see page 393).

poultry stock

There is more calcification in the bones of free-range, slow-growing poultry than in intensively reared birds, and consequently they make more and better stock. You can use the carcasses of roast chicken, duck or turkey in this recipe.

Makes about 1.5 litres/2½ pints

1 poultry carcass

1 bay leaf

a pinch of dried thyme

6 black peppercorns

4 sprigs of parsley

1 sprig of tarragon (optional, for European recipes)

Plus vegetables, chosen from:

2 onions, peeled and halved

3 celery sticks, roughly chopped

4 carrots, cut in half

1 fennel bulb, or its outer layers

2 leeks, cut in half

Put everything in a pan and cover with 1.75 litres/3 pints of water. Follow the cooking, straining and storing instructions for meat stock on page 115, but simmer for just 45 minutes–1½ hours.

game stock

Makes about 1.5 litres/2½ pints

1kg/2¼lb venison bones or 2–3 game bird carcasses

1 bay leaf

a pinch of dried thyme

6 black peppercorns

4 sprigs of parsley

4 juniper berries

Plus vegetables, chosen from:

2 onions, peeled and halved

3 celery sticks, roughly chopped

4 carrots, cut in half

1 fennel bulb, or its outer layers

2 leeks, cut in half

Put everything in a pan and cover with 1.75 litres/3 pints of water. Follow the cooking, straining and storing instructions for meat stock on page 115, but simmer for just 2 hours for venison, 45 minutes–1½ hours for game birds. Game stock tends to have more gritty 'bits', so strain the finished stock through a very fine sieve or a piece of muslin (available from hardware or haberdashery stores, or nursery shops).

slow-cooker stock

Slow cookers, those independent lidded pans that plug into the wall, have a real purpose in the rolling kitchen for cooks who are out all day and cannot wait around for stews and stocks to cook. They have undergone a small renaissance looks-wise, too – there are now sleek, chrome-covered pans with black ceramic linings and glass lids replacing the ubiquitous cream décor with a hideous brown ear-of-corn motif.

The slow-cooker method is only suitable for meat stocks, because they are the only ones that benefit from a long cooking time. The slow cooker gives them a beautiful clarity and intensity of flavour. You can also get more stock from the average amount of bones because it cooks for such a long time. There is one problem with slow cookers, however, and that is their distinctive, sour smell. It has no impact whatsoever on the finished stock but if you can place the cooker in a well-ventilated room, or even in an outbuilding with mains electricity, so much the better. I put mine in the utility room, where it competes with the smell of washing powder and the tumble dryer.

To make slow-cooker stock, use the ingredients specified in any of the meat stock recipes on pages 115–19. Before you put them into the slow cooker, start them off in a large pan. Add a tablespoon of vegetable oil and swirl around the vegetables as best you can over a high heat, followed by the bones. When the vegetables soften slightly, add the water and bring to the boil, skimming off the foam that rises to the top. Then transfer everything to the slow cooker and turn it to the highest setting. You will have lovely crystalline, flavoursome stock within about 6 hours. Most slow cookers have an automatic setting that allows you to set the stock to boil before you go to bed or out to work.

vegetable and fish stocks

basic vegetable stock

To make a broth from meat you need at least an hour, or even 4, but vegetable stocks need only about 30 minutes – they are last minute in comparison. This opens the door to a soup that would otherwise be impossible. You can have that risotto, the potato dish, or noodles with slices of leftover pork.

A store of a few useful vegetables, peelings and herbs is all that is needed. If you are cooking a meal with a lot of vegetable peelings, put them in a pan as you go, cover with water and simmer for a simple stock.

Makes about 900ml/1½ pints

60g/2oz butter

1 onion, chopped

1 carrot, chopped

1 celery stick, with leaves, chopped

trimmings from any of the following: mushrooms, fennel, leeks, green beans, lettuce, asparagus and broccoli (use as much or as little as you have)

a few parsley stalks

1 sprig of thyme, marjoram or oregano (or ½ teaspoon dried thyme or oregano)

10 fennel seeds

salt and freshly ground black pepper

Melt the butter in a decent-sized pan and stir in the vegetables and trimmings. Sweat, covered, over a low heat for 10 minutes, then add the herbs and fennel seeds. Cover with 1 litre/1¾ pints of water and bring to the boil. Reduce the heat, half cover the pan with a lid and simmer for 15 minutes. Strain through a sieve.

concentrated celery and leek stock

A thicker, greener stock that can be used as a base for sauces or cold dressings, such as the one on page 135.

Makes about 750ml/1¼ pints

30g/1oz butter
2 heads of celery, chopped
4 leeks, chopped
6 sprigs of parsley
1 sprig of thyme
1 bay leaf
salt

Melt the butter in a large pan and add the vegetables and herbs. Cover with about 1.75 litres/3 pints of water and bring to the boil. Simmer for 50 minutes. Strain through a sieve into a clean pan, pushing as much juice out of the vegetables as possible. Boil until the stock has reduced by half, then season with salt.

✳ kitchen note ✳

You can make a similar broth with fennel instead of celery and leeks. Return a few of the cooked fennel pieces to the stock after straining, liquidise and use as a broth to pour over fish. I had something similar with shellfish in Richard Corrigan's lovely restaurant, Lindsay House, in Soho, and have never forgotten it.

shellfish stock

This golden stock can be made from cooked North Atlantic prawns or from langoustines, using the 'toasting' method.

Makes about 900ml/1½ pints

prawn or langoustine shells and heads from about 1kg/2¼lb
shellfish (raw or cooked)
1 celery stick, chopped

Put the shells and heads in a large, dry frying pan and toast them until golden. Put them into a saucepan with the celery and 1 litre/1¾ pints of water and bring to the boil, skimming off any foam that rises to the surface. Turn down to a simmer and cook for 20 minutes – no more, or the flavour will spoil. Strain through a fine sieve.

✳ kitchen note ✳

Shellfish stock keeps best when frozen, for up to 3 months.

Fish stock

Use this in place of shellfish stock, for all fish soups and stews. If the fish supplier has any little oddities such as small crabs or gurnard, ask for them too – they provide a lot of extra flavour.

Makes about 1.5 litres/2½ pints

1kg/2¼lb non-oily sea fish bones, heads and tails (ask for the gills to be removed)
150ml/¼ pint white wine (optional)
1 onion, roughly chopped
1 carrot, roughly chopped
1 celery stick, roughly chopped
a sprig of thyme
4 sprigs of parsley
6 peppercorns
6 fennel seeds
10 coriander seeds

Wash any slime off the fish and put it in a large casserole with all the other ingredients. Cover with about 2 litres/3½ pints of water and bring to the boil, skimming away any foam. Simmer for 30 minutes, then leave to cool. Strain through a fine sieve and taste for salt.

❋ kitchen note ❋

Fish stock keeps best when frozen, for up to 3 months.

using stock in cooking
making gravy

The two recipes below are for making gravy after you have cooked a roast. You can use beef, lamb, pork, poultry or game stock, no matter which type of meat you have roasted.

thin gravy

Serves 6–8

1 glass of wine or sherry (optional)

600ml/1 pint meat stock

salt and freshly ground black pepper

Once you have removed the roast from the tin and put it in a warm place to rest, pour any fat out of the tin, leaving behind the bits that lurk and cling to its base. Place the tin over a low heat and allow it to sizzle. Add the wine or sherry, if using, or a ladleful of stock, and scrape with a wooden spoon to lift the bits off the tin (known to professionals as deglazing). Simmer for half a minute, then add the remaining stock. Bring to the boil and simmer for about 3 minutes. Season to taste.

thickened gravy

Children seem to like thicker, meatier gravy, so I always make it when I eat roasts with them.

Serves 6–8

1 tablespoon plain flour

600ml/1 pint meat stock

salt and freshly ground black pepper

Pour off the fat from the roasting tin, leaving approximately a tablespoonful behind, and set the tin over a low heat. Add the flour and stir with a wooden spoon, making a paste and scraping away at the bits on the bottom of the tin. Add the stock a little at a time, incorporating it to make a smooth sauce the consistency of single cream. Bring to the boil and simmer for 3 minutes, then season to taste. If there are any lumps, you can always push the whole lot through a sieve.

recipes using meat stock

ham hock and bean soup

A ham hock is a salted knuckle of pork, sold smoked or unsmoked. The bone enriches the broth, and there is plenty of sweet, lean meat under the rind. This soup, kept in the fridge, will provide a week of warming winter lunches.

Serves 6

1 ham hock, soaked overnight in cold water

2 tablespoons vegetable oil

2 onions, finely chopped

2 celery sticks, chopped

2 garlic cloves, peeled but left whole

1 can of chopped tomatoes or the equivalent of Tomato Sauce (see page 358)

1.5 litres/2½ pints meat stock

a pinch of dried oregano

3 cans of cannellini beans

salt and freshly ground black pepper

Put the ham hock in a large pan, cover with water and bring to the boil. Drain well, then cover the hock with fresh water and bring to the boil again. Turn down to a simmer and cook for about 1½ hours, until the ham begins to fall away from the bone. Remove the hock from the water and leave to cool, then chop the meat into bite-sized pieces.

Heat the oil in a large casserole and add the vegetables. Cook gently until soft, then add the tomatoes, stock and oregano. Bring to the boil and simmer for 40 minutes. Add the ham and beans and cook for 10 minutes. Season to taste with salt and pepper.

✳ kitchen notes ✳

✳ You can make this soup with a chunk of bacon and add lean Italian pork sausages or semi-cured chorizo.

✳ Beg the end of the Serrano or even Iberico ham bone from Spanish groceries and use in the soup.

noodle soup

Serves 4

Cook 200g/7oz Chinese dried egg noodles in boiling water for about 4 minutes, until soft but firm to the bite. Divide them among 4 bowls and pour 250ml/8fl oz meat stock (approximately 1 mugful) over each one. My children like this soup plain, but you can finish with freshly ground black pepper and perhaps some coriander leaves and a little chilli oil.

recipes using chicken stock

The gentle taste of chicken stock is the most versatile of all, but beef, veal, pork and game bird stock are pretty interchangeable.

vegetable broth with basil and garlic oil

A pool of bright green sauce floats above the simplest soup of clear chicken broth and soft vegetables. The French call the sauce *pistou*; originating on the southern coast, it is a relative of the northern Italian pesto.

This is a soup to eat when shop shelves are stacked with beans, peas and waxy little potatoes, but it converts to winter vegetables, too. Try celeriac, parsnips, celery, or thinly shredded green cabbage.

Serves 4

1.75 litres/3 pints chicken stock

2 courgettes, quartered lengthways and sliced into small pieces

4 tablespoons fresh or frozen peas

2 medium potatoes, boiled and cut into 1cm/½ inch dice

other optional vegetables: turnips, fennel, chicory or cooked flageolet beans – all but the beans finely chopped

salt and freshly ground black pepper

For the sauce:

4 tablespoons olive oil

2 garlic cloves, crushed to a paste with a little salt

6 sprigs of basil, torn to bits

Bring the stock to the boil in a large saucepan and add all the vegetables. Bring back to the boil and simmer for 5 minutes, by which time the vegetables should be cooked. Taste and adjust the seasoning.

Mix together all the sauce ingredients. The best way to do this is in a pestle and mortar, but without one, give them a good stir and mashing in a bowl with a wooden spoon.

Give everyone a bowl of soup, dropping a tablespoon of the sauce on to the surface.

smooth vegetable soup

I love thin, creamy, frothy soups with one primary vegetable flavour. The addition of crisp fried bacon or black pudding, or just a few drops of herb oil, makes them special, rather than ordinary. The following recipe fits all non-green vegetables.

Liquidisers make the best smooth soup, but a standard food processor will do. Once the soup has been made, never let it boil when reheating.

Serves 4 generously

30g/1oz butter

2 onions, roughly chopped

2 medium-sized white potatoes, roughly chopped

1 litre/1¾ pints chicken stock

500ml/16fl oz single cream or whole milk

salt and freshly ground black pepper

Plus one of the following vegetables:

1 large parsnip, diced

half a small cauliflower, broken into pieces

half a swede, cubed

2 large turnips, cubed

1 head of celery, the strings stripped away and chopped

4 medium-sized waxy potatoes, diced (omit other potato)

3 young green leeks, chopped

1 butternut squash or 2 thick slices of pumpkin, peeled, deseeded and chopped

Melt the butter in a large pan, add the onions and cook gently until soft but not brown. Add the potatoes and the vegetable you have chosen and cook for a minute, then pour in the stock. Bring to the boil and simmer until the vegetables are tender.

Cool slightly, then liquidise with the cream or milk until smooth. Return to the pan and reheat gently. Season to taste with salt and pepper.

smooth green vegetable soup

For the same soup made with green vegetables – peas, watercress, outer leaves of lettuce, spinach – follow the above method but add the primary vegetable 1–3 minutes before the end of cooking, allowing it to become just tender before liquidising.

things to add to soups

Lightly stir any of the following into the surface of the soup after you have put it into bowls.

* Olive oil flavoured with curry powder, or chopped parsley, garlic and basil, or red chilli (see page 91). These go best with potato, pumpkin or squash, parsnip and celeriac soups.
* Sautéed slices of black pudding or chorizo; chunks of dry-cured bacon. Best with potato, spinach and watercress soups.
* Fresh herbs such as thyme leaves or lovage. Best with soup made from outer lettuce leaves.
* Chilli pepper sherry, made by steeping fresh red chilli in sherry for about 48 hours. Best with lentil or barley broth (see page 134).
* Cream and crushed pink peppercorns. Best with lettuce, pea, watercress and celery soups.

a sauce for meat flavoured with mustard and white wine vinegar

This is a light sauce made from the juices in the bottom of the roasting tin or sauté pan – a great mopping-up sauce for pork, veal and chicken, eaten with mashed potatoes.

Pour away any excess fat from the roasting tin or sauté pan, place it over the heat and add a glass of white wine. Scrape away at the juices in the bottom of the pan with a wooden spatula, then add 2 tablespoons of Dijon mustard and 250ml/8fl oz chicken stock, plus the torn leaves from 2 sprigs of tarragon. Bring to the boil, stirring. Simmer for 1 minute, then add 2 deseeded and chopped tomatoes and a teaspoon of white wine vinegar. Adjust the seasoning and serve with the meat.

✳ kitchen note ✳

To make a good sauce for reheating cold poultry and meat, add 150ml/¼ pint crème fraîche or single cream to the sauce above, after adding the tomatoes and vinegar, and simmer briefly. Pour the sauce over the slices of meat and reheat in a covered dish in the oven. Eat with rice or mashed potato.

risotto

To make stock into something weightier than soup, use it for risotto. Risotto gets its character from short grain rice, which absorbs not only liquid but flavour, too. The basic principle of making risotto is the same whatever flavouring ingredients you use, but purists say you must not add more than two extra ingredients to the master recipe of rice, onion, white wine and stock.

Cooks argue about the texture of a good risotto. I have eaten runny, soup-like risottos with a spoon and tackled heaps of a more solid type with a fork. Awkwardly, I'd always go for a texture that is somewhere between; a soup you can eat with a fork. Ultimately it is up to you, the cook, how much stock you add just as the risotto reaches the point of being cooked, and how you personally like it.

Serves 4

1 heaped tablespoon butter

1 heaped tablespoon finely chopped white onion

360g/12oz risotto rice

90ml/3fl oz white wine

1.2 litres/2 pints or more chicken stock

2 tablespoons freshly grated Parmesan cheese, plus extra to serve

1 tablespoon cream or a knob of butter

salt and freshly ground black pepper

Melt the butter in a pan, add the onion and cook gently until soft. Add the rice and cook, stirring (preferably with a wooden fork), for a minute or so, then add the wine and simmer until evaporated. Over a medium heat, stir in the stock a ladleful at a time, allowing the simmering rice to absorb it before you add more. Continue until the rice has absorbed enough liquid and tastes cooked to the bite. Stir in the Parmesan cheese. Stop further cooking with the addition of the cream or a knob of butter. Season to taste and take straight to the table. The whole process should take about 35 minutes.

✳ kitchen note ✳

Risotto does not like to wait for people, it becomes stodgy and dry. If you prefer not to cook right up to the moment food is served, there is a 'nearly instant' risotto on page 59.

various risottos

✳ Saffron – Steep a pinch of saffron in some warmed stock, then strain and add at the end of the cooking. This is the classic risotto to eat with meat braises (see pages 216–17).

✳ Dried or fresh mushrooms – Steep dried mushrooms in hot stock for about 15 minutes, until soft, then drain. Add to the risotto at the end of cooking (the soaking liquid can be added to the risotto with the stock). Fresh mushrooms should be sautéed until tender in a separate pan and added at the end of cooking.

✳ Langoustines and clams – Steam the langoustines and/or clams in a covered pan with a little wine and add to the risotto just before serving.

✳ Beef bone marrow and parsley – You must order the marrow bones from a butcher. Cut out the marrow, wiping away any hard fragments of bone, then fry it in butter and add towards the end of cooking.

✳ Peas and broad beans – Simmer peas and broad beans in a little stock, pop the beans from their thin skins and add at the last minute. You can use frozen peas and broad beans with great success (see page 80).

✳ Squash – Peel, deseed and dice 1 butternut squash or 3 Gem squashes and add them with the onion.

✳ Use cheese, preferably Parmesan or the English equivalent, on all but seafood risottos. Make use of windowsill herbs, too, such as parsley, basil, chives and chervil.

duck and celery soup

We are back in the realms of 1930s country-house food – a shimmering duck soup with a few thin slices of celery, chopped celery leaves and wild mushrooms. Use wild or farmed duck for this recipe, left over from a roast.

Serves 4

1 large duck carcass or 4 mallard carcasses

a little dripping or butter

2 celery sticks, roughly chopped

2 carrots, roughly chopped

2 shallots, roughly chopped

2 juniper berries

salt and freshly ground black pepper

To serve:

4 tablespoons sherry

1 celery stick

8 wild mushrooms (chanterelles in autumn, morels in spring), very thinly sliced

Preheat the oven to 200°C/400°F/Gas Mark 6. Rub the carcasses with a little dripping or butter and roast them until golden. Transfer to a large pan, add the vegetables and juniper berries and cover with water. Bring to the boil, skimming off any foam, then turn down to a simmer and cook for 1–2 hours. Strain the stock and pass it through a very fine sieve or a muslin cloth. Skim off any remaining fat – although I like to see a bubble or two of it floating on the surface.

To serve, pour the stock into a clean pan, add the sherry and bring almost to boiling point. Pull the 'strings' from the celery and slice it very thinly across the stem. Add to the soup with the mushrooms. Season to taste and serve with Cheddar Crisps (see page 437).

game broth with barley or wheat and parsley oil

Use cooked pearl barley for this soup, or whole durum wheat, sometimes sold as Ebly. Add the flavoured oil the moment it goes on to the table.

Serves 4

1.5 litres/2½ pints game stock
200g/7oz pearl barley, cooked until tender
herb oil (see page 212)
salt and freshly ground black pepper

Bring the stock to the boil in a pan. Divide the cooked grains between 4 bowls and pour over the boiling stock. Add a drop or two of parsley oil and serve.

recipes using vegetable stock

Vegetable stock can be used in all the soups and braises in this book – substituted for meat, poultry or fish stock – so I will give no more recipes for it apart from this one, an intense, green dressing to pour over salads.

vegetable dressing

4 tablespoons concentrated celery and leek stock

8 tablespoons extra virgin olive oil

2 tablespoons very finely chopped parsley

8 basil leaves, very finely chopped

10 chives, very finely chopped

a few drops of lemon juice

salt and freshly ground black pepper

Put all the ingredients in a jar and shake until well blended. Alternatively, for a smooth sauce, pound them in a food processor or a pestle and mortar.

Make a salad using one or more of the following and dress with the sauce:

cooked artichokes

avocados

cooked new potatoes

cooked broad beans (skinned frozen broad beans are very good) or thin green beans

cooked beetroot (try to find yellow or stripy beetroot, as it does not bleed)

salad leaves

fresh cheeses

langoustines

North Atlantic prawns

recipes using shellfish and sea fish stock

spiced soup with mushrooms

A light, clear broth, sour and hot with lemongrass and chilli to clear the head. Add coconut milk for a richer soup.

Serves 4 as a starter, 2 as a main course

5cm/2 inch piece of lemongrass, outer layers removed

1 red chilli

1 green chilli

1 shallot

a large sprig of coriander, with root

1 tablespoon vegetable oil

1 litre/1¾ pints shellfish stock or fish stock

about 30 button mushrooms, sliced

Roughly chop the lemongrass, chillies and shallot, then crush them to a paste in a food processor or a pestle and mortar with the coriander root (keep the leaves until the end). Mix the paste with the vegetable oil.

Heat the stock in a saucepan and add the paste by degrees, tasting until you have the heat you want. Some like this soup as hot as they can take it. Add the mushrooms 5 minutes before you eat the soup, then the coriander leaves as it sits in the bowl.

aromatic soup with saffron and aniseed

This is very similar to the base for a French *soupe de poisson*. You can eat it as a broth with toasted day-old bread and *rouille* (see page 394) or you can use it as a base stock for a big-meal seafood soup.

2 tablespoons olive oil

1 fennel bulb, finely chopped

2 onions, finely chopped

4 garlic cloves, finely chopped

2 glasses of white wine

1 litre/1¾ pints shellfish stock or fish stock

a pinch of saffron threads

½ teaspoon fennel seeds

½ teaspoon coriander seeds

6 tomatoes, skinned, deseeded and chopped, or ½ tin of

chopped tomatoes

3 tablespoons Pernod

Heat the oil in a large pan, add the fennel, onions and garlic and cook until soft. Add the wine and cook for 1 minute, then add the stock with the saffron. Crush the fennel and coriander seeds in a pestle and mortar. Add to the soup with the tomatoes, then bring to the boil and simmer for 30 minutes. Stir in the Pernod just before you eat the soup.

shellfish soup with rice noodles, coconut milk and chilli

In Southeast Asia, this is called a *laksa*. There are some flavours from faraway shores that are so easy to adopt – think of Thai green curry and chicken tikka. The base paste for this soup is one of those. The quantities given below for the paste will make enough for at least 3 meals. Store the extra in the fridge for 2–3 weeks. Both the shrimp paste and dried shrimp can be found in Asian or Thai grocer's shops, or buy the Blue Dragon brand from a supermarket.

This is a fresh-tasting soup that you can cook from your stores by making sure you always have cans of coconut milk or a bar of coconut cream and some rice noodles in stock, perhaps peas in the freezer and a pot of mint on the windowsill.

Serves 4

600ml/1 pint shellfish stock or fish stock

600ml/1 pint coconut milk

2 teaspoons fish sauce (*nam pla*)

200g/7oz wide rice noodles

4 tablespoons frozen peas

leaves from 3 sprigs of mint

sea salt

For the *laksa* base:

2 onions, roughly chopped

5 large red chillies, halved and deseeded

2 teaspoons shrimp paste

1 tablespoon dried shrimp

2cm/¾ inch piece of fresh ginger, grated

2 lemongrass stalks, outer layers removed, chopped

1 teaspoon ground turmeric

2 teaspoons ground cumin

Put all the ingredients for the *laksa* base into a food processor and whiz to a paste.

Boil a kettle. Heat 2 tablespoons of the *laksa* base in a large saucepan until it bubbles, then add the stock, coconut milk and fish sauce and bring to the boil. Put the noodles in a large bowl and pour over the boiling water, then leave for a couple of minutes.

Add the peas to the simmering soup. Drain the rice noodles in a colander and divide them among 4 soup bowls. Scatter the mint leaves on to the noodles and pour over the soup with the peas. Put sea salt on the table; I find you need a tiny bit to bring all the flavours out.

✳ To make this soup from scratch with langoustines or prawns, use 20 raw crustaceans. Pull the meat from the shells (reserve it to add to the soup) and then put the shells in a dry frying pan to make stock (see page 122). Strain, chuck away the shells, and follow the recipe above. Add the raw crustaceans to the soup with the peas and cook until pink.

✳ If you make the soup with raw chicken thigh meat or thinly sliced pork, add it to the boiling soup before the peas. You can substitute runner beans, string beans, Thai yard beans – anything in the pea family – for the peas, if you want. You can see I cannot make up my mind with this soup – but that is its beauty.

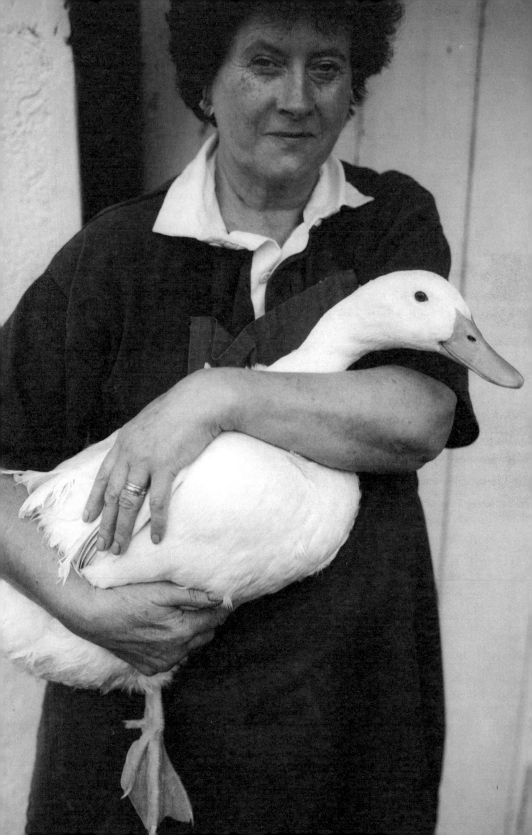

4
poultry

Chicken was my inspiration for this book. Long before I knew that the unwanted shells of langoustines made glorious broth, or that a hunk of stale bread had so many beautiful uses, I knew about chickens, good things and bad. The good news about the chicken is its recent renaissance. It is now so much easier to buy a bird that has been reared kindly, and whose well-calcified bones make gelatinous stock and many meals from it. The bad news was – and is still – the meat industry's ruthless exploitation of this once-valuable bird's suitability for factory farming. Sadly, the same can be said for other poultry – ducks, guinea fowl and turkey.

There are now two types of poultry available commercially: factory reared and naturally reared, with the latter costing up to three times more. This is the reason I cannot throw away the carcass of a chicken without making stock first. It's the reason I pick every bit of cold meat from it, even if only to make a small sandwich.

The naturally reared bird grows slowly, taking its exercise outdoors, where it pecks about and behaves as nature intended. It is fed on grains and plants, free of any growth-promoting drugs or animal protein. Its active lifestyle means it has plenty of muscle on long, strong bones. You'll know this when you eat it: the meat has more flavour than factory-farmed birds and is agreeably chewy. At the risk of sounding savage, the way this mature meat squeaks to the bite is utterly pleasurable.

The story of that other bird is a very different one.

poultry highs and lows

Talk to anyone who was around before the 1960s and they will tell you that a roast chicken was once a luxury that would appear on the table only for Easter lunches or other special occasions. Chickens may have made more frequent appearances on farmhouse tables but they tended to be male birds that were unwanted for procreation in the egg runs. Robust and strong, these were the birds that you braised with vegetables until their awesome meat fell off the bone. They were highly valued by farmers, and by anyone lucky enough to eat them.

Not so the contemporary broiler bird, jostling for space in a shed with a low roof, on bedding that is unlikely to be changed during their short lifetime – just over 40 days. Fed a high-protein diet – soya, sometimes fishmeal – they are also routinely given antibiotics in their feed to prevent the outbreaks of disease that occur frequently when birds are kept in such close contact. These are described as growth promoters, since no disease means the development of the birds will be uninterrupted. They reach the 'desirable' weight in time – the said fortyish days – and costs are kept low.

imported meat

There's also a major market for imported poultry meat in the UK, much of which finds its way into restaurants, ready meals, takeaway foods, office canteens, schools and hospitals. In Europe it is permitted to inject breast meat with protein-enhanced water to add weight and substance. For reasons of food safety – it can be very unhygienic – this meat is not permitted for sale in the UK, but there is no guarantee it does not find its way in. The food industry, like any other, has its cowboys.

the ultimate cost of cheap meat

All this makes for very cheap meat, but shoppers pay in the end. Numerous studies have concluded that putting antibiotics in animal feed affects the immune system of the people who ingest them. As bacteria become resistant to antibiotics, we are more likely to succumb to infections. And our ill health must be paid for – by loss of earnings, by the National Health Service, or by the purchase of pharmaceutical drugs. Ultimately we pay.

Factory farming thrives, however, because the industry will always persuade the government that the post-war generation must have cheap food. After 50 years of this, we have paid a very high price indeed for cheap food, and continue to do so. Worse still, it is the most vulnerable people – those on low incomes – who suffer the most because they are the chief consumers of intensively farmed meat. Banning the use of routine antibiotics in farming is the answer – but would the government do it? Would it upset the broiler industry? Or the supermarkets that make all that money from chicken breast meat? Would it ever.

chicken utopia

Let's imagine that it did or, even better, that it went all the way and abolished the broiler system, admitting that it is a revolting practice that is no longer acceptable to the public. Imagine a world where more farmers have diversified and free-range chicken farming – which even at its lowest standard is preferable to broiler houses – is commonplace in the warmer counties. Those loosely housed chickens are less vulnerable to disease and suffer little stress. Delicious chicken meat is there for everyone. But one thing is certain: the price of chickens has increased. Let's say it has doubled – and it is vital for cooks to know how to make the most of each chicken they buy.

you're the one with the money – vote for what you want

We'll be waiting a while for the utopia described above, but if consumers ask for it, it will happen. Retailers won't take action without a strong shove from shoppers. The alternative would be new legislation to improve poultry welfare but experience teaches that any such thing would be slow in coming and that consumer power has always been the short cut to change.

However, as I have said, it is possible to buy decently farmed birds, and hopefully the number will increase as more people become aware of the horrors of intensive farming. The more people avoid broiler chickens, the more farms are encouraged to adopt free-range systems. Vote with your wallet – the message will be heard.

where to buy naturally reared chicken

Every supermarket, and virtually every butcher, sells or has access to birds that have been naturally reared. Organic chickens are reared to the highest welfare standards of all, but they rarely come in at less than £12 each, which is why it is essential to make the most of them and treat them as a special-occasion food. Having said that, there are some farms that have developed extraordinary modern systems and have their own abattoirs; their organic chickens are better value than some of those in supermarkets (see the Shopping Guide).

Free-range chicken systems vary – once again you must ask the butcher, or read labels very carefully. The more they tell you, the better tends to be the news. The following guide will lead you to welfare-friendly chicken – don't forget to ask for the giblets.

✳ Buy direct from farms – There is a well-established number of poultry producers who pride themselves on their high standards. Many have websites with clear statements regarding feed, breed and welfare. The range is diverse, from co-operatives selling boxes of six good-value birds, to organic farmers, to producers of small, aristocratic French breeds that feed just two people (see the Shopping Guide).

✳ Butcher's shops – It is rare to find a butcher who does not offer free-range chickens. Again, ask where they are from, and how they are fed and reared.

✳ Farm shops – Poultry farms selling at the farm gate have two distinct advantages for the shopper: value for money and the chance to see the birds in their field.

✳ Farmers' markets – contact the National Farmers' Retail and Markets Association (tel: 0845 230 2150; www.farmersmarkets.net) to find out details of your local farmers' market. They are fun to visit and the farmers themselves enjoy the interaction with their customers.

✳ Supermarkets – Take your reading glasses, if necessary; it's time to scrutinise some labels. The words 'free range' are not enough. A well-bred chicken will have a lot more information on the label about its lifestyle and feed. Don't be afraid to ask questions at the customer service desk – they must respond and your curiosity will be noted.

look for new-old breeds

Poultry breeding was once all the rage, the pursuit of keen lady farmers, but now a chicken is a chicken, and rarely sold by breed. However, there is a growing number of specialist poultry farms reviving old breeds, or breeding crosses between such old varieties as Rhode Island Reds, White Rock and Cornish hens. The French farmhouse-style, black-legged chicken from Bresse is also back.

It's the same story with turkey. The Kelly family in Essex revived the Norfolk Bronze turkey, calling it the Kelly Bronze, and the rare, long-bodied Norfolk Black turkey is being raised again. Who knows, those American wild turkeys that stand chest high to men might make a comeback, too . . .

good economics in whole birds

It makes greater economic sense to buy a whole bird than chicken breasts. The breasts are the most valuable part – worth two-thirds of the total cost of the bird. Look at it this way: £4 of chicken breasts means £3 more to buy a whole, free-range bird. From that you will get a curry for two people from the thighs, while four small children will enjoy roasted chicken wings and drumsticks with some Corn Fritters (see page 357). That's two adults' and four children's meals for £3 – and all from a free-range chicken. Any butcher will joint a chicken for you for free. In supermarkets the cost of cutting it, however minimal, is built into the price of portioned chicken.

The same attitude can be taken with duck. Frankly it is easier to cook a jointed duck. Carving a whole roast duck is very difficult; it's much better to eat the roasted breasts from a large duck for one meal as they cook quickly and serve three to four. Then braise the legs very slowly with whole peeled potatoes that cook to a crisp as they absorb that lovely fat. When asking the butcher for a jointed whole duck, don't forget to ask for the carcass, so you can make a clear, sherry-shot broth flavoured with celery (see page 133).

Naturally reared turkey is available all year round (see the Shopping Guide).

the price of chicken

The cheapest high-quality naturally reared chicken is around £7 for a medium-sized bird but it is normal to pay £14 for a large, top-quality free-range or organic bird. The following table shows the economics of buying a £14 bird, based on a household of four people. A 2.5kg/5½lb chicken should yield just over 1kg/2¼lb meat.

one chicken weighing 2.5kg/5½lb

1st meal:	four 150g/5oz helpings of roast chicken
2nd meal:	four 90g/3oz helpings of cold meat in a salad
3rd meal:	two sandwiches made with the remaining cold meat
4th meal:	four helpings of creamed squash soup, made from 1 litre/1¾ pints of chicken stock
5th meal:	two helpings of mushroom risotto, made from 500ml/16fl oz stock

One £14 chicken goes into five meals, making 16 helpings at an average cost of 87 pence each.

storing chicken

Chicken must be stored in the fridge and cooked soon after purchase – a maximum of two days is safe. Raw chicken freezes well, however, and properly wrapped it will still be in good condition after three months. I have kept cold cooked chicken for up to a week, sometimes more, but five days is safe as long as you have followed the usual rule of cooling hot chicken quickly and getting it into a sealed container and into the fridge as soon as possible. If you have made poached chicken, for eating throughout the week, take it out of the fridge and bring it to the boil in its cooking liquor every other day.

a large roast free-range chicken with long, hard bones, squeaky, firm meat and skin like mature, burnished parchment

To accompany roast chicken in winter, I make creamy bread sauce, roast potatoes (because my children allow nothing else) and a big dish of carrots covered in butter and parsley. In summer, roast chicken sits beside a large pan of rice pilaff, couscous, cracked barley or wheat, or new potatoes. Herbs and spices are somehow essential in summer – allspice, ground coriander and my favourite herbs, mint, parsley, dill and coriander.

Leftover cold chicken goes into sandwiches but can also be shredded for spicy salads dressed with sesame or mixed with herbed mayonnaise. And yes, again the carcass will yield a nice brown stock with many uses. It will give real depth of flavour, real length to, perhaps, a green vegetable soup, ready in minutes to eat with garlic- and basil-flavoured olive oil, or creamy, frothy soups made from turnips, pumpkin, peas – whatever you choose. Any leftover stock can be stored in the freezer and used to make a smooth mustard, tarragon and tomato sauce (see page 130).

roast chicken

Serves 4–6

1 large oven-ready chicken, preferably with giblets

½ lemon

a walnut-sized lump of butter

vegetable oil

dried thyme or oregano

salt and freshly ground black pepper

If you can buy a chicken that contains giblets, put the liver in a bag and store it in the fridge to make a spread for toast (see page 156). Preheat the oven to 190°C/375°F/Gas Mark 5.

Untie the chicken if it is trussed. Put the heart – very recognisable among the giblets – in the cavity with a grind or two of black pepper and throw in some salt. Push in the lemon, giving it a squeeze as you do so, then add the butter. Pull away the fatty lumps on either side of the cavity opening. Rub the chicken with a little oil and season the surface with salt, pepper and a pinch or two of dried thyme or the gentler oregano, sometimes called wild marjoram.

Put the chicken in a roasting tin – you will not need further oil – and roast for just over 1½ hours. Test for doneness by stabbing a fork or skewer into the thigh, through to the breast. It is the thickest part of the meat and if the juices are clear, the chicken is cooked. If they are pink, it needs a further 10 minutes. Roasting a chicken slowly in this way allows a natural gravy to develop in the bottom of the tin. If you own one of those clever double-spouted gravy jugs that separate the juices from the fat, you will not need to make gravy.

Allow the chicken to rest for 10 minutes after roasting, so that the juices that have risen to the surface seep back into the flesh.

to carve the chicken

Remove the wishbone – you do not have to do this – but it makes it much easier to carve the breast. The wishbone is a loose, fork-shaped bone found at the wing end of the chicken, between the 2 breasts. Simply cut downwards on either side of it and hook it out. With a carving knife, cut the skin between the breast and leg. Use the knife to push the leg outwards. This should break the joint but if it doesn't, do so with the knife or twist the leg using a carving fork.

Slice the breast meat, then slice away the wings, again cutting through the joint or twisting it with the help of a carving fork. Underneath the chicken you will find two 'oysters' of lean brown meat in a recess. They can be easily prised out with a knife.

stuffing

I cannot see the point of stuffing a roasting chicken, nor any bird for that matter. You only end up overcooking the bird in pursuit of thoroughly cooked stuffing. There is, however, a clever way to stuff chicken that does enhance it. Make a stuffing based on chopped garlic and herbs, a little grated lemon zest, plus a few teaspoons of breadcrumbs made from old bread (or use toasted pine nuts) and season with salt and pepper. Run your fingers under the skin between the breast and the leg meat – you will find it lifts quite easily. Push the stuffing between the skin and the meat, then roast the bird as described above. The same can be done with a guinea fowl or turkey. If you are lucky enough to have a supply of real Perugia white or French black truffles, you can slip a few slices under the skin with butter. A true luxury – it will be nothing but bean soup for a month after!

to roast chicken drumsticks and wings

Browning chicken joints on the hob and then finishing the cooking in the oven is the quickest method, and ensures that the meat is well coloured on the outside and juicy within. Do invest in a good-quality roasting tin (see the Shopping Guide). Put some olive oil in a bowl and add a strip of lemon zest, a crushed garlic clove, some dried *herbes de Provence* or just dried oregano, and black pepper. Do not add salt. Roll the chicken joints around in this mixture; they can be cooked immediately or left to marinate for several hours.

Preheat the oven to 190°C/375°F/Gas Mark 5. Put the roasting tin on the hob over a medium-high heat. Take each joint out of the marinade, lay it gently in the tin and brown on each side. Put the tin in the oven and cook for 20 minutes.

✳ kitchen notes ✳

✳ This marinade can be used for barbecued chicken, too.
✳ You can also coat the chicken in the yoghurt marinade on page 421 and then cook it as described above. Alternatively, instead of marinating, you could breadcrumb the chicken joints (see page 33).

chicken thighs

It seems a sin to curry a naturally reared chicken, since the spices will obliterate the flavour of the meat. But curries are lovely and there is a part of every chicken that is perfectly suited to them: the brown thigh meat can be skinned and cut away from the bone, leaving you with meat that is so much more flavoursome in a curry than a dull, skinless chicken breast. Save the thighs if you are buying jointed whole chickens – or ask the butcher for them. You will need about two per person. The butcher will be happy to find a customer for them, so the economics are good all round and everyone's happy – except perhaps the person nibbling the umpteenth piece of chicken breast fillet they have had that week.

cold roast chicken

chicken sandwiches

Mayonnaise is a sauce to sit beside cold chicken, not drench it. Why drown good meat in egg yolks and oil? The return of the leggy, strong bird that thrives outdoors allows you to let its flavour stand almost alone. In a sandwich made from decent bread spread with good butter, a little lettuce and salt are all you need.

chicken with herb mayonnaise

Chop a few sprigs each of basil, tarragon, chives and parsley. Add to freshly made Mayonnaise (see page 393) and serve in a separate bowl with cold chicken, boiled potatoes and runner beans or canned flageolets – an immaculate outdoor lunch.

cold chicken with sesame sauce

The Chinese call this bang-bang chicken, and it has become a much-loved dish in many Chinese, specifically Sichuan, restaurants in the UK. Adjust the quantity of red chilli according to your own liking for hot food.

Serves 4

8 spring onions, shredded lengthways, then left in cold water to refresh

1 cucumber, peeled, halved lengthways, deseeded and sliced

360g/12oz cold chicken, shredded across the grain of the meat

2 tablespoons sesame seeds, dry toasted in a hot pan

1–3 red chillies, deseeded and chopped

For the sesame sauce:

a pinch of golden caster sugar

1 tablespoon rice wine vinegar

1 tablespoon soy sauce

3 tablespoons tahini (sesame seed) paste

a large pinch of Sichuan pepper

For the sauce, mix together the sugar, vinegar, soy sauce and tahini and season with the Sichuan pepper. Drain the spring onions well, mix them with the cucumber in a bowl and lay the chicken shreds on top. Zigzag the sauce over it, then scatter with the sesame seeds and red chilli.

poached stuffed chicken and the richest chicken soup

The most magnificent chicken recipe of all, and one that honours a really good-quality bird. You can make this recipe into a banquet, serving the soup with the chicken and a few poached leeks or carrots, or just eat the meat and save the soup for another day – perhaps with a few thin egg noodles. The chicken is stuffed with its own chopped liver and heart, plus morel mushrooms, pine nuts and stale breadcrumbs. Any leftovers will make a wholesome sandwich or salad the next day. Once the carcass has been stripped and all the stuffing eaten, return the bones to the stockpot containing the poaching liquor (if there is any left) and simmer for an hour to make a richer stock. This can be stored and used for soups, rice, potato and pasta dishes during the rest of the week. Any leftover stock can be used to poach another chicken the following week, and so on – this way, you will always have a supply of richly concentrated stock.

If you have a store of chicken livers or hearts in the freezer, use up to 3 of them in your stuffing.

Serves 6–8

2.25–2.75kg/5–6lb chicken, with giblets, the wishbone removed to help you carve (this is not difficult but a butcher will do it for you)
1 onion, cut into quarters
2 cloves
½ cinnamon stick
6 peppercorns
1 bay leaf
a sprig of thyme
8 sprigs of parsley
1 heaped teaspoon salt
8 small carrots, scraped
2 leeks, sliced

For the stuffing:
4 slices of stale or day-old bread
12 dried morel mushrooms
200ml/7fl oz milk
1 walnut-sized piece of butter
1 onion, finely chopped
1–3 chicken livers, chopped
1–3 chicken hearts, chopped
4 rashers of smoked back bacon, chopped

2 garlic cloves, chopped

1 tablespoon pine nuts

a pinch of grated nutmeg

1 egg, beaten

salt and freshly ground black pepper

To serve the soup:

1 slice of toasted baguette per person

extra virgin olive oil

crushed pink peppercorns

chopped chervil

First make the stuffing. Soak the bread and mushrooms in the milk for a few minutes, then squeeze dry and chop roughly. Throw away the milk. Melt the butter in a frying pan and add the chopped onion, liver, heart, bacon and garlic. Fry for a minute, then add the pine nuts, nutmeg and some salt and pepper. Remove from the heat and leave to cool. Mix with the bread, mushrooms and egg. Stuff the mixture into the chicken's cavity and tie it with string like a parcel so the stuffing cannot escape during cooking.

Put the chicken in a large pot with the onion, spices, bay leaf, thyme, half the parsley and the salt. Cover with water (or chicken stock, if you have any), bring to the boil, skimming away any foam with a slotted spoon, then turn down to a simmering bubble and cook for 60 minutes. Add the carrots and cook for a further 30 minutes, adding the leeks 10 minutes before the end.

Lift out the chicken and the vegetables, then strain the stock and reserve, keeping it warm in a pan. Untie and carve the chicken. Divide the meat and vegetables among plates, remembering to give each person a spoonful of stuffing. Spoon some stock over the chicken, chop the remaining parsley and throw it over.

If you want to turn the meal into a banquet, serve a bowl of the stock 'soup' ladled over the toasted bread before the chicken. Finish with a few dots of olive oil, crushed pink peppercorns and chervil. To make this a lunchtime soup, scatter a grated hard nutty cheese on to the bread and toast it before adding the soup.

poached chicken with leeks, tarragon and creamy stock

This is simmered chicken too – but this time with only minimal work. The sublime match between chicken and tarragon is shown off at its best in this dish – so lovely to eat in the colder months with bread fried in dripping or a buttery baked potato.

Serves 4

60g/2oz butter

1 chicken, jointed into 8 pieces

900ml/1½ pints chicken stock

3 leeks, cut into rounds

leaves from 4 sprigs of tarragon

250ml/8fl oz double cream

sea salt and freshly ground black pepper

Melt the butter in a casserole over a medium-high heat but do not let it burn. Add the chicken joints and brown them on both sides, then pour over the stock. Bring to the boil, skimming away any foam. Turn down to a simmer, cover and cook for about 45 minutes, until the chicken is tender. Add the leeks, tarragon and cream, season and cook for a further 10 minutes.

✳ kitchen note ✳

Once you have reached the seasoning stage, you can transfer everything to a pie dish and fit a pie crust over the top, following the recipe for shortcrust pastry on page 436. Bake the pie for 20–30 minutes in an oven preheated to 200°C/400°F/Gas Mark 6.

chicken giblets

Some naturally reared chickens come with their giblets. They can all be used for making stock apart from the liver, which you can use for the recipe below or the one on page 153. The hearts can be sliced and sautéed for salads.

chicken livers on toast with anchovies and capers

Save chicken livers in a container in the freezer. Don't forget to mark it with a pen – freezer amnesia is a common condition. How often have you stared at a solid lump of something covered in ice crystals and wondered what on earth it is?

Once you have a few chicken livers, make this soft, crumbly pâté to eat on toast. It is based on the traditional Tuscan version, eaten on toast.

Serves 4

1 tablespoon butter

1 onion, or 3 shallots, very finely chopped

6 chicken livers

8 anchovy fillets

2 tablespoons capers

1 small wine glass of red wine or stock

sea salt and freshly ground black pepper

Melt the butter in a pan over a medium heat, add the onion and cook until pale golden. Add the chicken livers and cook over a medium-high heat for 2 minutes, until coloured. Add the anchovies and capers and cook for 1 minute, then add the wine or stock. Simmer for 1 minute, then season with a pinch of salt and a few grinds of black pepper. Turn the whole lot on to a wooden board and chop finely (any liquid should be absorbed as you chop the ingredients). Transfer to a bowl; the mixture will keep for 3 days in the fridge. Serve it on toast as a starter, or spread thinly on small triangles of Melba Toast (see page 30) to eat with drinks.

✳ **kitchen note** ✳

You can use duck livers in the same recipe.

braised cockerel with trotters and red wine

Every now and again, I am offered a cockerel by my butcher or a local farmer. More often than not, he will have been an over-aggressive ex-companion to a flock of egg layers, and met his end before another vicious attack could happen.

It is best to braise rather than roast a cockerel older than 5 months. The French do this in their famous *coq au vin*. The following recipe is based on *coq au vin*, with the addition of juicy pig's trotter meat – an idea taken from Fergus Henderson's book, *Nose to Tail Eating* (Bloomsbury, 2004), which all meat-faithful people should own.

Ask your butcher if he can find you a cockerel, or try a farmer who keeps hens. The bird needs to be jointed into 10 pieces: 2 drumsticks, 2 thighs, 2 wings, 4 pieces of breast with bones attached – the parson's nose and the glands underneath must be removed.

Serves 6–8

1 large pig's trotter with knuckle, split in half

1 bay leaf

4 sprigs of curly parsley

2 sprigs of thyme

1 glass of brandy

1 bottle of red wine

750ml/1¼ pints chicken stock – you may need more

1 cockerel, jointed into 10 pieces (see previous page)

2 tablespoons plain flour

60g/2oz butter or dripping

20 small onions, peeled

2 celery sticks, very finely chopped

4 garlic cloves, chopped

4 tablespoons sunflower, groundnut or olive oil

20 chestnut mushrooms, or button mushrooms

sea salt and freshly ground black pepper

Put the pig's trotter in a pan with the bay leaf, parsley, a sprig of thyme, the brandy, wine and stock. Bring to the boil, skimming off any foam, then turn down to a simmer and cook for 2½–3 hours, until the meat is falling off the bone. Lift out the trotter and pick off the meat, setting it to one side in a large casserole. Strain the stock and wine mixture and discard the herbs, bones and skin.

Roll each piece of cockerel in the flour. Melt the butter or dripping in a deep frying pan over a medium heat and cook the onions, celery and garlic slowly until they turn pale gold in colour. Remove them with a slotted spoon and put them with the trotter meat in the casserole. Put the oil in the frying pan and turn up the heat. Brown the cockerel pieces on each side without burning them – you will not be able to fit them all in the pan, so do them in batches, setting the browned ones to one side with the vegetables. When they are all in the casserole, add a further sprig of thyme and grind some black pepper over everything.

Place the frying pan over the heat again and pour in some of the stock and wine mixture, scraping at the base of the frying pan with a wooden spoon. Pour this cooking liquor, through a sieve, over the meat and vegetables in the casserole, then add the remaining wine and stock. Cover with extra stock if necessary. Bring to the boil, skimming away any foam that rises to the surface, then reduce the heat, cover and cook slowly for 1½–2 hours, until the meat is tender. Add the mushrooms and cook for another 10 minutes. Season to taste with salt and serve with mashed potato.

✳ kitchen note ✳

If there is any cooking liquor left after the meat and vegetables have been eaten, strain it and add a little chopped tarragon and double cream for a lunchtime soup.

duck

The majority of ducks on sale in the UK have been reared just as intensively as chicken, but some butchers and specialist meat companies sell free-range or organic ducks. Duck breeds include Barbary and Aylesbury, with some new farms developing their own strains. It is peculiar how the welfare of farmed ducks has not caught the public imagination in the same way as chickens. It may not be something eaten regularly at home but vast amounts are consumed in Chinese restaurants. The welfare of farmed ducks is now very much in question. The charity, Compassion in World Farming, reports that approximately 90 per cent of the 18 million ducks reared each year in the UK are factory farmed; with up to 10,000 at a time reared indoors with little room to move and no access to that element they so love – water. Drinking water is given but ducks fundamentally need a pond in which to exercise, dive for food, and as a place to clean themselves. Traditionally ducks were farmed in small, loosely stocked flocks, with constant daytime access to outdoor water. They should be fed naturally and allowed to grow slowly to develop flavour.

where to buy duck

Be on the lookout for cowboy outfits, who rely on your assumption that all ducks flap around farmyards, sploshing in puddles. Always ask for the hearts and liver, plus any spare fat for making confit (see page 253).

* Buy duck direct – As with chickens, there is a growing range of welfare-friendly farmed duck available by mail order (see the Shopping Guide). As usual, ask questions about welfare. Do not listen to excuses about lack of water (some producers cite it as a hygiene threat).

* Butchers, farmers' markets and specialist shops – All may sell free-range duck, and labels or staff should provide you with the information you need.

* Supermarkets – Some supermarkets are moving towards selling genuine free-range duck but be wary. Brands such as Gressingham are marketed as sticking to high standards of welfare but in fact rear the ducks indoors without access to water.

how to get more from a duck

The average free-range duck costs about £10–12, which seems quite a bit when a whole roast duck serves three, barely four. I prefer not to roast them for this reason and instead ask the butcher to joint them, leaving 2 boneless duck breasts, 2 legs, and the carcass with 2 wings, both with a little bit of meat on them. Once added to other ingredients, the breast will go far in a salad or can be fried, sliced and eaten with a fruity sauce. The legs can be added to a bean casserole with some lean sausages. Store any duck livers in the freezer, collecting enough to use in a pâté (see page 156, and use instead of chicken livers). Keep any fat and roast potatoes in it – a dish in itself.

duck breasts with lentils, watercress and redcurrants

Duck tastes lovely at room temperature, or slightly warm. This is essentially a salad, but can be eaten as a main course for dinner.

Serves 4

2 duck breasts

4 helpings of cooked lentils (see page 65)

2 bunches of watercress, leaf end only (keep the stalks for soup –

see page 129)

about 120g/4oz redcurrants

1 teaspoon pink peppercorns, crushed in a pestle and mortar

soft crystal sea salt

For the dressing:

1 tablespoon Dijon mustard

2 tablespoons red wine vinegar

1 teaspoon brown sugar

1 tablespoon water

8 tablespoons olive oil

½ teaspoon salt

Heat a ridged grill pan or a heavy-based frying pan until moderately hot and fry the duck breasts for about 6 minutes on each side for rare meat, 10 minutes for well done. Transfer to a wooden board.

To make the dressing, put all the ingredients in a jar and shake until emulsified. Put the lentils on a plate with the watercress, pour over half the dressing and mix well. Slice the duck and lay the slices on top of the lentils, followed by the redcurrants. Spoon the remaining dressing on top, and scatter over the crushed pink peppercorns with a little soft sea salt.

✳ kitchen note ✳

The redcurrants make this a summer dish but you could use pomegranate seeds in late summer, blueberries in autumn, clementines or blood oranges, cut into segments with the membranes removed, in winter.

duck legs and potatoes

In this simple pot supper, the potato edges become crisp and caramelised as they absorb the duck fat. It takes a while, but you hardly need to look at it once it's on the go. A good, heavy casserole dish, something on a par with Le Creuset, is virtually essential, although you could use an anodised roasting tin (see the Shopping Guide). Eat the duck and potatoes with something cutting and peppery, such as a watercress or rocket salad.

Serves 4

4 duck legs, the skin pricked with a skewer
8 medium-sized old potatoes, peeled and halved
salt and freshly ground black pepper
lemon wedges, to serve

Season the duck legs with salt and pepper. Place them in a casserole over a high heat and quickly brown them on both sides. Add the potatoes, stir to coat with the fat, then turn down the heat and cook for about 50–70 minutes, until everything is golden and crisp. Turn the potatoes and duck from time to time. Serve with lemon wedges – sometimes the duck can be a little rich and the acidity of lemon juice will correct this.

roast salt duck

Duck will crisp beautifully during cooking if you salt it first. Rub breast or leg portions with salt and leave for 8 hours. Carefully wipe off the salt and prick the meat with a fork. Preheat the oven to 230°C/450°F/Gas Mark 8. If using duck breasts, sear them in a heavy-based pan on the hob, then transfer to the oven and cook for 20–30 minutes, depending on size, until crisp outside and pink within. Leave to rest in a warm place for 10 minutes before serving. Legs can be placed straight in the oven and roasted for 40–50 minutes, until crisp on the outside and well done inside.

keeping duck fat

Store duck fat that has been rendered from a roast, or from frying duck breasts, in a jar in the fridge. It keeps seemingly for ever and has a very high smoking point, making it useful for browning meat as you start a casserole or for roasting vegetables.

duck, sausages and beans

A big meal for 2 hungry people that is very easy to make. It contains a generous amount of beans, so you can add stock to them and eat them on other days as a thick soup. Choose very lean sausages; ones that have been partly cured, such as Denhay, are good. Garlic lovers should go for Toulouse sausages.

Serves 2

4 tablespoons duck fat or lard

2 duck legs

4 sausages

2 garlic cloves, crushed

2 onions, sliced

2 cans of cannellini or haricot beans, drained

1 teacupful of Tomato Sauce (see page 358), or 1 tablespoon tomato purée

600ml/1 pint meat stock

a sprig of thyme

1 teaspoon dried oregano

a small sprig of rosemary (or 1 teaspoon *herbes de Provence*)

sea salt and freshly ground black pepper

Heat the fat in a casserole, add the duck legs and sausages and brown them all over – it's not necessary to cook them through. Add the garlic and onions and swish them about a bit. Add the beans, tomato sauce, stock and herbs and season with a pinch of salt and a few grinds of black pepper. Bring to the boil, turn down to a low, bubbling simmer and cook, partially covered, for 20 minutes or until everything is tender.

crispy duck pancakes

Chinese groceries sell authentic, thin, wheat-flour pancakes for Cantonese or Peking duck in their freezer sections, usually packed 50 at a time. Use them to wrap the leftover dry, crisp skin of the duck from a roast and any pickings of meat – even the smallest amount will have a big effect.

Try to find good-quality plum sauce, made with natural ingredients (see the Shopping Guide).

Serves 4 as a starter or snack

About 180g/6oz leftover cold duck, or 2 raw duck legs

12 wheat flour pancakes

½ cucumber, cut into thin strips

4 spring onions, cut into thin strips

1 jar of plum sauce

If you are using raw duck legs, preheat the oven to 230°C/450°F/Gas Mark 8. Season the duck legs, prick them with a fork and roast for 40–50 minutes, depending on size. Leave until cool enough to handle, then cut, scrape and pull every last bit of meat and skin from them. Shred the meat and skin into thin strips. If using leftover duck, simply shred it into thin strips.

Heat the pancakes by steaming them in a colander over a pan of boiling water. Put some duck meat and skin, cucumber and spring onion in the centre of each pancake, spoon over a little plum sauce and roll it up.

guinea fowl and quail

The air of exotic luxury that hangs over alternative poultry such as guinea fowl and quail hides the fact that much of it is indoor reared in cramped conditions very similar to broiler chickens. It's very hard to tell, unless specified by the butcher or on the packaging, exactly how these birds are reared, especially when so many of them come from France. All supermarket birds, as far as I'm aware, are intensively reared. A few good sources of welfare-friendly exotic poultry farms are emerging, however (see the Shopping Guide).

turkey

Christmas or Thanksgiving, the same issues apply. Naturally reared turkeys are premium luxury meat. Wide grained, juicy, savoury tasting, they yield outstanding, golden-brown, gamy stock. I am always happy to see the back end of the Christmas carcass and a freezer stacked with cartons of this nectar. But with Christmas being such a drain on everyone's expenses, it is hard to suggest paying £40 for a turkey. However, if you love turkey but hate the woolly, factory-bred birds, buy a smaller, free-range Bronze turkey via mail order (see the Shopping Guide). Even a small bird yields a lot of meat and a lot of stock. If you are a large party and you have been dumped with the cooking and shopping, I cannot see what is wrong with a whip-round.

And think of this: small turkey, less cooking time, more time having fun and no getting up early to cram the beast into the oven. And for those of you who feel that way, just imagine: *no leftovers*. But don't say I said so.

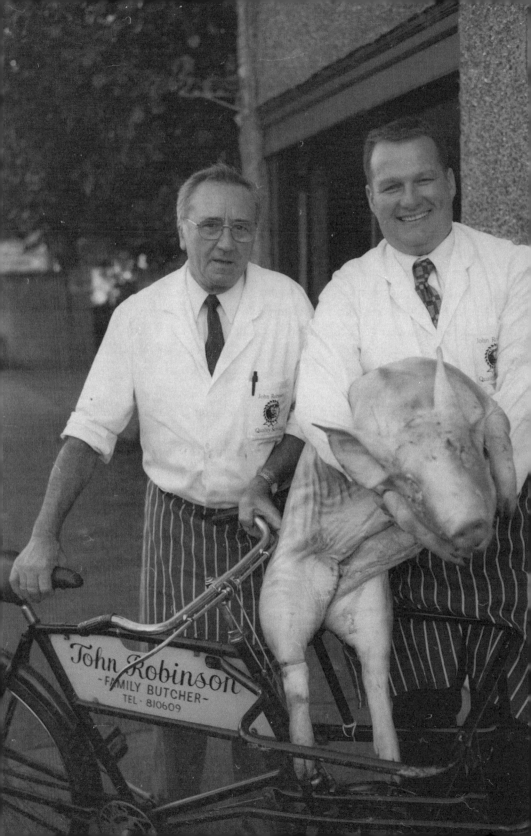

5

beef, pork and lamb

Every meal made with meat comes with the present of one and sometimes two or three meals more. A simple roast gives you cold meat for lunchtime sandwiches. A lean fillet leaves behind a bone to enrich soups and braises. Even the rind and fat have their uses: a spinach salad with soft-boiled eggs and crunchy pork crackling is just the kind of food I want to eat every day.

It makes good economic sense to spend more up front, because the better the meat's quality, the more you can get out of it. This kind of food management results in other good things. Realising food's full flavour potential should also boost your confidence when approaching less popular cuts, which cost less but come packed with possibilities. The more people choose naturally reared meat the more it encourages traditional methods to flourish. And if you start to choose different cuts, you will take some of the pressure off a meat industry that currently has a hard time selling anything that is not a chicken breast fillet, sirloin steak or loin of pork.

the art of cooking meat

Embrace meat and discover its infinite variety. The true world of meat is one of a hundred different cuts and ten times as many recipes. Cooks and their butchers are at their most artistic when they create with meat. The ingenuity behind some recipes is astounding, and the ability to make them is a virtue to value. But skill with meat is a fading art and a declining asset. It is, however, very easy to revive – with a little tuition. And there's an excellent motive for bringing back that knack of knowing what to do with cuts beyond the steak.

Using a wide range of cuts helps to solve the great contemporary carnivore's dilemma: should we eat cheap meat from intensively reared animals, or should we pay more for better meat? Answering yes to the second question is the braver response, because committed fans of fillet steak and loin chops will see their grocery bills double. But if you seize the challenge to be creative, you are at the beginning of discovering dozens of new cuts from each type of meat. Once you know what to do with them, good meat will be yours and you will be better, not worse off.

a new revolution in eating meat

Meat scares dominated the end of the twentieth century. But the positive outcome has been an increase in consumer interest in high-quality meat, inspiring farmers to promote their high standards of animal welfare and natural rearing techniques. The best-handled livestock ends its days in the least stressful manner, on short journeys to the remaining local slaughterhouses, then goes to careful butchers who take time to hang meat on the bone and pay a great deal of attention to ensuring its eating quality. This development has created a new predicament. Such meat is much more expensive, putting daily doses of rump steak far beyond the reach of anyone on an average income, so it is now necessary to learn how to make meat affordable within your means. My mission is to show you how easy this can be.

the price of meat

The cost of naturally reared beef, pork and lamb is approximately twice that of standard meat sold in supermarkets (meaning, that which is not labelled free-range, organic or similar). In supermarket promotions you may find some that costs only a third of the price of its naturally reared equivalent. Gram for gram comparisons are also misleading as intensively reared meat invariably shrinks more during cooking, so the portion itself will be smaller. The naturally reared beef, pork and lamb that supermarkets sell isn't always the bargain it's hyped up to be. It is frequently more expensive than similar meat sold direct from farms by mail order, at farmers' markets and farm shops. So the big four supermarkets' greatest claim – that their prices are unbeatable – can be untrue.

The four major supermarket chains are engaged in a price war as they fight to increase their share of the market. This means that the price of intensively reared meat is likely to fall, for promotional reasons if nothing else. And this price drop will frequently be borne by the producer.

The price of naturally reared meat, however, is likely to rise. The running costs of a small-scale livestock farm are much higher than those of larger farms, and new rules and regulations that have followed the recent spate of meat scandals will increase the farmer's costs. Similarly, small-scale abattoirs and butchers are suffering from the growing costs of our current regulatory regime. Again, if their output is small, these costs are disproportionately greater for them to bear.

what good meat can do for you

I'd like to outline the economics of eating good, naturally reared meat. The initial price may make you gulp, but you can roll really flavoursome meat into many meals. The tables overleaf show what even the premium cuts of beef, lamb and pork can make you, quite aside from the cheaper cuts mentioned towards the end of this chapter. Bear in mind, when putting these tables to practical use, that meat loses variable amounts of weight during cooking, which will marginally affect the result.

one leg or loin of pork weighing 2kg/4½lb plus extra bones

1st meal:	four 200g/7oz helpings of roast pork, crackling and gravy
2nd meal:	two helpings of salad with remaining crackling crumbled on to salad leaves, plus a poached egg
3rd meal:	four 90g/3oz helpings of shredded cold pork with noodles, sesame and vegetables
4th meal:	four 90g/3oz helpings of cold pork added to a spiced lentil stew
5th meal:	two sandwiches with remaining roast pork and watercress
6th meal:	four helpings of mushroom risotto made with 1 litre/1¾ pints stock from the roasted bones
7th meal:	two bowls pea soup, made with remaining 500ml/16fl oz stock

One £25 piece of prime pork goes into seven meals, making 22 separate helpings at an average cost of £1.14 each.

one forerib beef (four ribs) including rib bones weighing 4kg/9lb

1st meal:	six 200g/7oz helpings of roast beef and gravy
2nd meal:	dripping on toast, with mustard and cress
3rd meal:	six 120g/4oz helpings of cold beef, to eat with salad
4th meal:	six 120g/4oz helpings of beef with lime and rice noodles

5th meal:	six helpings of meat and potato pie made with 400g/14oz minced once-cooked beef
6th meal:	four helpings of Italian meat sauce made with 300g/10oz minced or chopped cooked beef
7th meal:	four helpings of noodle soup made with 1 litre/1¾ pints beef stock
8th meal:	six helpings of smooth vegetable soup made with 1 litre/1¾ pints beef stock

One £56 forerib of beef goes into eight meals, making 38 helpings excluding the dripping on toast, at an average cost of £1.49 each.

one leg of lamb weighing 2.5kg/5½lb

1st meal:	six 200g/7oz helpings of roast leg of lamb
2nd meal:	four 90g/3oz helpings of lamb pilaff
3rd meal:	two 90g/3oz helpings of lamb and butternut squash hash
4th meal:	six helpings of braised lamb made with 1.5 litres/2½ pints stock

The £25 leg of lamb goes into four meals, making 18 helpings. Discounting the braise, each helping has an average cost of £2.08.

respect for meat

So why should you pay more for your meat? There are many reasons why the time has come to change our ways of buying meat. The first and most significant motivation for me to start writing about food was the contradiction inherent between the almost daily food 'scare' stories that dominated the news pages, and the unending celebration of lean prime cuts in cookery features sections. While tales abounded of the appalling conditions in which chickens, veal calves and pigs were kept; of how cattle were fed meat and bone meal to produce cheap beef, the cookery columns seemed to dictate that readers use only chicken breasts, best end of lamb and loin of this, loin of that – cuts which constitute only a small fraction of the actual animal. And what happened to the rest – the bones, the braising cuts and offal? Well, we do know that much of it was processed to provide the very cheapest burgers, fertiliser, and yes, it re-entered the animal food chain and was brewed into feed, mainly for the dairy sector, with catastrophic consequences. Our desire for cheap, 'easy' meat unwittingly perpetuated a vicious circle of leftover cuts being fed to animals in order to produce more cheap, easy meat, which creates more leftover cuts. And so on and so on.

empowerment and a better quality of life

Those who love meat must take some responsibility for the way cheap meat is produced and discourage intensive farming techniques by using the power in their wallet. This will encourage more good meat on to the market. I will, I know, be accused of preaching – but at least it's preaching for empowerment, and a better quality of life. For a healthy attitude to meat, look back to when meat was considered by all to be a luxury and cooks were very clever in their use of it.

the welfare of the animals

There is no doubt that feed, lifespan, travel and stress affect the quality of meat, but quite apart from that, I feel uncomfortable eating meat when I know the welfare of the animal that produced it was questionable.

Animal stress and the eating quality of meat are closely related. It is by no means purely altruistic to be interested in livestock's welfare. Animals that travel long distances or live in overcrowded conditions suffer stress. Even if their suffering were not of concern, there is scientific proof that stressed animals produce meat of poor eating quality. The pH balance in a stressed animal's body is altered, which makes for tougher meat.

Naturally fed, slowly grown animals that are not stocked in high densities are far more resistant to disease and can therefore reach the end of their lives without ever being treated with medicines apart from vaccines which have been cleared as safe (organic meat will not have been vaccinated).

the end matters

If animals travel short distances to a slaughterhouse with a straw-bedded, quiet rest area where the sexes are not mixed, they suffer little stress. There was once a vast network of small slaughterhouses, which meant that animals travelled short distances and suffered as little stress as possible before slaughter. These were the slaughterhouses that supplied butcher's and farm shops. Sadly, the supermarkets, or perhaps it is their meat suppliers, are not into the culture of the local small-scale slaughterhouse, preferring that animals are processed in the abattoir of their choice. These are usually vast state-of-the-art plants to which the animals must sometimes travel hundreds of miles. Farmers that care about their animals are not fond of such places; most say they would prefer to use a local abattoir. But the supermarkets argue that the meat they buy must fit their specifications. I have interviewed many slaughtermen from local abattoirs and have not met one who would not – within reason – work to supermarket specifications, and likely improve upon them. But they are not being given the business. Economics has a lot to do with it. High-throughput modern abattoirs can slaughter more for less.

the cost of regulations

The Ministry of Agriculture, now renamed the Department for Environment, Food and Rural Affairs (Defra), has not helped the cause for reducing animal stress. Slaughterhouses must bear the costs of frequent inspections, and pay for any changes they are asked to make to the premises in the name of food hygiene. Paranoia abounds at Defra after the BSE scandal when much blame for the catastrophe was heaped upon the Ministry. Now they operate according to a mantra of 'ever-increasing standards'.

Common sense would say there is a cut-off point: a food is either safe, or it isn't. It isn't feasible to continue raising standards for ever, nor can you make any food 100 per cent safe. The cost of the constant demands made by hygiene inspectors falls heavily upon the smaller slaughterhouses. These businesses, minuscule in scale, operate local services for farmers and are intrinsic to the fragile web of artisan meat companies in rural areas. They are vital to the organic sector, and they are essential if we are going to continue to enjoy the flavour of great meat.

the politics of the national farmers' union and meat

Three words come to mind when mulling over the National Farmers' Union: out of touch. I concede that the NFU is an odd thing to brood on, but the gnashings of small-scale farmers' teeth when you raise the subject should not be ignored. For so long solely concerned with farm incomes, the leaders of Britain's only farmers' union realised rather too late that there were consumers worried about food production.

It fascinates me that over half the NFU's members (124,694 in 2004) aren't actually farmers, but members of NFU Countryside – mainly people who operate non-farming businesses in rural areas. In 2002 Defra reported there were 163,800 full-time farmers, which supports the view that many have abandoned the NFU. The cost of farmers' subscriptions is calculated on the amount of land they own; big British 'agribusiness', those arable farmers with acres and acres of land, therefore contribute a vast percentage of the NFU's income (in 2003 they had an income of £25.8 million, and £22.1 million of this came from membership fees). Even though such businesses make up less than 10 per cent of the membership, it is clear that claims that they exert an undue influence on the NFU are not without foundation.

Historically, lobbying for small livestock farmers has not been a priority at NFU headquarters, although regional NFU branches in poorer farming areas do their best for their membership. During the 2001 foot-and-mouth outbreak, for example, specialist meat producers and organic farmers (who had been thriving) begged the government to consider vaccination at a time when the outbreak was relatively confined and 300,000 animals had been slaughtered. The NFU was vehemently opposed to vaccination and the experts who advocated it, even going so far as to dismiss the views of respected scientists who were doing their best to persuade government to use it. Interviewing the then president at the time, Ben Gill, at the NFU's headquarters was a memorably deflating experience. The NFU chiefs appeared to some to be taking the side of those large-scale meat dealers who hide behind the name of 'farmer', for whom mass slaughter meant millions in compensation from the government and tax-payer. Vaccination was not adopted, with the result that in excess of six million animals were slaughtered. Government inquiries since the outbreak have suggested that vaccination must be used in future outbreaks. The influence of the NFU might have made all the difference.

Countless livestock farmers I have interviewed over the years have complained they have been let down during times of crisis. The union did not lobby for them when the smaller abattoirs started closing due to over-regulation and red tape. Now the NFU pays lip service to the success of farmers' markets, but they remain in thrall to big meat exporters and will not challenge the Big Four supermarkets who, they correctly point out, sell 75 per cent of food produced in Britain. They do not protest when supermarkets seek ever-bigger profit margins – at the expense of the farmer. On the other hand, they say farmers should co-operate more, and they are right. But a co-operative has no power unless it can produce something exclusive that the supermarkets and their customers cannot do without.

natural growth

The meat industry has many tricks and one of the most successful, in its eyes, has been the discovery of ways to make animals grow fast. A variety of innovations work together to make for fast-growing animals: selective breeding, protein-rich feeding regimes, and the use of antibiotics that promote growth and mitigate against the effects of confining many animals together. (Growth-promoting antibiotics are not permitted for lamb, but widely used in the intensive farming of pigs; beef can be subject to such treatment, although this is discouraged by retailers.)

A commercial pig in a high-tech Danish farm, for example, can reach 90 kilos in five months, while a traditional pre-Second World War breed like Middle White reaches just 45 kilos during the same period. Imagine if you were bred to grow fast, fed large quantities of protein and carbohydrate to fatten you up, plus drugs to speed your growth further. Sounds like a childhood obesity epidemic, but that's another topic entirely. In America animals are routinely fed hormones to promote growth. Thankfully meat from these animals is banned from sale in Europe, but US meat company lobbyists would love to see that ban lifted.

tasting the new-old breeds

On a happier note, some farmers are once again interested in the traditional breeds or seeking to breed animals with traditional characteristics for what is known as the value-added market. When it comes to flavour, first and foremost, breed matters. There is a new understanding that a natural rate of growth produces meat and poultry with improved taste and texture, and which cooks well. Meat from slow-grown animals costs more, which is why it is essential to get the most out of the meat you buy, and operate with the assumption that each cut will become at least two meals.

hanging and the cut

Two other factors have a significant impact on meat's taste and cookability: maturity and butchery. Traditionally, meat was hung on the bone (the whole or half side of a carcass suspended from a hook) at a cool temperature, between two and three degrees centigrade. In the past, all meat was hung, even poultry, which was left for a few days with the guts in, in effect flavouring the meat. Really good beef is hung for between three and five weeks to mature. This process slowly tenderises the meat, relaxes the muscle and allows the flavour to develop. Much mass-market beef is now matured for half that time in sealed plastic bags in a fridge, which keeps down costs but in no way produces the same flavour as a piece of beef that has been allowed to oxidise at a suitable temperature. It is an artificial process and the difference is noticeable when the meat is on the plate.

Hanging meat for the maximum amount of time is particularly pertinent with the forequarters, the part of the carcass that provides the cheaper cuts. The longer they hang, the more tender they are, which is essential to cut the cooking time for a braise, and achieve greater success with the hammered meat recipes on pages 205–7.

The art of cutting meat is also vital. Good butchers take the time to cut carefully, seaming between muscle sections, which helps to seal in the juices as the meat cooks. But hasty production-line cutting can halve the time it takes to divvy up a side of beef. This may leave too much fat on the steak: there is money in the extra weight, but it does nothing to improve a grill. They might not have time to remove that piece of gristle, which is a nuisance when you carve, or use electric cutting tools, which leave bone fragments on the surface of the meat and mash the flesh.

Butcher's artistry may be an oxymoron, but it matters that it remains available to meat lovers who understand its value. That value is high and reflected in the price.

In 1997, pregnant with my daughter Lara, I had it fixed in my mind that I should learn to cut meat. The excellent butcher in Battersea's Northcote Road, Bob Dove, offered to initiate me and I staggered over there three days a week with swollen ankles. I remember the pre-election fever. Politicians of every persuasion kept walking into the shop begging for 'the vote of local business'. Since both Bob and myself agreed that no post-war politician had done the slightest bit of good for butchers we shook our cleavers and chased each one out of the shop.

Butchers suffer from the sad but typical malaise of the high-street shop. The supermarket down the road can undercut them on price, if not on quality, and many small butchers have been driven out by rising rents and the cost of keeping up with every new slab of food hygiene laws.

a lamb with four back legs

The lorry from Wales that brought the lamb to the butcher in Northcote Road was a weekly spectacle. Bob was an HGV enthusiast and encouraged the drivers to do three-point turns in the narrow market street so he could judge their turning skills. The resulting traffic jams were worthy of the Turin scenes in *The Italian Job*. The delighted Bob ignored enraged drivers and stallholders: he was himself enraged by something else connected to this delivery. Out of the back of that lorry came 20 lamb carcasses, and 40 extra legs of lamb. It was explained to me that the desire for 'prime' roasting and grilling cuts of meat meant buying extra legs. No way, he said, would he be able to sell all the cuts of 40 lamb carcasses, in spite of the successful pie business run by his wife at the back of the shop. We boned the shoulders and minced the bellies for her, but still could not sell the cheap cuts. In newspapers the row about the prospect of genetically modified food raged on, and yet here were consumers effectively demanding lambs with four back legs.

where to buy meat

✳ When it comes to buying beef, pork and lamb you have a great deal of choice.

✳ Butcher's shops – Butchers need your support, providing they are the type that will happily answer questions about their wares' origins, livestock breeds, and animal welfare, as well as know how to hang their meat well – that is, not wrapped in plastic but in temperature-controlled rooms where the air can reach the meat.

✳ Home delivery – There are also many high-quality meat companies and farms who sell direct, and will deliver to your door.

✳ Farm shops – These can be a good source: you should be able to see first-hand how well they care for their animals.

✳ Organic – Organic farms are also renowned for their high standards of animal welfare, but many must still make headway on hanging and cutting. Farmers' markets are well worth supporting. Not only are they another source of good meat, but they boost the incomes of struggling small farmers.

✳ Supermarkets – Wherever you buy your meat, the best way to ensure its quality is to ask informed questions: has it been naturally fed and had access to the outdoors? Even supermarkets are obliged to answer those questions because you are the most important person to them. In recent years all supermarkets have changed their meat-selling practice – to a degree. Almost all have widened the choice, including free-range and organically produced meat among the intensively reared options. But reading the label carefully is essential when buying supermarket meat. It is up to you, the person they really care about, to demand from them the best British-reared, slow-grown, naturally fed, drug-free, locally killed, well-hung, beautifully butchered meat available. For this you will have to pay more, which is, I know, a lot to ask. My aim is to offer a positive way round the problem.

cheap cuts

Many recipes in this chapter are based on some of the most expensive, prime cuts which can be cooked fast – either fried or roast. But most of an animal's meat traditionally requires slow cooking, such as braising. This flesh comes from the muscle that gets more exercise, the forequarters and lower parts of the leg, and will cost around half the price of prime meat. I have discovered that you do not always have to cook the cheap cuts slowly, however. There is a section devoted to recipes for this technique later in this chapter (see pages 204-7).

beef

breeds

It is only when you try, maybe for the first time, beef that is truly wonderful that you will understand the difference. It will be tight-grained rather than loose, deep in colour, have a texture that allows the beef literally to fall apart in the mouth, and a flavour that delivers a long, savoury taste, bringing to mind the variety of grasses and cereals eaten by the steer. Steers – the boys – have the finest-textured meat, but a heifer that has grown slowly can be very good too.

The golden age of British beef came in the eighteenth and nineteenth centuries when the great breeders perfected the native British breeds: the Herefords, Aberdeen Angus, Beef Shorthorns, Lincoln Reds, South Devon, small Dexters and ghostly White Park cattle. These breeds produce the compact, flavoursome joints that are ideal for classical British cooking – the roasts, steaks and slow braises. The meat sold by supermarkets is rarely pure-bred, even if the label names a specific breed. Aberdeen Angus, for example, can take that name even if it is half-bred. Why does this matter? Because the cross-breeding is usually with large Continental cattle – Charolais, Simmental and Belgian Blue, which have enormous backsides, meaning more meat and more money. However, the cross-bred calves can be so large that a native-breed mother has trouble giving birth. Indeed, pure-bred Belgian Blue calves are often delivered by caesarean section, something that farmers are reluctant to admit. A secondary and no less disturbing consequence of this practice is the tragic loss of the national herd. Two millennia of cattle-breeding are in danger of being wiped out.

Continental beef is often eaten young, as veal, and the Continental breeds are ideal for this purpose: they prefer the indoors, have thin skins and grow fast. Native British breeds are thick-skinned, hardy types that thrive well grazing outdoors. Not all year round, mind. They like to be brought into barns during the winter months – free-range is a phrase that applies only to summer, in the mind of the caring farmer.

Since the BSE crisis, all cattle in the UK, bar a few select varieties, must be killed at 30 months. This is not enough time for the native outdoor-reared breeds to grow to their full size. Crossed with a Charolais bull there will be plenty of meat on the bone by 30 months. There is nothing wrong with meat from such animals when it is expertly matured and cut, although for me it lacks the character and flavour of the native breeds. The good news is that the Meat and Livestock Commission expect the 30-month ban to be lifted for all breeds by the time this book is published. This is good news as farmers will once again be able to grow native breeds at normal rates and will not be forced to cross-breed.

good roasting cuts for beef

✳ Forerib – Four ribs serve six, with meat to spare; there is usually lots of fat on the forerib, giving you delicious beefy dripping.

✳ Sirloin – Very expensive; you are unlikely to have much meat left over but ask the butcher for the bones and rib trim (pieces of meat between each bone) to make a small stew or a pie.

✳ Fillet – The priciest of all, meltingly tender, but lacking the flavour of sirloin or forerib.

✳ Boned rolled topside – A tougher cut coming from a more active muscle, this must be carved very thinly; you will need a sharp carving knife. It makes excellent carpaccio, if you can cut it thinly enough (chill or put in the freezer for an hour, and use a very sharp knife).

roast forerib of beef

To roast 4–5kg/9–11lb beef (about 4 ribs), heat the oven to its highest temperature. Put the beef in a deep roasting tin and rub with vegetable oil or dripping. Scatter over 2 pinches of dried thyme or sprigs of fresh thyme. Season well with black pepper and sea salt. Put the beef in the oven and cook for 20 minutes, then turn the heat down to 190°C/375°F/Gas Mark 5. Cook for another 40 minutes, then test for doneness (see below). Before carving, leave the meat to rest in a warm place, covered with foil, for 15 minutes. Meanwhile, make the gravy (see page 124). Serve with Yorkshire pudding, if liked (see page 183).

the skewer test for doneness

Once you know how to do this, you will never look back. My sister, Sam Clark, taught me it. Up to that point I had operated on the principle that all average-sized roasting joints – beef, lamb, pork, venison – took 1 hour 20 minutes; a guess that is not actually far off. But the skewer test is failsafe – unless you wait too long to do it, in which case your meat will be ruined. Besides beef, you can use this method to test lamb and venison, which should be pink in the centre, pork and ham, which should be well done, and veal, which should be somewhere between the two.

Take a long steel skewer, stick it into the centre of the deepest part of the meat and leave it there for 1 minute. Pull it out and test the temperature of the part of the skewer that would have been roughly at the centre of the meat. The best testing place is your lower lip.

* The skewer is cold: the meat is very rare and bloody in the centre.
* The skewer is just above blood temperature: the meat is reddish-pink in the centre, perfect for those who like rare beef.
* The skewer is hot, bearably so: the meat is well done on the outside and pink in the middle.
* The skewer is very hot: the meat is well done all the way through.

yorkshire pudding

The key to a good Yorkshire pudding is patience. Early attempts to make it left me trying to pass off the result as that early Nineties mealy meal phenomenon, polenta. But I have since learnt – or I would not dare provide the recipe – that Yorkshire pudding needs plenty of time to strut its stuff. In my oven it takes a good 45 minutes, not the average 30 minutes of cookbook lore. Use strong white flour; it has definite 'rise to the occasion' qualities.

Serves 6

240g/8oz strong white flour
a pinch of salt
3 eggs
400ml/14fl oz whole milk
100–200ml/3½–7fl oz water
a little dripping

Put the flour and salt in a big bowl, make a well in the centre and add the eggs. Using a whisk to stir, gradually add the milk and water, beating it in until you have a batter with the consistency of single cream. If your eggs are very large, you will need only 100ml/3½fl oz of the water.

Melt some dripping in a large roasting tin over the hob until you see the first smoke rise off the fat. Pour in the batter and put the tin in the oven with the roast. Cook for about 45 minutes, until it is well puffed up – don't keep peeping, you will only let that valuable heat out of the oven. Serve immediately.

sauces to go with roast beef

horseradish cream

The fire in fresh horseradish is released when you cut it, and there is nothing like the heat of the real thing to match the gentle but distinctive taste of good beef. You can buy grated horseradish vacuum-packed in jars, which is not bad, but it is better to buy a whole root when you see one and freeze it, wrapped in clingfilm, in 5cm/2 inch chunks.

Serves 6

2 tablespoons fresh horseradish, finely grated

6 tablespoons double cream

1 teaspoon mustard powder

a squeeze of lemon

Combine the horseradish with the cream and mustard. Add a squeeze of lemon to thicken the mixture.

summer green sauce for beef

Serves 6

5 sprigs of parsley, chopped (or chervil, if you can find it)

3 sprigs of tarragon, chopped

4 sprigs of basil, chopped

about 2 tablespoons chopped chives

2 anchovies, rinsed and chopped

1 heaped teaspoon capers, rinsed and chopped

1 teaspoon Dijon mustard

6 tablespoons olive oil

salt and freshly ground black pepper

Mix all the ingredients together, seasoning with salt and pepper to taste.

extra-hot mustard

Only make as much as you need. The quantity below will get you through Sunday lunch for 6.

2 heaped teaspoons Colman's mustard powder

5 shakes of Tabasco sauce

1 teaspoon vegetable oil

Mix the ingredients together in an eggcup or mustard pot with enough water to make a soft paste. The oil will prevent a skin forming.

dripping on toast

Save your dripping carefully, tipping all leftover fat and juices from beef roasts into an earthenware bowl. The juice sets to a thick jelly, the fat to a dense, buff paste that is surprisingly non-greasy. A little of the fat, and slightly more of the jelly, is lovely spread on toast or Melba toast (see page 30). A little watercress on the toast makes it an almost grand thing to eat with drinks on winter evenings.

beef dripping sandwiches

Spread good fresh bread rolls with dripping and place a slice of beef inside each roll with sliced cucumber and some sea salt.

cold beef

There is always something left over from a joint of roast beef, and a meal of cold meat is not one to sniff at. I roast large pieces of meat with the sole purpose of eating them cold, especially when I need to feed a lot of people. There will always be enough, though, for an honest beef sandwich.

beef sandwiches

Butter 2 slices of bread – rye is especially good for a beef sandwich. Spread one side with your favourite mustard. Put a slice of rare beef on top with some peppery salad leaves such as rocket, mustard and cress or watercress, season with soft sea salt crystals and a grind or two of black pepper, then slap the other slice on top.

cold beef with lime and sesame dressing

The dressing for this beef is based on those citric Thai salads that are lovely on hot nights.

Serves 4

1 carrot, pared into thin strips with a potato peeler

4 handfuls of young spinach leaves

4 slices of cold roast beef, cut into thin strips

For the dressing:

3 large, mildly hot red chillies, deseeded and chopped

2 sprigs of coriander, chopped

2 sprigs of basil, torn to shreds

2 sprigs of mint, chopped

2 teaspoons soy sauce

juice of 1 lime

1 teaspoon Thai fish sauce (*nam pla*)

1 heaped tablespoon brown sugar

1 tablespoon sesame seeds, toasted in a dry pan until golden

Mix together all the ingredients for the dressing. Put the carrot and spinach on serving plates and pile the beef on top. Pour over the dressing.

✳ kitchen note ✳

For a more substantial course, serve over rice thread noodles. You can buy them, with all the dressing ingredients, from Southeast Asian supermarkets.

cold beef with watercress and winter sauce

The sauce here is a close relative of the one made famous by Harry's Bar, home of the original carpaccio. Harry's Bar is a fantastically expensive restaurant in Venice but it understands how to create luxury out of everyday foods. Its customers can consume caviar by the bucketful, if they wish, but they can also choose to eat a fine egg sandwich or a plate of risotto seasoned only with saffron.

Serves 4

8 thin slices of cold roast beef

1 bunch of watercress

For the winter sauce:

200g/7oz Mayonnaise (see page 393)

3 tablespoons chicken stock

a few drops of Tabasco sauce

a dash of Worcestershire sauce

a pinch each of salt and pepper

1 tablespoon mustard of your choice – English or French

Whisk all the ingredients for the sauce together until you achieve the consistency of double cream. Arrange the beef on a plate with the watercress. Zigzag the sauce over the top.

soup noodles with rare beef, spring onions, pak choi and coriander

When I am at home for lunch and cannot face another sandwich, I fill a huge bowl with Chinese egg noodles that have been boiled for 4 minutes, pour piping-hot beef or other meat stock over them and then lay slices of leftover rare roast beef on top. With a few shredded spring onions, some pak choi leaves, the leaves from a couple of sprigs of coriander, a splash of soy sauce and a drop or two of chilli oil, I am my own noodle bar.

braised once-roasted beef

If you want to save roast meat to use in other dishes, chop it after the roast has cooled, using an old-fashioned hand-cranked mincer or a food processor. Do not overchop or the finished sauce will have an unpleasant smooth texture. Without either gadget you can simply cut leftover meat into 1cm/½ inch chunks to make a lovely rustic sauce. Wrap it and put it in the fridge, away from raw food.

Even a little leftover meat will surprise you with the quantity of braised meat sauce it can make. This one contains grated root vegetables, giving it all the benefits of their flavour while remaining invisible – an effective strategy for feeding children vegetables. The recipe is from Sarah Husband, a hero of mine. She cooks dinners at a school in North Yorkshire, and has committed the school kitchen to serving only locally reared meat and fresh vegetables, using the recipes of Nigel Slater and the River Café. She has banned vending machines, removed the daily chips from the menu and has so far converted many pupils to her way of thinking. It is uphill work, but when I visited the school most children were scoffing this beef braise with green (not grey) peas – yes, it's a school – poured over Yorkshire puddings. Lovely. Just thinking about it makes me want to eat some now.

Serves 6–8

2 tablespoons olive oil

1 large onion, finely chopped or grated

900g/2lb chopped or minced roast beef or lamb

20 button mushrooms, grated

2 carrots, grated

about 4 heaped tablespoons grated root vegetables – parsnip, turnip, swede, celeriac (mix them, if you wish)

1 heaped teaspoon English mustard powder

1 litre/1¾ pints beef stock

3 tablespoons Worcestershire sauce (optional)

sea salt and freshly ground black pepper

Heat the oil in a large casserole, add the onion and cook until lightly browned. Add the beef and all the vegetables and cook, stirring, over a medium heat for 1 minute. Add the mustard, stir a few times and pour over the stock. Bring to the boil, then reduce the heat to very low and simmer for about 40 minutes–1 hour, until the beef is tender and the juices much reduced. Season to taste with salt and pepper, then add the Worcestershire sauce, if using.

beef and parsnip pasties

Makes 4

240g/8oz shortcrust pastry (see page 436)

2 parsnips, diced

1 tablespoon butter

2 sprigs of parsley, chopped

8 tablespoons Braised Once-roasted Beef (see page 188)

1 egg, beaten

Roll the pastry out on a floured board to 5mm/¼ inch thick and cut it into 4 squares about 15 x 15cm/6 x 6 inches. Leave to rest in the fridge for half an hour to relax the pastry and prevent shrinkage during cooking.

Put the parsnips in a pan of salted water and bring to the boil. Simmer until soft, then drain well and mash with the butter. Allow to cool, then stir in the parsley.

Preheat the oven to 200°C/400°F/Gas Mark 6. Put 2 tablespoons of the meat and a tablespoon of the parsnip mash in the centre of each square of pastry. Brush the edges of the pastry with beaten egg, then bring up the corners into the centre and pinch them together to seal. Brush the pasties all over with beaten egg, place on a baking sheet and bake for 20–25 minutes, until golden.

meat and potato pie

Preheat the oven to 200°C/400°F/Gas Mark 6. Spoon Braised Once-roasted Beef (see page 188) into a shallow ovenproof dish and cover with 2.5cm/1 inch thickness of mashed potato or slices of peeled waxy potatoes. Bake until the top has browned. If you beat a little melted butter or double cream into the mashed potato, it will form a lovely crust.

italian meat sauce

This is the sauce, known in Italian as *ragù*, to use between layers of lasagne or over tagliatelle in the Florentine way. If you use the chicken livers, they will give it a velvety richness.

Serves 4

2 tablespoons olive oil

1 large onion, finely chopped

1 celery stick, finely chopped

a pinch of dried rosemary

a pinch of dried thyme

1 bay leaf

240g/8oz minced or chopped cooked beef

4 rashers of dry-cured green streaky bacon, finely chopped

2 chicken livers, chopped (optional)

1 glass of white wine

90g/3oz canned chopped tomatoes, or 1 heaped tablespoon tomato purée

450ml/¾ pint meat stock

salt and freshly ground black pepper

Heat the oil in a pan and add the onion and celery. Cook over a medium heat until soft, then add the herbs with the chopped beef, bacon and chicken livers, if using. Cook, stirring, for 1 minute, then add the wine, tomatoes and stock. Bring to the boil and simmer very slowly for 1 hour, until the meat is completely tender and the juices much reduced. Season to taste with salt and pepper.

pork

Pork from breeds of pig that have been grown slowly, outdoors or indoors with access to pasture, have recently made a comeback. Anyone who grew up in the 1970s will remember the sizzling 'Danishhhh!' telly adverts. That all-too-appetising noise spelt not only the advent of cheap pork, but the demise of the slow-grown pig. Commercial pig farming took off in the 1960s. Pig farmers receive no subsidies under the Common Agricultural Policy, and Danish and Dutch farmers led the way in breeding pigs that grew to their bacon weight at an exceptional rate. British farmers followed suit. Methods have changed little in Denmark and the Netherlands. To force five litters in two years from one sow reared entirely indoors on a commercial pig farm, her piglets are weaned in three weeks. Having been weaned early, the piglets suffer low immunity – one reason why antibiotics are added to their feed, along with flavour enhancers for their meat and large amounts of protein to boost speed of growth.

These practices continue – to a lesser extent – in the UK, in spite of changes to the pig welfare rules in Britain at the end of the twentieth century. The rules are meant to be adopted by all European member states in due course, but British farmers got them early due to Defra's eagerness to improve British farming's image after BSE. Thanks, Defra. We got better welfare but in your haste to do so you put many of our pig farmers out of business.

The new rules forced farmers to put the price of British pork up, and it was abandoned by retailers, who chose instead to buy cheaper imports. One positive outcome was that British pig farmers sought a new, value-added market, bringing about a revival in free-range pig farming and many of the traditional, or hybrids of the traditional, slow-growing breeds for which consumers are happy to pay a premium. Thirty per cent of British pork is now farmed free range.

Imported pork is still everywhere, however. The catering trade, who do not need to label food with its country of origin, take advantage. The same lame excuse is trotted out by motorway cafés and others. 'The British only want large rashers of bacon and British pigs tend to be small,' the spokesman of one catering giant once told me. I don't believe it. People who love bacon will eat it at any size. Of course, big rashers from Denmark and the Netherlands are very cheap – a big 'come hither' for caterers and their accountants. For the low price of this bacon you get poorer than British-standard animal welfare and a watery meat that bleeds white salty liquid as it cooks. In any event neither bacon nor pork – even from the finest pigs – is a highly priced meat. The important thing is to make the most of the pork you buy. Every little bit – right down to the tail.

every bit of the pig

Prime cuts of pork are the roasting joints, and they also come with a treat, like no other roast, that brings real tears of joy to the eyes of everyone without expensive dentistry in their mouths: crackling. But pork is unique in that the meat found on the cheaper cuts – the extremities, as Jane Grigson used to call them – is almost more delicious than the pricier prime cuts. And it is not difficult to bring out the best of these extremities.

roast loin of pork

The loin is the tender meat that runs the length of the pig's back. It comes coated in rind, which you must ask the butcher to score with a knife for the crackling. Ask your butcher to bone the loin for you, too. You can then roast the meat in a cradle of the rib bones and make stock with them later (see page 114).

Roast loin of pork is a great dish for a big party – you can buy 2 whole loins direct from the farmer and have enough crackling and pork for 50 people. You might have to cut them up to fit them into your oven, however.

Serves 4–6

1 piece of pork loin, with 6 ribs

1 teaspoon salt

a little vegetable oil

a pinch of dried oregano

Preheat the oven to 230°C/450°F/Gas Mark 8 and boil a kettle. Place the pork in a metal colander in the kitchen sink and pour the boiling water over the rind; this will open out the score marks on the skin so it 'crackles'. Rub the salt thoroughly into the rind. Rub the meat and bones (but not the crackling) with oil and scatter over the oregano. Place the meat in a roasting tin and roast for 15 minutes, then reduce the heat to 180°C/350°F/Gas Mark 4 and cook for a further hour. Pork is best served well done – test with a skewer (see page 182).

Remove the pork from the oven and leave to rest in a warm place for 15 minutes to allow the juices that have risen to the surface to sink back into the joint. Meanwhile, make the gravy (see page 124). Before carving the meat, cut away any string and remove the crackling by sliding a knife under it. It should come away easily. Put it beside the pork on the dish. It is easier to cut up the crackling using scissors than with the carving knife. Slice the pork downwards across the grain and serve, with the gravy, Apple Sauce or Apple and Onion Sauce (see below), or Cornichon, Egg and Herb Sauce (see page 196).

✳ kitchen note ✳

If the pork is ready but the crackling not quite done, turn up the oven, cut away the crackling (see above) and place it in the oven on a dry roasting tray while the meat is resting. It should crisp up given the extra time.

roast leg of pork

This is available on or off the bone; prepare and cook as for loin.

roast pork belly

The meat from pork belly is melting and sweet flavoured but it needs longer cooking to allow the fat to render (melt away). Choose a piece weighing about 1.5kg/3¼lb. Prepare and cook as for loin of pork, putting it on a rack in the roasting tin and giving it 1½ hours after the initial 15 minutes. The surplus fat can be stored in the fridge; it's very good for roast potatoes.

sauces for roast pork

apple sauce

Peel, core and chop 8 eating apples, place in a pan and cook over a low heat with a knob of butter and 1–2 tablespoons of water until they reduce to a soft, smooth sauce to serve cool with roast pork.

apple and onion sauce

Make as for apple sauce, above, but substitute 2 onions, peeled and chopped, for 2 of the apples. Cook very slowly for about 45 minutes.

cornichon, egg and herb sauce

I put this sauce on the table with roast pork, leftover cold pork, new potatoes or artichokes, or serve it with brawn (see page 226) or pork terrines.

Serves 4–6

10 cornichons (baby gherkins)

4 semi-soft-boiled eggs (see page 380)

4 sprigs of tarragon

4 sprigs of parsley

about 20 chives

olive oil

salt and freshly ground black pepper

Chop the cornichons and put them in a bowl. Chop the eggs and the herbs and add them to the cornichons. Stir in enough olive oil to make a thick sauce, then season to taste.

spare crackling

Is there any such thing? Probably not on the roast but there is a lot of skin on a pig and butchers cut much of it away. Ask your butcher to give you any spare. Pour boiling water over it, as for roast pork loin (see page 194), then roast it at 230°C/450°F/Gas Mark 8 until crisp and brittle. Leave to cool, then break it up roughly. Grind a little black pepper over the pieces – this will combat any saltiness – and serve in small bowls with drinks.

crackling with salad leaves and semi-soft-boiled eggs

For each person, prepare a bowl of salad leaves, the crisper the better, and dress them with a vinaigrette made with Dijon mustard. Cut a peeled semi-soft-boiled egg in half lengthways and lay it on top. Scatter over pieces of crackling.

✳ kitchen note ✳

You can also use cold pork in the following recipes in the beef section: Cold Beef with Lime and Sesame Dressing; Cold Beef with Watercress and Winter Sauce; Soup Noodles with Rare Beef, Spring Onions, Pak Choi and Coriander; Beef and Parsnip Pasties; and Meat and Potato Pie.

lamb

Some states of affairs just progress contentedly along, no matter that there is no common sense applied to them. Meet the world of lamb. The meat industry and logic rarely go hand in hand, but with lamb, I sometimes feel like the only person who has spotted the emperor is naked. I look in the chiller cabinet of the supermarket. New Zealand lamb looks back. And on the road I see the eyes of sheep peer balefully through the open slats of lorries destined for Europe. It's hard to meet their gaze.

The foot-and-mouth disease outbreak in 2001 summed up, on a horrifying, daily basis, everything that was wrong with the industry: the long-distance movement of meat, the vast numbers of animals being shunted across continents and the needless cruelty of exporting live animals.

The highest concentration of foot-and-mouth was grouped around Britain's main motorway corridors, up and down which thousands of sheep travelled every day. We now know that early vaccination would have saved millions of animals, but the authorities took the decision to protect the export industry, despite its low worth to the farming economy apart from a handful of extremely wealthy livestock dealers. Worried that vaccination would leave us with a sheep export ban lasting 12 months after the end of the outbreak, the government, backed by the NFU, decided to opt for mass slaughter. The export market was worth just under £230 million in 2001, whereas at the end of the outbreak six million animals had been slaughtered at a cost of £3 billion for killing them and compensating farmers – money that was taken from the tax-payer. Our cheap meat has cost us dear. Vaccination would have saved both money and loss of life, and has since been recommended by the European Union as a solution in any further outbreak, echoing the view of most animal health experts and scientists. In any case, even with the slaughter policy, exports resumed only one year and eight months after experts had begged the government to give the go-ahead to a vaccination programme – a longer delay than if vaccination had been pursued. Neither the lost lives nor compensation were necessary.

In 2002 the total amount of lamb imported into Britain was 101,000 tonnes; our exports in the same year came to 55,200 tonnes. So why are we importing when we have so much lamb on our doorstep? The lambs we send to Europe are the hill and mountain breeds. Smaller lambs that suit Southern European dishes: charcoal grills, skewers, slow braises with pulses . . . Recognise any of these? Yes – they are the kind of lamb dishes we are now very much into turning out of our own kitchens. Why do we send all this lamb away? Because, the industry tells us, we like young, mild-flavoured lamb all year round. This is their excuse for shipping in New Zealand lamb from September on. But I disagree. I like the way lamb from the British Isles changes colour, size and flavour through the seasons and I like the way it influences the way I cook. Nor do I believe that other consumers would mind it either, were they aware of the crazy contradiction in shipping in quantities of lamb when we ship so much out.

It seems that only a few meat dealers benefit from lambs being transported to and fro. Farmers would do better if they could sell them to the domestic market, the lambs would be better off not travelling on journeys of up to 70 hours, and we would be better off by having more interest and variety in the lamb we eat.

In spring British lamb is small, delicate and pale pink. In summer you can buy salt-marsh grazed lamb and other large lowland breeds. In September there are the so-called light lambs, normally destined for the *tavernas* of Greece. I buy ready-cut half lambs from the butcher, or via home delivery, and store the pieces in the freezer: this gives me a leg, a shoulder, a half rack, a few chops, a bit of neck and neck fillet and a kidney to wrap in a piece of bacon and stuff inside a baked potato. I also buy shearling, hogget and wether: big, strong-flavoured lamb from older animals that would once have been called mutton. Older lamb makes outstanding braises and shepherd's pies.

roast lamb

I like cooking roast lamb the French way, over a layer of chopped vegetables, then chucking in a little water or stock near the end of cooking. You end up with juicy lamb that is pink in the centre, plus a rich, clear, russet gravy. Raymond Blanc cooks lamb this way in his book, *Cooking for Friends* (Headline, 1991), a second-hand copy of which is well worth seeking out for its wonderful recipes for home cooking.

Suitable roasting joints include a leg or half leg of lamb, or a boned and rolled shoulder.

Serves 6

4 tablespoons olive oil

a few lamb bones (the butcher should be only too happy to give them to you)

1 large onion, finely chopped

1 large carrot, finely chopped

2 celery sticks, finely chopped

3 garlic cloves, chopped

2kg/4½lb leg of lamb

a large pinch of dried rosemary, or 1 sprig of fresh rosemary

a large pinch of dried thyme

3 tomatoes, chopped

600ml/1 pint water or meat stock

1 glass of white wine (optional)

sea salt and freshly ground black pepper

Preheat the oven to 200°C/400°F/Gas Mark 6. Heat the oil in a roasting tin on the hob and brown the lamb bones in it. Add the vegetables and garlic and mix well with the oil. Rub the lamb with a little more oil and place it on top of the bones and vegetables. Season with salt and pepper and scatter the rosemary and thyme over everything.

Transfer to the oven and roast for 40 minutes. Remove from the oven, tilt the roasting tin and spoon out any excess fat. Add the tomatoes, water or stock and the wine, if using, and return the tin to the oven. Reduce the heat to 180°C/350°F/Gas Mark 4 and cook for a further 50 minutes. Remove from the oven, put the lamb in a dish and leave to rest in a warm place for 20 minutes, covered with foil.

Strain the juices from the roasting tin into a warm jug, discarding the vegetables and bones. Add any juices that seep from the resting joint of lamb. Serve the lamb with the juices.

cold lamb

shepherd's pie

So much the better for making use of already-roasted lamb, this dish is one my husband, Dominic, takes charge of. Frugality runs in his family, and our old hand mincer, bought at a boot sale, brings tears of joy to his eyes.

This, I remind myself mid tug of war, as I try to get a moth-eaten sweater of his into the bin, is the man who makes his own windscreen-wiper washer. A hideous amalgam of water, washing-up liquid and methylated spirit, it sends fumes through the air vents of the car with one push on the squirt button. Having said that, he makes great shepherd's pie – and insists it is essential to season the meat with the Worcestershire sauce last.

Serves 4

1 tablespoon vegetable oil or lard

2 onions, chopped

2 carrots, chopped

1 celery stick, chopped

240g/8oz minced leftover roast lamb

300ml/½ pint lamb stock or poultry stock

1 bay leaf

1 heaped tablespoon tomato purée

Worcestershire sauce

½ quantity of Mashed Potato (see page 75)

a knob of butter

salt and freshly ground black pepper

Heat the oil or lard in a pan, add the onions, carrots and celery and cook over a medium heat until soft. Add the lamb and stir over the heat a few times. Add the stock with the bay leaf and tomato purée and simmer for 35–45 minutes, then taste and season with salt, pepper and Worcestershire sauce to your liking.

Preheat the oven to 230°C/450°F/Gas Mark 8. Spoon the meat into a shallow ovenproof dish, spread the mashed potato on top and scratch it with a fork. Dot with the butter and bake until the pie is bubbling and the surface has browned.

pilaff with cold meat

This may not be the strictly authentic way to make a pilaff but it's a good method of using up the last bits of cold meat from roasts, however tatty. It's based on Elizabeth David's recipe. She called hers the most 'comforting dish in the world', which it is. We eat this dish so often that I now make sure all the ingredients are in the fridge or store cupboard at one time.

Serves 4

1 heaped tablespoon pine nuts or shelled pistachios

2 tablespoons lard, dripping or vegetable oil

1 onion, chopped

4 tomatoes, deseeded and chopped

1 heaped teaspoon ground cumin or a pinch of ground allspice

leftover roast meat, chicken, duck or pheasant, chopped

8 tablespoons cooked basmati rice (see page 53)

salt and freshly ground black pepper

chopped parsley and mint, to garnish

Greek yoghurt, to serve

Dry-toast the nuts in a frying pan until lightly browned, then tip them into a bowl and set to one side. Melt the fat in the same pan and add the onion. Cook gently until golden, then add the tomatoes with the spice. Cook until the tomatoes are soft, stir in the meat and heat it through. Add the rice, season and stir well until thoroughly heated. Scatter the nuts and herbs over the pilaff and serve from the pan, with a bowl of yoghurt to one side.

lamb and butternut squash hash with cumin and coriander

I buy butternut squash thinking, how useful, and then it sits for weeks on the side. They are very forgiving, however. There is always enough juicy, orange flesh left under its hard skin for this late-night fry-up.

Serves 2

1 butternut squash, peeled, deseeded and cut into 1cm/½ inch
pieces
1 onion, chopped
oil for frying
leftover roast lamb, cut into chunks
1 teaspoon ground cumin
1 teaspoon ground coriander
a pinch of cayenne pepper
1 egg, beaten
4 sprigs of coriander, chopped
salt and freshly ground black pepper

Cook the squash in a pan of boiling water for about 10 minutes, until soft. Drain and leave on a cloth or kitchen paper. While it cools, fry the onion in a little oil until golden. Put it into a bowl, add all the rest of the ingredients, including the squash, and combine them into a well-amalgamated hash.

Heat some oil in a large frying pan and tip the hash into it. Press it down with the back of a spoon and fry for about 4 minutes on either side, until browned. Eat with mango chutney.

✳ **kitchen note** ✳

You can also use cold beef in this recipe.

cheaper cuts of beef, pork and lamb

Most cookbooks suggest you use prime roasting or grilling cuts of meat for frying. But I have discovered that you can get away with using the cheaper cuts, with a little preparation. They may be slightly more of a chew, but good, well-hung meat will make that a very good chew.

turning cheap cuts into fast food

Slice the pork, lamb or beef approximately 1cm thick. Place each slice between two sheets of greaseproof paper and put on a wooden chopping board, then pound with a rolling pin or the smooth side of a meat hammer. The meat can be fried whole, as escalopes, or cut into slivers for stir-frying. The rule of the day is *not* to add any liquid to the pan with the meat: it must be scooped out before you make the sauce or it will revert to a rubbery texture.

The following cuts are suitable for frying with this method:

* Beef – Chuck steak, blade steak or shin.
* Lamb – Neck fillet, chump, shoulder and leg steaks (a little goes a long way)
* Pork – Shank steak, shoulder chop, chump chop (cut away bone and fat)

✳ kitchen note ✳

Ask the butcher if he will slice your meat thin for you – he has the benefit of very sharp knives and the skill needed to do this.

lamb in a pan with peas, mint and butter

Serves 4

750g/1½lb lamb slices, prepared as on page 204
90g/3oz butter
2 small onions, peeled and quartered
200ml/7fl oz white wine or meat stock
480g/1lb frozen peas
1 tablespoon vegetable oil
leaves from 4 sprigs of mint
salt and freshly ground black pepper

Season the lamb with salt and pepper. Have a warmed dish ready. Heat all but a walnut-sized piece of the butter in a pan, add the onions and stew until soft. Add the wine or stock and bring to the boil. Add the peas and boil for 1 minute, then transfer the mixture to the warmed dish.

Dry the pan by placing it over the heat briefly. Add the remaining butter and the oil, bring almost to smoking point, then throw in the lamb. Cook the lamb quickly, turning it frequently, for 2–3 minutes, until browned. Place it on top of the peas and scatter over the mint.

fried lamb escalopes with flageolet beans

Serves 4

750g/1½lb lamb slices, prepared as on page 204
60g/2oz butter

4 shallots, finely chopped

2 cans of flageolet beans, drained

1 glass of white wine

1 tablespoon vegetable oil

salt and freshly ground black pepper

Season the lamb with salt and pepper. Have a warmed dish ready. Melt the butter in a pan and add the shallots. Cook until soft, then add the flageolet beans and wine. Simmer for 5 minutes, season to taste and transfer to the warmed dish. Dry the pan by placing it back over the heat. Add the oil, bring to smoking point and quickly fry the lamb on both sides. Serve the lamb with the beans on the side.

beef with garlic greens

Serves 4

4 slices of beef, prepared as on page 204

2 heads of spring greens, thick stalks cut away

120g/4oz butter

8 garlic cloves, peeled and cut in half

a large pinch of grated nutmeg

1 tablespoon vegetable oil

salt and freshly ground black pepper

Season the beef with salt and pepper. Have a warmed dish ready. Slice the greens into thin shreds. Heat the butter in a large pan, add the garlic and cook gently until softened, then stir in the greens and cook for 2–3 minutes, until they begin to soften. Season with the nutmeg, remove from the heat and set aside.

Heat the oil on a grill pan or in a heavy-based frying pan until smoking, then quickly sear the beef on both sides, pressing it down hard with a spatula. Serve the beef with the garlic greens to the side, accompanied by French mustard. A dish of mashed potato or parsnip would be good, too.

pork with wood-roasted peppers and hot potato salad

If you have access to some of the more flavoursome types of new potato, such as Jersey, La Ratte or Shetland Black, they make this an even more interesting dish.

Serves 4

600g/1¼lb small salad potatoes

4 shallots, sliced

2 tablespoons sherry vinegar

7 tablespoons olive oil

4 slices of pork, prepared as on page 204

4 canned wood-roasted peppers (see the Shopping Guide)

cut into strips

2 sprigs of parsley, chopped

salt and freshly ground black pepper

Boil the potatoes in salted water until tender but still waxy. Drain well, slice them 1cm/½ inch thick and put them in a dish. Mix the shallots with the sherry vinegar and 6 tablespoons of the olive oil and set to one side.

Heat the remaining oil in a frying pan and quickly stir-fry the pork until cooked through. Add the peppers and parsley, stir again, then mix with the potatoes, pouring the dressing over the top.

burgers and patties

Butchers make mince from the parts of beef, lamb, pork and veal that are difficult to cook whole on account of having too much fat or gristle.

With the exception of beef burgers, which I think should be made from leaner meat, fattiness is an advantage: meatballs and minced lamb Middle Eastern-style patties taste better because the fat is absorbed into the breadcrumbs or wheat used in these recipes, and enhances the flavour of any added vegetable, herb or spice (see page 443 for Veal Meatballs).

burgers

It is years since I ate a McDonald's. The cunning of the popular fast-food chains is in the addictive nature of their food. Certain aromas and flavours stick in your mind for ever. I disagree with the idea that the burgers are disgusting: they are not and that is the problem. I have a greater grumble with their marketing strategies. I have lost hours being pestered for McDonald's food by my children because the latest Disney film character toy is included in their Happy Meals. A meeting with Eric Schlosser, author of *Fast Food Nation* (Allen Lane, 2001), further convinced me of what I had always suspected. The effect of fast food on society is negative, whether you are one of their workforce, obese as a result from eating it, a farmer forced to sell his produce on the cheap, or just someone who remembers real family meals.

One burger in a while is a great meal but one a day is going to ruin your appetite for a diverse and healthy diet. It is worth, then, making the odd great burger at home, and dressing it up with delicious gherkins, salad, mayonnaise and relish. The best burger I have ever eaten was in a restaurant on California's staggeringly beautiful coastal road, Highway One, which runs through Big Sur. The restaurant was named Nepenthe, after the herb recommended by the ancients for forgetting sorrow, and sure enough, this place was manned by ageing hippies, with grey hair and beards down to their waists. We sat side by side at tables positioned at the optimum angle to watch the grey whale migration north, washing down the burgers with dry martinis. At Nepenthe they sandwich the burgers in crisp French bread, toasted on the inside. Sheer bliss.

French and Italian butchers are in the habit of mincing meat to order, in front of you – a practice I like because you can be absolutely sure of what meat you are buying. An alternative is to buy the meat you want, and chop it yourself in a food processor.

beef burgers

Makes 4

480g/1lb well-hung rump steak, or a mixture of chuck and rump steak

4 pinches of celery salt

2 tablespoons vegetable oil (if frying the burgers)

freshly ground black pepper

To serve:

either 4 thick chunks of baguette, split open and toasted lightly on the cut side (I do this in a frying pan while I cook the burgers);

or 4 soft baps (easy for children with wobbly teeth)

Trimmings – choose from the following:

thin slices of cheese – Malvern, Durras or Oxford Blue would be good

sweet German mustard (or your favourite mustard)

tomato chutney or ketchup

Cos or romaine lettuce

sprouting seeds (see page 69)

chopped coriander

cornichons, thinly sliced lengthways

good-quality bought mayonnaise (home-made is just not as good with burgers)

Cut the meat into 2cm/¾ inch pieces and chop in a food processor, being careful not to process it to a paste. Transfer to a bowl and mix with the celery salt and some black pepper. Shape into 4 round patties.

Cook the burgers either on a barbecue or indoors. To cook them indoors, heat the oil on a large ridged grill pan or in a heavy-based frying pan until it begins to smoke. Put the burgers in the pan and turn the heat down to medium. For a rare burger, cook for about 2 minutes on each side; for a well-cooked burger, cook for about 4 minutes per side. To test, prise open the centre of a burger with a sharp knife and take a look. Don't worry if this spoils the appearance, the burger will soon be inside the bun. If you are making a cheese burger, put a slice of cheese on the burger while it is still in the pan, approximately 2 minutes before it is ready.

To assemble the burgers, spread one side of the bread with mustard and tomato chutney or ketchup. The burger goes on top, followed by the salad ingredients, then mayonnaise.

lamb patties

These little patties made from minced lamb and bulgar wheat are known as *kibbeh* in the Lebanon, and are best cooked on a barbecue. They are very good served cold. Eat them with a herb salad of parsley, mint and dill, dressed with plenty of olive oil and lemon juice as *kibbeh* are characteristically quite dry.

Makes at least 16

240g/8oz bulgar wheat
480g/1lb lamb – neck fillet or shoulder meat
1 onion, grated
½ teaspoon freshly ground black pepper

Soak the bulgar in cold water for 10 minutes, then squeeze out the water. Cut the lamb into 2cm/¾ inch pieces, discarding any hard skin, and put it in a food processor. Process until nearly smooth, then add the bulgar with the onion and black pepper. Process again until you have a soft paste. Shape into patties 1cm/½ inch thick and cook on a barbecue. Alternatively you can grill or fry them indoors.

slow, slow cooking

The perception that cheaper cuts of meat mean a load of boring brown food could not be further from the truth. Imagine the soft meat from a pink ham hock, resting in a clear juice with small white beans and an olive oil and parsley sauce. Picture braised lamb shoulder with the greenest peas and heavenly scented mint, or a crisp baked potato, burnished with olive oil and stuffed with a buttered kidney wrapped in bacon. Think of burgundy slices of silverside with a mustard and caper sauce, brawn speckled with pink peppercorns, potato soups flavoured with spiced sausages, or coarse sausages with duck legs and pink beans, spare ribs rubbed with chilli and salt, meatballs on pasta, pâtés and terrines . . . I could go on. There is nothing dull about this type of home cooking. All these dishes, irrespective of their origins, we can call our own. They belong to a colourful and aromatic range of contemporary food – food which has its roots in tradition.

braised lamb with potatoes and parsley oil

When lamb cooks slowly it sweetens, and needs only a few vegetables to bring out its flavour. For this stew you could use lamb stock instead of water, if you have some.

Serves 4

12 pieces of neck of lamb, both middle neck and scrag end

8 small onions, peeled and halved

8 small carrots, scraped but left whole

12 small potatoes, peeled but left whole

900ml/1½ pints water

2 sprigs of thyme, or a pinch of dried thyme

salt and freshly ground black pepper

For the parsley oil:

10 sprigs of parsley

125ml/4fl oz olive oil

1 garlic clove, peeled (optional)

Brush the surface of the meat to remove any bone splinters and trim off excess fat. Put this fat in a large frying pan and render it down over a gentle heat. Remove it from the pan, leaving the melted fat behind. Turn up the heat, add the meat to the pan and brown on both sides.

Layer the meat, onions, carrots and potatoes in a large casserole. Pour a little of the water into the frying pan and bring to the boil, scraping up the juices from the base. Pour this liquid over the casserole with the remaining water and season with salt and pepper. Tuck in the thyme, place the casserole over the heat and bring to the boil. Cook on a low simmer for 1–2 hours, until the meat is tender – do not cook for longer than necessary.

In a pestle and mortar, or in a food processor, blend together the parsley, oil and garlic, if using, with a little salt until smooth. Serve the braised lamb with the oil zigzagged over the top.

✳ kitchen notes ✳

✳ Other suitable cuts for this braise include chump chops, knuckle or shanks, and shoulder meat.

✳ White haricot beans could be substituted for the potatoes. Soak the beans overnight and cook for 1 hour before adding to the casserole, or add 2 drained cans of beans 30 minutes before the lamb is ready.

simmered salt silverside and tongue with watercress dumplings

This was my mother's Easter dish. She loved brined meat and went to the trouble of finding a butcher who could do the job well. Some traditional butchers keep a brine tub on the go but if you order a week in advance, most will be able to provide the cured beef and tongue needed for this recipe.

You can make this dish for a smaller number with just a piece of either tongue or beef. Rolled boned brisket is a good alternative to the leaner silverside, but make sure the butcher cuts away any tough gristle. The first time I used brisket, no one could get their teeth through it no matter how long it simmered.

Serves 10–12

1 brined ox tongue, the skin on and the root bones removed

2.25kg/5lb brined piece of silverside

2 carrots, peeled but left whole

2 onions, peeled and quartered

2 celery sticks, sliced

1 bay leaf

8 black peppercorns

1 star anise

1 litre/1¾ pints good beef stock

Worcestershire sauce

chopped parsley, to garnish

For the watercress dumplings:

180g/6oz self-raising flour

90g/3oz grated beef suet, dried or fresh

a pinch of salt

leaves from 2 bunches of watercress, finely chopped

Put the ox tongue and silverside in a large pan, cover with cold water and leave to soak for a few hours. Drain well, then return the tongue to the pan, add the vegetables, bay leaf, peppercorns and star anise and cover completely with fresh water. Bring to the boil, skim away any foam that rises to the surface and simmer for 1½ hours. The liquid in the pot should bubble slowly with the surface barely moving or the meat will be dry and tough. Add the beef and cook for a further 2 hours at the same, very slow boil. Test the beef for doneness by cutting a sliver from the edge; cook for another 30 minutes if it isn't tender enough. Remove the tongue and allow to cool for a few minutes. Skin it, using a small knife to peel the membrane away. Place the tongue and beef (removing any string) on a warmed serving dish and cover with foil.

Mix all the dumpling ingredients together and bind to a soft dough with a little cold water. With floured hands, form into walnut-sized balls and place on a floured board. Bring the meat pan back to the boil, add the dumplings and simmer them in the liquor for 10 minutes. Meanwhile, heat the beef stock to boiling point and add a splash or two of Worcestershire sauce for flavour.

Lift out the dumplings and arrange them around the meat. Pour over a little of the stock, leaving the rest in a jug for the table. Throw some chopped parsley over the meat and bring to the table, hopefully to gasps of admiration. Carve at the table, size permitting.

caper and mustard sauce for boiled meat

This is a lovely sauce to eat with hot poached silverside or brisket, or with hot roast ham (see page 218).

Serves 10–12

4 egg yolks

4 hard-boiled egg yolks, pushed through a metal sieve until crumbled

2 heaped tablespoons Dijon mustard

2 heaped tablespoons capers, soaked in water for 10 minutes, squeezed dry, then chopped

150ml/¼ pint olive oil

6 sprigs of parsley, chopped

1–2 tablespoons red wine vinegar

salt and freshly ground black pepper

Combine the raw and cooked egg yolks with the mustard and capers, then stir in the olive oil gradually with a wooden spoon. Mix in the parsley, season to taste and add 1 tablespoon of the vinegar; taste and add more if necessary.

sliced cold silverside and tongue

Any leftover meat can be eaten the next day, on buttered malty brown bread or alone, with the sauces for cold beef on pages 186 and 187.

ribs and rib trim

Back to the butcher, this time to ask when you buy rib of beef if he will save the trim between the ribs for you. Not all butchers do this but if you know one that trims meat the French way, he will know what you mean. Rib trim is extraordinary when braised. The fat melts and can be skimmed away and the meat left behind has a flavour close to sirloin.

braised beef

This is the big stew we eat at weekends in winter, with baked or mashed potatoes and Sprout Tops with Cream, Lemon and Rosemary (see page 341) on the side, or watercress dumplings (see page 214) for a real treat. The added trotter makes a luscious gravy. Ask the butcher for any of the following cuts: rib trim, shin, neck, chuck, skirt, blade, forerib, flank. It is a good, basic, adaptable recipe (see variations below) that suits a wide range of meats, including pork, lamb and game such as venison and hare.

Serves 6–8

5–6 tablespoons olive oil or dripping

2 garlic cloves, chopped

2 onions, finely chopped

2 celery sticks, finely chopped

2kg/4½lb braising beef, cut into 4cm/1½ inch chunks

1 pig's trotter, split lengthways in half

1 bay leaf

a pinch of dried thyme

2 glasses of red or white wine

1 heaped tablespoon plain flour

beef or other meat stock to cover

salt and freshly ground black pepper

Heat about a third of the fat in a large, deep-sided pan and gently cook the garlic, onions and celery in it until soft. Remove the vegetables with a slotted spoon and set aside. Add more of the fat to the pan, turn up the heat and brown the beef on all sides, cooking it in batches and setting it aside as you go. Add more fat as necessary. Brown the pig's trotter briefly, then remove from the pan. Add the herbs and wine to the pan and bring to the boil, scraping away at the base of the pan with a wooden spoon. Return the meat and vegetables to the pan, sprinkle with the flour and stir well. Add enough stock to cover, then stir and bring to the boil, skimming off any foam that rises to the top. Turn down the heat to a slow bubble and cook for 1½–2 hours, until the meat is tender. Pick the trotter meat, discarding skin and bones, and return it to the stew. Season with salt and pepper to taste.

various braises

This recipe can be adapted by making various substitutions for the meat, vegetables, liquor and/or other accompaniments.

* Pork, dry cider and chicken or pork stock, with prunes added 15 minutes before the end.
* Pork, red pepper, lemon zest, canned tomatoes, chicken or pork stock, celery and cumin, with green lentils added in the last 45 minutes and fresh coriander at the end.
* Beef, kidneys, red wine and/or beef stock, with field mushrooms added 15 minutes before the end – a great base for a pie.
* Beef, stout, wild mushrooms (dried or fresh) and beef stock.
* Lamb, cumin seeds, aubergine, canned tomatoes, white wine and lamb stock.
* Lamb and lamb stock, with spring vegetables (small carrots, small onions, mangetout and French beans) added in the last 20 minutes.
* Venison, red wine, venison or pheasant stock and dried wild mushrooms.

hot sugared ham

A ham in the house is the answer to feeding large numbers without too much fuss or boredom. The feast begins with a hot sugared ham, served with Pickled Cucumber (see page 95), Cumberland Sauce (page 219) or Caper and Mustard Sauce (page 215), and mashed potato. The leftover cold ham can be used in sandwiches, tarts, baked with eggs, or as a flavouring in numerous dishes. One of the things I like best about having a roast ham in the house is having a slice for breakfast with a piece of semi-soft cheese such as Ashmore. A whole ham will keep for about 10 days in the fridge.

You can buy whole or half hams, preferably on the bone for flavour – and for stock. The ham will come covered in rind, which you remove for the last part of the cooking. Seek out hams from naturally reared, slow-grown pigs; mail order often offers the best value (see the Shopping Guide).

boiling the ham

I part boil hams to keep them juicy inside, then roast them for the last 30 minutes to give them a good glaze. If possible, soak the raw ham overnight to extract excess salt, then drain. If you are short of time, just cover the ham with water, bring to the boil, then drain and discard the water.

Bring the ham to the boil in a large pan of fresh water. For hams weighing up to 2.25kg/5lb, boil at a slow bubble for 30 minutes per 480g/1lb; for hams weighing 2.5–5kg/5½–11lb, cook for 15 minutes per 480g/1lb; for hams weighing over 5kg/11lb, cook for 10 minutes per 480g/1lb. Top the pan up with water from time to time, if necessary; the ham should remain covered. To test for doneness, stick a long skewer into the deepest part of the flesh, leave it for 30 seconds, then pull it out. If the part of the skewer that was roughly at the centre of the joint is hot, the meat is done.

glazing the ham

If you want to finish the ham by glazing it, remove it from the pan half an hour before the end of cooking. Preheat the oven to 190°C/375°F/Gas Mark 5. Slide a knife under the ham rind, leaving as much fat as possible on the joint, and peel the rind away. Stud the ham fat with cloves, in rows 2.5cm/1 inch apart. Spread English mustard all over the fat, then cover with demerara sugar, pressing it on with your hand. Place the ham in a roasting dish and roast for half an hour, until the glaze is golden and caramelised. The ham is ready to carve immediately.

cumberland sauce

This is my favourite sauce to eat with hot ham and mashed potato.

Serves 6–8

1 orange
3 tablespoons redcurrant jelly
2 small glasses of red wine (or port)
freshly ground black pepper

Pare the zest from the orange with a potato peeler, then slice it into thin slivers. Put it in a small saucepan with the jelly and red wine. Place the pan over a low heat and bring to the boil. Simmer for 5 minutes, remove from the heat and leave to cool. Season with black pepper.

✳ kitchen note ✳

Use Seville oranges when in season (see page 342).

ham broth

This is the warming winter broth, made with lentils, whole wheat or barley, that I eat for lunch in the winter. Serve with a spoonful of herb- or chilli-flavoured oil (see page 91). I sometimes beg or buy the bones of dry-cured Spanish hams from delis to pop into this simmering broth, giving it real, deep-down, depth of flavour.

Serves 4

2 tablespoons olive oil

2 onions, finely chopped

1 celery stick, finely chopped

1 large carrot, finely chopped

1 mug of green lentils, whole wheat (see the Shopping Guide) or pearl barley

1 ham bone or roast pork bone

1.5 litres/2½ pints meat stock – pork, lamb or beef is best

4 sprigs of parsley, chopped

salt and freshly ground black pepper

extra virgin olive oil, or herb- or chilli-flavoured oil to serve

Heat the olive oil in a large pan, add the onions, celery and carrot and cook until soft. Add the lentils, wheat or barley and swirl them around in the oil for a moment. Add the bone and stock and bring to the boil. Simmer for 1 hour or until the grains are cooked to the bite. Taste for seasoning and add salt only if needed. Scatter with the chopped parsley and add a dash of oil.

a ham broth for autumn

You can season the above broth with garlic and saffron powder, adding them with the lentils, wheat or barley. Add chopped squash or marrow 10 minutes before the end of cooking and serve scattered with mint.

sausages

Almost every country in the world produces some sort of sausage or other, and it has traditionally been the butcher's way to use up the cheaper and fattier cuts. It all went wrong when sausage manufacturers began to use mashed bone, gristle and endless flavourings and preservatives to bulk out sausages for the mass market. That textured, lean, sage-flavoured banger became a tube of artificial skin containing an unidentifiable pink paste. But good sausages made from high-quality, naturally reared British meat are back in many forms – cured, dried or fresh. I love them plain, but there are one or two more interesting things to do than eat them with mash.

braised sausages with cider and hot potato salad

My Aunt Dariel showed me how to make this. It became my economical party standard.

Serves 8

16 large, meaty pork sausages

about 300ml/½ pint dry cider

2kg/4½lb new potatoes, scrubbed or scraped

4 spring onions, chopped

6 tablespoons olive oil

2 tablespoons cider vinegar

salt and freshly ground black pepper

Preheat the oven to 230°C/450°F/Gas Mark 8. Place the sausages in a roasting dish and pour in enough cider to half-submerge them. Put them in the oven and bake for 20 minutes, until coloured. Turn over the sausages and bake for a further 20 minutes, until done.

Meanwhile, boil the potatoes until just tender – they should be slightly waxy in the centre. Drain well, then add the spring onions, oil, vinegar and some salt and pepper and give them a big stir. Serve with the sausages, using the cooked cider as gravy.

black pudding, dry-cured sausage and bacon with leaves

A light, fast means of using up odd sausages and all the cured meats, chicken giblets and cooked potatoes that lurk in the fridge looking for a home.

Serves 4

4 large handfuls of salad leaves – Cos, watercress, rocket and spinach are ideal
4 cooked potatoes, peeled and diced – leftover baked or roast potatoes and boiled new potatoes are fine
2 tablespoons olive oil

Plus at least 4 of the following:
black pudding, cut into 2cm/¾ inch chunks
chorizo or other dry-cured sausage, cut into 2cm/¾ inch chunks
plain pork sausage, cut into 2cm/¾ inch chunks
bacon or ham, cut into 1cm/½ inch chunks
chicken livers and hearts, sliced
lamb's kidneys, sliced

For the dressing:
125ml/4fl oz olive oil
juice of ½ lemon

4 sprigs of dill, chopped

salt and freshly ground black pepper

Put the salad leaves in a big bowl with the potatoes. In a frying pan, sauté the different meats in the olive oil, beginning with the raw meats and adding the cooked or cured ones at the end just to heat through. Allow to cool slightly, then mix with the salad leaves. Shake over the olive oil, lemon juice and some seasoning and throw over the chopped dill.

✳ kitchen note ✳

For a richer salad, put a peeled semi-soft-boiled egg (see page 380) on top of each helping.

barbecues

Locally made charcoal is making a comeback thanks to the efforts of woodland managers who are trying to revive what is a very ancient practice. Ask at local garden centres, or look on the internet for suppliers (see the Shopping Guide). It feels good to use a fuel that has not travelled miles when you have already made the effort to buy locally reared meat.

offal

The pork on sale in the English market in Cork, southern Ireland, is a revelation. Tails, ears and snouts; hands (forelegs), knuckles, bellies, ribs . . . The cooks of Cork have handed down knowledge of how to handle every less valuable part of the pig – and for a very good reason. Cork was a provisions city, the last stop for ships before they prepared to cross the Atlantic. The meat workers who cut and prepared the salt beef and pork for the ships' long voyages were paid in offal, sparking a taste for these things that has never died. If only this trend were more widespread.

Health scares have done nothing to help sales of offal, and butchers must now pay to have much of it collected and disposed of. There are some types of offal, connected to the spinal cord of cows, which are known, in relation to the disease, BSE, as specified risk material (SRM). It is compulsory for this to be removed at the abattoir.

I grew up eating offal. It was not always welcome and a natural childish squeamishness would sometimes make me push it around the plate. But by some gradual osmotic process I grew to love it. That first oxtail stew! I used to love the way the dark threads of meat fell away from those knobbly bones. Then there was hot, poached tongue, with its gentle flavour and a texture similar to fillet of beef. Later in life Jane Grigson's writing taught me to love terrines made with pork and pork liver, and the delicate meat from a pig's head set in a natural jelly sweetened with wine. This transformation of something unappetising and faintly disturbing into a refined, delicious dish is for me what offal cookery should be about. I now put pig's trotters in braises, to enrich the sauce and add whatever meat they yield; on the other hand, I have to say, boned, stuffed pig's trotter is what restaurants are there for. I buy a lot of pâté and meat pies from places that make them with traditionally reared meat in the traditional way. You still have to think twice before serving offal for dinner unless you know your guests' tastes back to front, but with the emerging popularity of offal in restaurants like St John in Smithfield, London, attitudes are slowly changing.

Butchers react with delighted surprise when asked for lamb sweetbreads, pig's heads, trotters and tails, pork fat, tripe and marrow bones. They are less astonished to be asked for liver and kidneys, both of which are also available in supermarkets, although not at present those originating from naturally reared animals. Unlike meat, offal needs no maturing and should be eaten quickly. Freshness is essential. Check it for dryness or discoloration.

kidneys

Beef (sometimes sold as ox kidneys) or pig kidneys should be diced, the white, threadlike ducts cut away, and added to beef braises. Fry them with the beef and continue with the braising process (see page 216).

lamb kidneys

These small kidneys are lovely fried. Simply cut them in half lengthways and snip the white ducts away with kitchen scissors. Season with salt and pepper and fry on both sides. Note that they will shrink as they brown.

potatoes stuffed with lamb's kidneys and bacon

When I buy a lamb box with half a lamb, there is usually one lone kidney to use up. Here is a way to stretch it for a meal for 2.

Serves 2

2 baking potatoes

a little olive oil

1 lamb's kidney

2 rashers of green streaky bacon

60g/2oz butter

2 sprigs of parsley, finely chopped

Preheat the oven to 230°C/450°F/Gas Mark 8. Prick the potatoes with a fork and rub them with oil. Bake for up to 1 hour, until the skin begins to feel soft to the touch.

Cut the kidney in half and snip away the fatty threads inside using scissors. Put each kidney half on a rasher of bacon with the butter and parsley and wrap the bacon round it. Cut off the top third of each potato. Use a spoon to scoop out a hole large enough to hold the bacon-wrapped kidney. Stuff the kidney into the potatoes, put the tops back on and wrap each potato in greaseproof paper. Return them to the oven for 30 minutes. Serve with butter and chopped parsley.

lamb sweetbreads

Sweetbreads – another good offal name – are taken from the thymus gland or pancreas. Their delicate white meat, with a texture of young chicken or shellfish, is sublime substituted for lamb in Lamb in a Pan with Peas, Mint and Butter (page 205). Make sure you remember to blanch them first.

sautéed sweetbreads

Serves 4

Soak 480g/1lb sweetbreads in cold water for an hour, throw away the water and bring them to the boil in fresh water. Simmer for 5 minutes, drain and leave to cool. Remove the skin and the ducts or tubes attached to them and slice each sweetbread into 3 or 4 pieces. Sauté in butter for 3–5 minutes, until firm, then season to taste. Serve with chopped pan-cooked spring onions, spinach, peas, broad beans or new potatoes.

brawn

Now here's an adventure not to be undertaken lightly: the meat from a pig's head, including the ears, cheeks and tongue, is extracted after a long slow simmer, then the cooking liquor is reduced with wine to a stock that will set, with the meat, to a crystal jelly. This is one for my husband, preferably when the children are at school and not likely to encounter the vision of a pig's snout poking out of a saucepan.

In the UK we call this dish brawn, or head cheese, but the French call it *fromage de tête* – a prettier-sounding name. French names for meat dishes always sound more elegant. It is worth remembering that after they invaded, nearly 1,000 years ago, the Normans gave us the word *boeuf*, or beef, which we were crassly calling cow; *porc*, or pork, for pig; venison (from *venaison*) for deer; and mutton (from *mouton*) for sheep. It is a pleasing reminder that we have always been a little sentimental. Even as enthusiastic carnivores we prefer not to confront the memory of the living thing once it is on our plate.

This recipe is an adaptation of the one in Jane Grigson's book, *Charcuterie and French Pork Cookery* (Michael Joseph, 1967). Brining the pig's head is what gives this dish its beauty. Grigson wrote, when lamenting that no one ate anything but expensive cuts of pork any more, that 'lack of proper care, above the statutory requirements of hygiene, and insensitivity to flavour make many manufactured dishes in England uneatable'. She pointed out that it is not that cheaper cuts are more 'difficult or tortuous' to cook but that 'they require judgement and care over detail'.

If you ask any good butcher for a pig's head, they should be more than happy to sell it to you very cheaply.

480g/1lb sea salt

360g/12oz brown sugar

3 litres/5 pints water (Grigson specifies rain water, but I have made this without!)

1 pig's head, split in half

1 pig's trotter, split in half

2 onions, roughly chopped

2 carrots, roughly chopped

2 leeks, roughly chopped

2 garlic cloves, roughly chopped

2 bay leaves

2 sprigs of parsley

2 sprigs of thyme

8 black peppercorns

2 tablespoons wine vinegar

a small pinch each of ground allspice, cloves and nutmeg

½ bottle of white wine

lemon juice

For the spice bag:

1 teaspoon juniper berries

a piece of nutmeg

1 bay leaf

3 sprigs of thyme

1 teaspoon black peppercorns

4 cloves

To serve:

Summer Green Sauce for Beef (see page 184)

some salad leaves, parsley and dill, dressed with olive oil and

lemon juice

To brine the head, tie all the ingredients for the spice bag up in a square of muslin. Bring the salt, brown sugar and water to the boil in a large stainless-steel pan, then allow to cool. Submerge the pig's head and the trotter in the brine, using a weight in a plastic bag to keep the meat below the surface. Leave in a cool place for 24 hours.

Remove all the meat from the brine. Put the vegetables, garlic, herbs, peppercorns and vinegar in a pan with the brined head and the trotter. Cover with water and bring to the boil, skimming away any foam that rises to the surface. Simmer for about 5 hours, topping up the water as necessary; the meat is cooked when it drops easily off the bone. Lift out the head, leave to cool, then remove the brains and set to one side (see below). Begin to pick all the lean meat from the trotter and head, including the cheeks and ears. Remove the tongue and peel it. Chop it by hand into 1cm/½ inch pieces and set to one side, seasoning it with the allspice, cloves and nutmeg. Strain the cooking liquor through a muslin square and put 500ml/16fl oz of it into a pan with the wine. Boil until the volume has reduced to 500ml/16fl oz again. Taste and season with salt and lemon juice. You must be absolutely happy with the flavour; Grigson reminds us that cold food loses flavour, so keep this in mind, as this is a dish served straight from the fridge.

Add the picked meat to the pan of reduced stock and simmer for 20 minutes. Check the seasoning once more. Separate the meat from the stock. Put half the meat into a straight-sided dish, lay the chopped tongue on top and put the remaining meat on top of that. Spoon over the liquid until it just covers the meat. Leave to set in the fridge. To serve, cut the brawn into slices about 1cm/½ inch thick and serve with Summer Green Sauce and a simple salad of lettuce, parsley and dill. Pour yourself an enormous glass of wine to congratulate yourself. You are now the ultimate meat cook.

economics of brawn

A conservative costing for the ingredients brings them to £7.20 if using meat from naturally reared pigs. With nominal energy costs, 12 good servings of pork heaven come in at 60 pence each.

pig's brains

Saving the brain from the poached pig's head will give you another meal. Slice it into strips, fry in butter until brown, then serve with butter flavoured with pink peppercorns, chopped chervil and capers – or try the Summer Green Sauce for Beef on page 184 or Cornichon, Egg and Herb Sauce (page 196). Treat as a hot terrine, with toasted bread to one side.

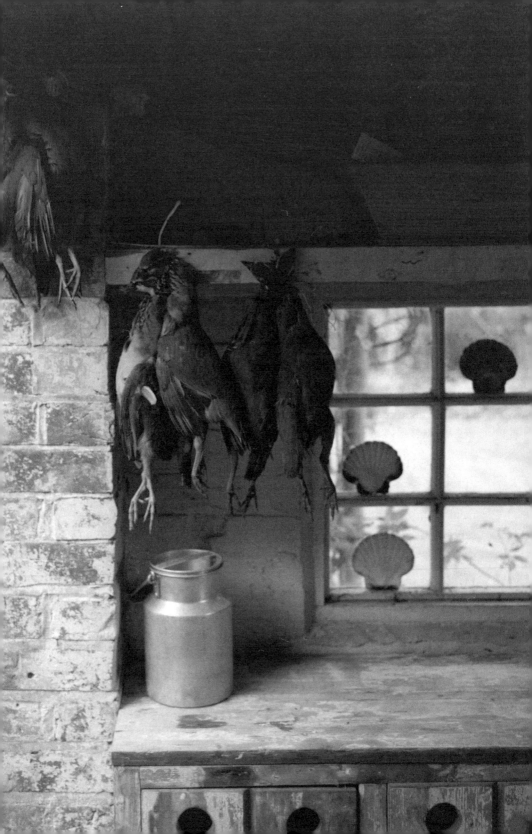

6

game and wild meat

All the while excuses have been made for the need to farm animals intensively there has been a source of meat that is diverse, delicious and which can be cheap, too. Outside country kitchens and city restaurants game and wild meat are avoided, and yet if a plate of it were put before you, you'd probably love it. Eating more game will, in a small way, release a little pressure from the food supply chain, and will also, by virtue of being unusual, enhance life itself.

Game, cooked typically on a cooler autumn or winter night in enjoyably robust recipes, has a rightness to it – a natural and irresistible appeal. Being part of an afternoon's shoot, with the smell of cordite and wet leaves in a November fog, is a rite of passage to a mushroom-infused braise for dinner, or perhaps a juicy roast beside a pool of bread sauce.

wild meat emotion

Wild meat provokes feelings in people that farmed meat does not. It is perceived as 'cruel' because it is shot rather than slaughtered in an abattoir. Rabbits are popular pets and cartoon characters – think Thumper – so eating them is a tricky proposition for parents to square with the kids. Some wild meat also has associations with class and false grandeur; it's perceived as something eaten only in gentlemen's clubs or in manor houses. And other wild meat went out of fashion because it was associated with bad times. I have heard people who ate a lot of rabbit during the Second World War say they will never touch it again.

It's a pity there is such reluctance, when there are so many positive reasons to eat wild meat. It is in plentiful supply, and when it is overlooked by cooks it simply goes to waste. That is why it has a place in the New English Kitchen.

While game is a rich subject for cookery, there's an urgent need for cooks to know more about it. Game's rich history and grand recipes have been celebrated in many good books, leaving many questions unanswered. How and why it is produced are less well-known, but for me these are crucial to understanding the reasons and methods for cooking and eating game.

the sensual case for eating game

If you choose not to eat wild food, this is what you miss: shoulder of venison braised with wild mushrooms; hare, slowly cooked with wine and garlic, heaped over buttered fresh egg noodles; rabbit stewed with lemon and garlic, or a juicy young pheasant with creamy bread sauce. Roast partridge needs little more than fried breadcrumbs, scented with parsley and lemon, mallard likes fruit, and wood pigeon breast goes best with green cabbage. The one grouse I eat each year is stuffed with two raspberries and a knob of butter, and sits on top of fried bread.

reasons to eat game

There is a real environmental need to eat game, especially those species that, either for natural or artificial reasons, are a little bit too plentiful. Pheasant and venison come to mind. If the countryside sport of game shooting is to be justified, then the meat of the quarry must find its way to the table. And from the cook's point of view, getting into game opens up a whole new larder of delicious meat for meals that can roll effortlessly into each another.

the economics of game

Like all meat, most game can be recycled. Pheasant bones make wonderful broth, venison likewise, although I find rabbit and hare do not. Cold cooked game can be used in versions of the various chicken, beef and lamb salads, pilaff and the hash recipe on page 203.

a brace of (two) whole oven-ready pheasants weighing 750g/2½lb each

1st meal:	four 150g/5oz helpings of roast pheasant and gravy
2nd meal:	two 375ml/12fl oz helpings of pheasant broth with egg noodles
3rd meal:	two sandwiches made with the remaining cold meat

Two £3 pheasants goes into three meals, making eight helpings at an average cost of 75 pence each.

The price of venison is very variable. There are several different breeds with different seasons; they are interchangeable for the recipes, although timing may vary according to size. Do not confuse farmed venison with wild, and always choose to eat wild over farmed because there are too many deer in the countryside and they need eating. For me, they taste more interesting than the farmed product. Make allowances for weight loss. Venison typically loses up to 20 per cent of its weight during cooking, depending on the age, sex and breed of deer.

one 5kg haunch of wild fallow deer, with about 3.75kg/7lb 13oz of meat

1st meal:	eight 200g/7oz helpings of roast venison and gravy
2nd meal:	eight helpings of Venison and Mushroom Pie made with 1.2kg/2½lb cold meat and 1.5 litres/2½ pints venison stock
3rd meal:	six 90g/3oz helpings of thinly sliced cold venison
4th meal:	four helpings of creamed mushroom soup, made with 1 litre/1¾ pints venison stock

One £45 haunch of wild fallow deer goes into four meals, making 26 helpings at an average cost of £1.73 each.

what is game?

Meat from wild animals is almost always dubbed game, on the basis that it is killed as part of a sporting pursuit. But it is a complicated subject: some game is from wild animals that were born and bred in the wild, other comes from farmed animals that have then been released into the wild. And not all game is shot purely for sport; there are instances where culling is necessary. Deer, for example, have no predator in the UK. Culling controls their numbers, and so benefits the health of the herd and the environment.

farmed game

Farmed game seems something of an oxymoron, but venison, rabbit and 'wild' boar are farmed routinely. There's even been a limited return to pheasant farming, a practice originally brought to Britain by the Romans, but rarely followed since. As with any farmed animal, farmed game should be reared with sufficient space to move around, access to the outside, water and natural feed that's not designed to speed up growth (feed is also an important factor when it comes to flavour). A good salesman should know whether what he's selling has been farmed intensively, so don't be afraid to ask. Be particularly wary when buying farmed rabbit.

Farmed game lacks the intensity of flavour of the wild animal. While you can use the recipes in this chapter for farmed game, my main aim is to give you enough information about wild meat and game for you to buy it and cook it confidently.

how game birds are reared

The two species of game bird most often reared and released into the wild are pheasant and French red leg partridge. They are reared in a similar way, although the rarer English grey leg partridge is rarely hand reared; if they turn up in the bag they are most likely to be from the wild population.

An estimated 38 million pheasants are reared and released into the wild in Britain each year. During the season from 1 September to 31 January 20 million are shot, and it is thought that only 10 per cent of those derive from the fully wild population. As animal rearing techniques go, that of the pheasant is all right. The poults are con- fined indoors for approximately 10 days. They are then given an increasing amount of access outdoors before being transferred into release pens. For 500 game birds, this will typically be in a grassed pen measuring perhaps 9 by 12 metres (30 by 40 feet). Release pens offer them some protection from vermin, but they can naturally 'escape' when they are mature enough to fend for themselves. By the age of three months, these hand-reared pheasants are living fully in the wild.

Pheasants are territorially aggressive, so gamekeepers may put a soft plastic clip on their beaks to prevent them damaging other birds in the smaller pens. The aim, as one gamekeeper told me, is to produce a healthy, totally wild bird capable of fending for itself.

The detractors of game shooting say pheasant rearing techniques are highly contrived, its supporters say it protects the young from predators, which in the wild can easily take 80 per cent of a brood. Moreover, they argue, it encourages biodiversity and the rural environment, and it makes good economic sense to the shoot. One thing is certain: unless game is eaten, it cannot be justified in any sense.

If the idea of farmed game birds troubles you, compare the minimum life cycles: a pheasant may live for six months, of which two weeks maximum are spent indoors, while broiler chicken may last six to eight weeks, all of them spent indoors. And ask yourself which is more problematic in terms of the creature's welfare.

The real surprise is that while game is sold for top prices, it is in fact an inexpensive meat. Even supermarkets, who now mercifully sell game birds and wild venison in certain stores, mark it up handsomely as a luxury product, and in so doing deny it to many people.

At the peak of the season in November and December, pheasant is too abundant. There is actually a pheasant mountain now that the French, Germans and Belgians, who used to take 80 per cent of our game – mainly pheasant and venison – now buy game birds extra cheap from other European countries, including pheasants from crafty Eastern European farmers who rear the wretches in cages. Before the foot-and-mouth outbreak and ensuing export ban in 2001, 85 per cent of wild venison was sold abroad, whereas now it is more like 80 per cent, which indicates a rise in domestic consumption (it can, for instance, be bought in Sainsbury's between October and late February). In Britain country people can buy pheasants direct from shoots, for the right price. I paid 60 pence per bird at peak season last year, but even then, city dwellers must pay through the nose for it.

game shooting controversy

The acceptability of game shooting is, for me, defined by its scale. Shoots can be small, cheery farm affairs, run to entertain the locals over the winter; then there are the responsibly run, medium-sized commercial shoots where every care is taken for welfare and conservation. There are also controversial commercial shoots with record-breaking bags, run in the name of sport, but some of which have become hard for shooting's supporters to justify. A 450-bird day may be a great sporting event for some, but for me it's a repulsive number of birds to shoot in one small area during one day. A small farm shoot would consider a bag of 80 birds large.

The body count from highly commercial shoots floods the market during the peak season. At the extreme end of the scale, large shoots release vast numbers of birds, sometimes more than can be sold once shot, to give the paying 'guns', or shooters, a better chance of a big bag. This type of shooting is wrong: it is intensive, putting animal welfare in question, and too many pheasants released into farm and woodland can damage not benefit the environment. These shoots give a bad name to a countryside tradition that is in many ways beneficial. The government may well be more receptive to campaigns for banning shooting if the large-scale shoots don't change their ways.

the true value of game

Two hundred game birds a day is an acceptable average bag for a commercial shoot. The gun pays about £25 for each bird he or she shoots, although only a couple of these will be taken home for supper. The bulk of the birds end up on the wholesale market with a value of between 60 pence and £1.20 each to game dealers, according to season, and the price to the consumer should be no more than £3 a bird. A brace of oven-ready pheasants should cost less than one good-quality, naturally reared chicken. The economics of all this may be somewhat skewwhiff, with shoots essentially subsidising the price of oven-ready pheasants in shops, but game shooting does not exist to make money out of meat. Sales of meat supplement the shooting economy and provide a financial opportunity for those connected to the shoot.

more good things about game

The actual good done by responsible shoots is multifarious. Game shooting generates around £3.2 billion for the rural economy and provides a much-needed source of money for those farmers who have no winter income. It also benefits the environment because farmers tend to leave stubble in fields over winter and grow a number of crops to give the game birds some cover and extra food, with the incidental effect of attracting wildlife. And socially, it is very important to the farming community, for whom the winter can be very long and dark. Farmers have the fourth-highest suicide rate among the professions. The Rural Stress Network strongly advocates the continuation of shooting as an ideal way for rural people to socialise, not to mention exercise. And fortunately not all shooting is commercial. The countryside is peppered with well-run farm shoots. They may only yield a small bag, but everyone involved has a good time and most laugh about how many they miss.

The game shooting organisations, worried for the sport's image, have issued guidance to all shoots asking them to follow a new code of good shooting practice, which sets standards for rearing, feeding regimes, environmental guardianship, and the conduct of those who go shooting. The controversial anti-parasite drug Emtryl has been withdrawn from sale in Britain after fears that traces of the drug in pheasant meat could cause cancer in humans. The drug enabled game farms and keepers to rear birds intensively, so this can only be a good thing. If game farmers and shoots stick to the new code, the future of British game shooting should see fewer, higher-quality birds on the market.

is game a clean meat?

Game is natural, but not organic. Both pheasant and partridge are routinely given a drug (Avatec) to control coccidiosis, a disease caused by a parasite. Avatec is not an antibiotic. However, with good husbandry, clean bedding, plenty of water and extra vitamins in the feed, loosely stocked birds should remain disease free, reducing the need for treatment. Keep in mind that all free-moving animals forage for whatever is in their locality. If that means gleaning corn from a field that has been sprayed with chemical fertilisers, pesticides and fungicides, the game bird on your table is not exactly going to be organic. Nevertheless, much of its diet will have been taken foraging in clean woodland and moorland.

when to buy game

Most of the year there's a season for something going on. Game is not – as you would imagine – just a November thing. There is fresh wild rabbit and wood pigeon available all year round and venison all the year except the March breeding season, as well as various game birds in different periods from high summer until February.

In spite of an ancient law that prevents the sale of fresh pheasant after the season ends, not every game supplier takes notice of it and it is possible to buy frozen pheasant fillets between the third week of February and October. Do buy it if you can; it's the best curry and pilaff meat.

where to buy game

✳ Mail order – If you live in a city, home delivery is best. The National Game Dealers' Association and the Countryside Alliance were involved in setting up the Game-to-eat campaign to encourage game cookery. Their website recommends a few reliable mail-order services (see the Shopping Guide). It is possible to order oven-ready birds, jointed rabbits, hares and venison, plus many other species, cut any way you want, via overnight mail in cold boxes. Mail-order game services will also give telephone advice on portions, preparation and even cooking, so do pick their brains. Note also that venison suppliers who send the meat mail order often offer good value 'boxes' containing non-roasting cuts (see the Shopping Guide).

✳ Butcher's shops – Butchers that are licensed to sell game are another good source. They sell all types and can joint and cut it for you to order (see the Shopping Guide).

✳ Supermarkets and game – Let's just say they are getting there. The supermarket buyers' reaction to news about the wonderful nature of wild food is 'can we control the supply?' They dislike variability in game birds' age, sex or size, want to be able to stock it all year round, don't want to take meat containing shot, and some game suppliers are obliged to use metal detectors to find and pick it out. If you like game, ask your supermarket customer services desk why they don't stock it from a local supplier when it is in season (see the Shopping Guide).

road kill – the rules

The exception rather than the norm, I know, but I have eaten the occasional pheasant or rabbit road kill, providing it is in good shape. My husband will eat any road kill, and there has been the odd tussle while I try to throw bits of them away. The rule on road kill is that technically you may only pick up something that someone else has hit – in other words, hunting with cars is banned. Even then there are some who argue that the carcass belongs to the highway authority, although they're not known to enforce this rule.

Don't try to get involved in roadside animal welfare. I know a man who tried to put an injured deer on the roadside out of its misery with a shovel, only to be viciously attacked by an outraged woman, who leapt out of a passing car believing the animal was the victim, not the patient.

fear of cooking game and wild meat – and the rules for doing it right

The tendency to eat game and wild meat 'out' in restaurants may well be a consequence of unsuccessful attempts to cook it. Lots of us love eating it – and yet we feel negative about actually cooking it. In reality, game isn't difficult to cook, but it needs different treatment from ordinary meat. After all, this is something that was not reared by a farmer, but largely in the wild. Depending on the time of year, and the animal's breed, age, sex and feed, each piece of meat or bird will taste slightly different. Being good at game cookery means understanding a few of its characteristics and following a couple of rules.

All game is almost fatless meat of an uncertain age. It needs gentle cooking with added fat for basting and a long resting time in a warm place after cooking. It also helps to buy game from a trusted source – someone who can answer any questions you might have about its background and how to cook it.

flavours of wild meat

Gaminess, the flavour attributed to all wild meat, is attributed to breed, feed and the way in which the meat is matured or hung in order to tenderise it. It is vital that it is handled hygienically. Game must be kept cool, cleanly plucked, and arrive at the shop looking like something ordinary people would like to eat. The tenderness of game birds generally comes from being hung in a chilled, fly-proof environment, as with venison, but wild rabbit should be eaten very fresh. While some game birds have a gentle flavour, others can be powerful. A grouse that has hung chilled for seven days will have a powerful fragrance and resonating flavour, whereas a partridge can taste only slightly less mild than a chicken. While I will eat a pheasant that has been hung on the feather in cold weather for a week, I get no kick out of the macho pursuit of eating really high birds.

shot

Birds that look as if their assailant had some sort of vendetta against them and are peppered with shot should not find their way to butchers.

Too much shot lodged in the meat is obviously unpleasant to encounter. It is also a sign of a badly shot bird that should not have been sold. A little shot will not hurt, though. A Dorset friend who used to beat at local shoots for a living had an MRI scan to investigate a pain in her back. They found nothing more sinister than a regular occurrence of shot, sprinkled throughout her gut (unrelated to her back pain). Rosie loved cooking game.

preparing game

The scenario: you have just been given a brace of two whole pheasants that are far from oven-ready, or a dead rabbit with its fur and head still on. You may well wonder what on earth you're meant to do. Shave it? Wax it? Chuck it out of the window and hope the neighbours' cats eat it?

Well, you could pluck your own game birds or skin your own furred game, but I favour going to the butcher. Most will pluck and dress game to be oven-ready for a small fee. You should freeze rabbit if you can't get them skinned within two days of receiving them. Ask the butcher to hang the pheasants in their cold room for five days to a week before plucking and gutting them. You can do this yourself, but bear in mind that you need dry cold weather for the desired result.

storing game

Oven-ready game stores well in the fridge for about five days. It never seems to spoil in the freezer, even if left for five months, because there is so little water or fat in the meat that it freezes very hard and does not weep as it defrosts. Cooked meat should be cut from the bone and cooled quickly before being stored in the fridge in a sealed container.

recipes for wild meat: venison, hare and rabbit

venison

Much of the countryside, particularly where there is woodland, is overrun with deer. They damage crops and trees, and their only predator is man. Unless they are culled – males at one time of the year, females at another time – it upsets the balance of the herds.

I once went deer stalking. It is extraordinarily difficult to track an animal so highly attuned to danger that they can smell or hear you if you misjudge your position or the wind direction. If they get the slightest hint you are there, they're off. If they do not and the stalker shoots the animal accurately with his rifle, they will never know anything about it. On the day I went stalking we walked 16 miles, were out until dark, and did not succeed in shooting a single stag.

Venison is a catch-all term for the meat of four main types of deer: roe, sika, fallow and red. The last is a very large deer and by far the hardest to roast unless you can be certain it is a young beast. The other three are easier to cook, and all four make lovely braises and a beautiful clear stock.

There are deer farms and parks all over the country. I have tasted this meat and cannot get as excited about the prospect of eating it as I do when it comes to wild meat. There's nothing exactly wrong with it, but it has the standardised flavour beloved of supermarkets, who generally sell it in preference to wild. There was a crisis after the 2001 outbreak of foot-and-mouth disease, when the countryside was literally overrun by deer and an export ban meant that tonnes of meat was going to waste. Game dealers' representatives successfully lobbied the supermarkets, who came to the rescue and started putting wild venison on shelves. I'm glad to say it's still there (see the Shopping Guide).

roast venison

Each time you roast venison, keep an open mind. The age and breed of the animal will have an impact on its cooking time. If possible, ask your supplier for younger beasts for roasting. The breed will determine the size of the leg, loin or saddle. Cooking a joint of any venison should not be difficult, however, if you baste it well and use the beef skewer test to check that it is cooked yet still pink in the middle (see page 182).

Make sure the serving plates are hot because venison contains very little fat and cools quickly. I have never noticed that venison really improves with marinating in wine, unless you are going to braise it.

Serves 8–10

1 haunch of young venison (sika, red, roe or fallow), weighing 3kg/7lb (or more)
90g/3oz softened butter
1 sheet of pork fat, approximately 30cm/12 inches square
leaves from 1 sprig of rosemary
salt and freshly ground black pepper

For the gravy:
250ml/8fl oz game stock or other meat stock
2 tablespoons rowanberry jelly (or redcurrant jelly)
2 tablespoons soured cream or crème fraîche

Preheat the oven to 190°C/375°F/Gas Mark 5. Rub the joint of venison all over with the butter, put it in a roasting tin and season with salt, pepper and the rosemary leaves. Cover with the sheet of pork fat and roast for about 1¼ hours. Test with a skewer for doneness (see page 182). It will probably need another 15–30 minutes but ideally it should still be pink in the centre. Once cooked, remove from the oven and leave, covered, in a warm place for 20 minutes; the juices that have risen to the surface of the meat during cooking will run back into the centre of the joint, preventing it becoming dry.

To make the gravy, tip the fat out of the roasting tin, place the tin over the heat and add the stock. Bring to the boil, stirring the bits from the base of the tin with a wooden spoon, then add the rowanberry jelly and simmer until it has dissolved. Stir in the cream. Heat until it bubbles, then adjust the seasoning and pour the gravy into a warmed jug. Carve the venison at the table and allow everyone to pour their own gravy. Serve with buttered shredded cabbage.

✳ kitchen note ✳

Loin or saddle (the two loins attached to the bone) makes a good roast. Cook as above, checking for doneness in the same way and bearing in mind that these joints usually take less time. If the butcher takes the loin off the bone, take the bone home with you and make it into stock (see page 114).

hot venison and mushroom pie

Use any leftover cooked venison in a hearty pie, with big field mushrooms.

Serves 4

15g/½oz butter

1 onion, finely chopped

1 celery stick, finely chopped

1 tablespoon plain flour

500ml/16fl oz venison or beef stock

600g/1¼lb leftover cooked venison, cut into chunks

300g/10oz field mushrooms, thickly sliced

300ml/½ pint double cream

1 quantity of shortcrust pastry (see page 436, or use bought pastry)

1 egg or egg yolk, beaten with 2 tablespoons milk, to glaze

sea salt and freshly ground black pepper

Melt the butter in a large casserole, add the onion and celery and cook until soft. Add the flour and stir to a paste. Cook for a minute or two, then slowly add the stock, stirring all the time, and bring to the boil. Add the venison, simmer for 15 minutes, then add the mushrooms and cream. Season to taste. Pour the mixture into a pie dish, putting a pie funnel or upside-down eggcup in the middle to support the pastry. Leave to cool.

Preheat the oven to 200°C/400°F/Gas Mark 6. Roll out the pastry on a floured board to 5mm/¼ inch thick. Brush the rim of the pie dish with the egg wash and lay the pastry on top. Trim the pastry around the edge of the dish, leaving a 1cm/½ inch overlap. (Be creative – decorate the pie with shapes cut from leftover pastry, stuck on with egg wash.) Leave to rest for about 20 minutes to prevent the pastry shrinking during cooking. Brush the whole surface with egg wash and bake for 40 minutes or until the crust is crisp and nut brown.

✳ kitchen note ✳

In an industrious mood, you could make several small pies in foil pie dishes, freeze them and use for weekday suppers.

venison sautéed with spring cabbage

A quick way to cook venison.

Serves 4

8 slices of venison, cut across the grain from the leg, shoulder, haunch or loin

2 smoked bacon rashers, chopped small

45g/1½oz butter

1 head of spring greens, very thinly sliced

2 tablespoons meat stock

a few black onion seeds (nigella)

1 tablespoon vegetable oil

salt and freshly ground black pepper

Place the venison slices between 2 sheets of wax paper or baking parchment and bash them with a meat hammer or a rolling pin until 5mm/¼ inch thick. Set aside.

In a large frying pan, cook the bacon in 30g/1oz of the butter until crisp, then add the greens and stock and cook, stirring, until the greens are tender. Season to taste, transfer to a warm dish and scatter a few onion seeds on top.

Heat the oil and the remaining butter in a large frying pan. Season the venison, add to the pan and fry over a medium-high heat for about 30 seconds–1 minute on each side, depending on whether you like your meat pink or well done. Eat beside the greens.

braised venison with wild mushrooms and real ale

This can also be used as a base for a game pie, adding stewing cuts from other species – pheasant, wood pigeon and rabbit.

Serves 4

4 tablespoons vegetable oil

1kg/2¼lb venison meat, cut into 4cm/1½ inch pieces

2 onions, finely chopped

4 garlic cloves, finely chopped

2 tablespoons plain flour

300ml/½ pint real ale

60g/2oz dried wild mushrooms, soaked in 500ml/16fl oz hot
game stock

salt and freshly ground black pepper

chopped parsley, to garnish

Heat the oil in a large casserole and sear the meat on all sides, cooking it in batches. Remove from the pan and add the onions and garlic. Cook until soft, then return the venison to the pan with the flour. Stir constantly while you pour in the ale, followed by the stock and mushrooms. Bring to the boil, stirring, then reduce the heat to a slow simmer. Partly cover with a lid and cook gently for 2 hours or until the meat is tender. Season to taste, then throw over some chopped parsley.

venison shanks with white wine and tomatoes

Treat shanks of red deer (see the Shopping Guide) as you would osso buco (shin of veal), eating them with mashed potato or saffron risotto (see page 132).

Serves 4

60g/2oz butter

4 venison shanks (or use 12 pieces of venison shin, cut 3cm/1¼
inches thick)

2 glasses of white wine

6 ripe tomatoes, skinned, deseeded and chopped

500ml–1 litre/16fl oz–1¾ pints game stock or other meat stock

6 sprigs of parsley, finely chopped

zest of 1 lemon

salt and freshly ground black pepper

Melt the butter in a large casserole, add the venison pieces and brown on all sides. Pour over the white wine and bring to the boil. Simmer for a minute, then add the tomatoes. Cover with the stock and bring to the boil, skimming away any foam. Reduce the heat to a simmer and cook for 1½–2 hours, depending on whether you are using shin or shanks, until the meat is very tender. Season with salt and pepper, then serve with the parsley and lemon zest scattered on top.

✳ kitchen note ✳

Shoulder of venison is also suitable for this dish. Ask your butcher to cut it into manageable pieces. Alternatively, use veal shin for a classic osso buco (see page 439 for information on veal).

venison sauce for pasta

This is an excellent way of using up leftover venison. Serve it with egg pasta – it's especially good in lasagne or over tagliatelle.

Serves 4–6

2 tablespoons olive oil

1 onion, finely chopped

2 celery sticks, finely sliced

1 garlic clove, chopped

2 streaky bacon rashers, chopped small

a sprig of thyme

240g/8oz minced cooked venison

2 chicken livers, chopped (optional)

1 glass of red wine

90ml/3fl oz Tomato Sauce (see page 358)

125ml/4fl oz game stock or other meat stock

salt and freshly ground black pepper

Heat the oil in a pan and add the vegetables, garlic and bacon. Cook until the vegetables are soft, then add the thyme, venison and chopped chicken livers, if using. Cook for a minute, then add the wine. Bring to the boil and add the tomato sauce and stock. Return to the boil and simmer for 45 minutes. Season to taste.

wild rabbit

The sight of chocolate Easter rabbits wrapped in gold foil always makes me smile. This great pagan symbol of fertility, later adopted by Christians, has been a victim of its talent for procreation. While we merrily give each other chocolate bunnies in recognition of the traditional mating season at Easter, few real wild rabbits simmer in pots with garlic, wine and the zest of a lemon. In part this is because over a thousand years after its introduction to Britain by the Normans, its number was deliberately decimated. So sick were farmers of the devastation wrought on their crops by millions of rabbits that they welcomed the Australian cure, which was to give wild rabbits a disease: myxomatosis.

What irony there is in the fact that myxomatosis was introduced to Britain in 1953, the year before rationing ended. Wild rabbit, you see, is a food for hungry people. Post-war Britain had found new ways to produce lots of meat very quickly: plump chickens in a matter of weeks; meaty cows or lambs; and very big fat pigs. Who needs to go to the bother of organising men, ferrets and guns to catch rabbits when you can shut a herd of pigs indoors and throw high-protein feed at them to make them grow fast? But waging germ warfare on an animal that had given a millennium of devoted service to this country's inhabitants seems more than a little ungrateful.

down to earth

There are now, fifty years on from the introduction of myxomatosis, plenty of healthy wild rabbits in the countryside, whose meat is clean and uncontaminated. Farmers would like to see the back of them because they can do extraordinary damage. Wild rabbit does not need to hang and must be bought and eaten as fresh as possible, so it is a good idea to buy it direct (see the Shopping Guide) or pre-order it from a butcher with a game dealer's licence. A whole wild rabbit costs about £2, and will serve four. This is cheap meat that has been produced with no stress to the animal.

using farmed rabbit

All the recipes below can be adapted to farmed rabbits, although you will have to double the quantities of other ingredients as farmed rabbits are around twice the size of wild. Do be fussy when choosing farmed rabbit (see the Shopping Guide). Welfare standards vary greatly from farm to farm, and yes, there is such a thing as intensively reared rabbit. I don't really like eating it because it tastes bland.

roast wild rabbit with figs and vinegar

I tend to put rabbit with garlic and something sweet, something sour, to remind me of the places around the Mediterranean where it is still valued. Serve with whole wheat, sometimes called pasta wheat, or bulgar.

Serves 2

1 young rabbit, jointed into 2 saddle pieces and 2 legs
1 tablespoon butter

2 streaky bacon rashers

4 dried figs, halved and soaked in 4 tablespoons white wine for about 1 hour

½ tablespoon aged sherry vinegar, or to taste

For the marinade:

250ml/8fl oz white wine

1 garlic clove, halved

1 onion, sliced

1 bay leaf

1 tablespoon olive oil

Mix together all the ingredients for the marinade, add the rabbit and leave to marinate for 1 hour. Lift out the rabbit pieces, reserving the marinade, and pat dry with a towel.

Preheat the oven to 200°C/400°F/Gas Mark 6. Rub the rabbit pieces with the butter. Place them in a roasting tin and lay the bacon on top. Roast for 45 minutes, basting every 15 minutes with the marinade and the fat in the bottom of the tin.

Put the roasted rabbit pieces on a warmed plate. Place the roasting tin over a medium heat and pour in any remaining marinade. Bring to the boil, deglazing the tin by scraping up the bits from the base with a wooden spoon. Add the figs and wine and simmer for 5 minutes. Add the vinegar to taste and spoon the sauce around the rabbit.

rabbit with lemon

This is the rabbit of French hillsides, bathed in herbs, wine and tomatoes and scented with lemon. The lemon removes the slight mustiness from rabbit that is a few days old or previously frozen – the very taste that puts people off rabbit.

Serves 4

4 tablespoons olive oil

2 rabbits, each jointed into 2 saddle pieces and 2 legs

2 onions, chopped

4 garlic cloves, chopped

2 celery sticks, chopped

2 carrots, chopped (you can chop all the vegetables finely in a food processor)

1 teaspoon dried *herbes de Provence*

2 glasses of white wine

1 can of chopped tomatoes

salt and freshly ground black pepper

To serve:

leaves from 8 sprigs of parsley

pared zest of ½ lemon, chopped

1 garlic clove, finely chopped

Heat the oil in a large pan, add the rabbit pieces and brown them all over. Stir in the vegetables and herbs, followed by the wine and tomatoes. Bring to the boil, turn down to a slow bubble and cook, partly covered, for about 1 hour, until the rabbit is tender. Season to taste, then eat with the parsley, lemon and garlic thrown over the stew, and a big bowl of mashed potato or rice.

rabbit confit

This will keep for ages in the fridge and can be revived to eat with boiled potatoes or substituted for duck legs in Duck, Sausages and Beans (see page 163).

Serves 2

4 rabbit legs

1 teaspoon dried thyme

8 tablespoons goose or duck fat (available canned – see the
Shopping Guide)

salt and freshly ground black pepper

Put the rabbit legs in a non-metallic container and sprinkle over about
1 tablespoon of salt. Add the thyme and twist over some black pepper.
Roll the legs around in the container to cover them in the seasonings,
then leave for 4–6 hours, until the meat weeps out a little liquid. Lift out
the legs and wipe off the seasoning. Put them in a heavy-based casserole
and cover with the goose or duck fat. Cook, tightly covered with a lid
or foil, over a very low heat for 45 minutes–1 hour, until just tender
when poked with a sharp knife. The meat should be poaching in the fat,
not frying. Transfer to a container and seal. It will keep in the fridge for
3–4 weeks.

To cook the confit, scrape off the fat and fry gently in a tablespoon
of fresh duck fat until golden all over. Eat with boiled potatoes, dressed
with a vinaigrette (see page 221).

✳ kitchen note ✳

Use the same method to confit duck, pheasant or turkey legs.

wild rabbit for curry

As part of my quest not to use chicken breasts in every curry, I buy fresh
young rabbit and take the meat off the bone. If you buy direct from a
butcher or by mail order, they might do this for you. You can then use
the meat with your favourite spice paste for Thai, Afro-Caribbean or
Indian curries, or in the recipe on page 360 – and one less broiler hen is
needed. It's curry with a clear conscience!

cold wild rabbit and cucumber salad

Shred leftover roast rabbit and mix it with half slices of peeled, deseeded cucumber (see page 93). Dress with a vinaigrette made from 1 tablespoon of Dijon mustard, 1 teaspoon of brown sugar, 1 tablespoon of aged sherry vinegar, 1 tablespoon of water and 5 tablespoons of olive oil. Scatter a few thin slices of sweet onion and some mint leaves over the top.

potted wild rabbit

Serves 6–8 generously

about 8 thinly cut streaky bacon rashers, rind removed

480g/1lb rabbit meat (about 2 young rabbits), cut into small chunks

120g/4oz ham, finely chopped

240g/8oz pork belly, minced

4 tablespoons sherry

a pinch of ground allspice

1 teaspoon pink peppercorns, crushed

1 teaspoon salt

Preheat the oven to 180°C/350°F/Gas Mark 4. Line an oval earthenware pot, about 20cm/8 inches long, with the bacon. Mix the rabbit, ham and pork belly with the sherry and pack into the pot, scattering the spices and salt over the mixture as you go. Cook for about 1½ hours, until the mixture springs back when pressed with a finger and has shrunk away from the edge of the dish. Remove from the oven, cover with a small plate that fits just inside the rim of the pot, and weight it down – I use cans of beans. Leave to cool, then place in the fridge for several hours.

Serve cut in thick slices, with Cornichon, Egg and Herb Sauce (see page 196) or egg and herb sauce (see page 395), plus watercress salad and toast.

✳ **kitchen note** ✳

You could substitute pheasant, duck or pork for the rabbit.

hare ragu

I think of hare as a sumptuous rarity because we see so few of them in Dorset, although I know other areas of Britain have plenty of hares. If I find a road kill, or an accidental kill by an errant local lurcher, I take all the meat off the bone and cut it into small cubes. With celery, a little tomato sauce and stock, it becomes a pure, down-to-earth sauce to eat with pasta. No cheese is needed – just flat-leaf parsley and good flat egg pappardelle.

When I first made this dish, I could not understand why I didn't like it until I realised it was the texture. Minced hare has an unpleasant quality, while cubed chunks make a great match for the robustness of the flavours. The same goes for rabbit and venison, which can be substituted for the hare in this sauce.

Serves 4–6

3 tablespoons olive oil

2 onions, finely chopped

2 garlic cloves, chopped

4 celery sticks, chopped

the meat from 1 hare, cut into 1cm/½ inch cubes

2 bay leaves

4 tablespoons Tomato Sauce (see page 358)

2 wineglasses white wine

up to 1 litre/1¾ pints game stock or other meat stock

leaves from 4 sprigs of flat-leaf parsley

salt and freshly ground black pepper

Heat the oil in a large pan and add the onions, garlic and celery. Soften them in the hot oil but do not allow them to brown. Add the hare and cook for about 5 minutes, then add the bay leaves and tomato sauce. Add the wine and enough stock to cover and bring to the boil. Turn down to a slow bubble and cook, partially covered, for about 1 hour, until the hare is tender. Add more stock if the dish dries out. Season well with salt and pepper. Eat with pasta, scattered with the parsley.

wild game birds

Wood pigeons may not make great stock, but they are a good source of inexpensive meat that appears luxurious on the plate. Their cold meat makes an excellent substitute for duck. And they show that game birds need not be served in the gentlemen's club style with endless bread sauce.

wood pigeon breasts with watercress, cobnuts and toasted sourdough bread

In Dorset, a familiar late-summer sight is wood pigeons gleaning the corn after the harvest. For gamekeeper Johnny Langdown it is the perfect time to hide behind a cobnut tree for hours, shotgun in hand, waiting and waiting.

Serves 2 as a main course, 4 as a starter

8 wood pigeon breasts

a little dripping or oil

4 slices of sourdough bread

2 bunches of watercress, the stalks removed (save them for soup or sauce – see page 129)

2 tablespoons shelled fresh cobnuts (in September) or hazelnuts, lightly crushed

a few drops of pumpkinseed oil (optional)

salt and freshly ground black pepper

For the dressing:

2 tablespoons sherry vinegar

1 shallot, thinly sliced

4 tablespoons olive oil

Mix the dressing ingredients together, season to taste with a little salt and then set aside. Season the wood pigeon breasts with salt and pepper. Heat the fat in a large, heavy-based frying pan until it sizzles when a drop of water is thrown in (at arm's length). Add the wood pigeon breasts and sear for 1 minute on each side. Transfer to a warm place and leave to rest for 5 minutes.

Toast the bread on both sides in the frying pan and put it on serving plates. Slice the wood pigeon breasts across the grain and put them on the bread with the watercress and cobnuts, then pour the dressing over. A few drops of pumpkinseed oil finishes an autumn salad such as this one perfectly.

grouse

Like pheasant, grouse are shot either during highly organised game shoots or 'walked up' by a row of men with dogs. But unlike most pheasant, they are a totally wild bird, living on the uplands of Britain. Their numbers fluctuate depending on the quality of management on the moors where they live, and a complex cycle of natural diseases.

Just one grouse a year is all I ask, hung for no more than one week (I have never been one for chasing game around the kitchen to get it into the pan). Rare, totally wild and expensive, this is a luxury you deserve after all the economies you've made in the New English Kitchen.

roast grouse

Serve 1 bird per person. Preheat the oven to 190°C/375°F/Gas Mark 5. Put 4 raspberries or 4 cranberries inside each bird with a teaspoon of butter and some salt and pepper, then rub some softened butter into the breast. Roast for 35–45 minutes, depending on how rare you want it to be, basting once during cooking. Leave to rest in a warm place for about 15 minutes – this allows all the juices that have rushed to the surface of the bird in the short cooking time to work their way back to the centre. The result will be a much juicier grouse. Serve with fried breadcrumbs (see page 31), rowanberry jelly and fried potatoes.

✳ kitchen note ✳

Grouse is nice served on a piece of bread fried in duck fat – all you will need on the side is a watercress salad.

braised beef scented with grouse

Add the carcass from a roast grouse to an ordinary beef stew (see page 216) with the stock and simmer with the meat. When the beef is tender, the gravy will be deliciously scented with the grouse.

grouse sandwiches

I find that people often leave a lot of meat on game birds, particularly the legs. Once the grouse is cold, strip the flesh from the bone, taking every tiny bit, and eat in a little sandwich with redcurrant jelly and cress. Bliss. It is also very good with cold pheasant, wild duck or partridge.

cold grouse with runner beans

In my quest to eat as many runner beans as possible in August while they are tender (and so I am not tempted to freeze them), I love to serve them dressed with a little oil and dill. Shredded cold grouse is a seasonally perfect addition.

pheasant

The pheasant is one of game's most flexible birds. Buying one brace gets you a roast, a little cold meat for special sandwiches, and delicious stock to pour over noodles. While I love roast pheasant in December when they are at their best, the meat from these birds, which originate from the foothills of the Caucasus mountains in Asia, is as good any other time in the season fried with oriental spices.

roast pheasant

One bird will serve 2 hungry people. Preheat the oven to 190°C/375°F/Gas Mark 5. Put a little butter, salt and pepper in the cavity of each bird, rub the skin with oil and place a strip of pork fat or unsmoked bacon on top to baste. Roast for about 45 minutes. Eat with gravy, bread sauce or fried breadcrumbs.

cold pheasant

Cold pheasant makes very good sandwiches, with watercress and a good curried chutney, or chop it finely and eat with sesame sauce (see page 152).

pheasant soup

My 9-year-old son, Jack, loves pheasant stock (see page 118) poured over egg noodles. For myself, I like to add more: some young cabbage or pak choi, coriander leaves, red chilli, straw mushrooms and a dash of soy sauce. Pheasant stock is also useful when making a rice dish to eat with partridge.

pheasant breasts, or fillets

Towards the end of the season, there are so many pheasants around that removing the breast meat without plucking the whole bird is justifiable, not wasteful. Pheasant breast meat can be used in curry recipes, or the whole fillets gently fried in a generous amount of butter and oil, before slicing and using in a pilaff (see page 202).

breadcrumbed pheasant

Cut the breasts from a fresh pheasant and slice into strips 1cm/½ inch thick. Dip first in seasoned flour, then beaten egg, then fresh bread-crumbs (see page 33). Shallow-fry in sunflower or olive oil, then serve with a squeeze of lemon, and maybe a little melted butter seasoned with tarragon or pepper.

pheasant with spring greens, ginger, sherry and soy

Echoing my sentiments about using fresh rabbit meat for curries, I also recommend eating pheasant meat in stir-fries because it, too, provides a nice change from endless chicken breasts. Pheasant is, after all, an Asian bird. Ask the butcher in advance if he will strip the meat off the bird, then stir-fry it with shredded fresh ginger, sliced garlic and spring onions, plus spring greens. Dress with light soy sauce, toasted sesame seeds, sherry and a little lemon juice.

partridge

Roast partridge has a gentle taste, so it's a good meat for game bird novices. But with their origins in the Southern Mediterranean, French red leg partridge (the type most often available) are more exciting when eaten in the style of that place: with rice, saffron and maybe a few strips of wood-roasted sweet pepper.

There's enough meat on a partridge to make one person very happy, so don't hold out for much in the way of spare pickings. Stock made from the carcass is a treat, though, (see page 118) and can be used as for any poultry stock.

roast partridge

You will need 1 bird per person. Preheat the oven to 180°C/350°F/Gas Mark 4. Put a little butter, salt and pepper in the cavity of each bird, rub the skin with oil and place a strip of pork fat or unsmoked bacon on top to baste. Roast for 25–30 minutes. Eat with fried breadcrumbs (see page 31).

partridge and freshwater crayfish with rice

Away from the sea, a dish that is reminiscent of a hunter's paella. I have always wanted to add snails to it but sadly they are hard to get, unless you are happy to open a can.

Serves 4

4 partridges

a little butter

4 strips of pork fat or rashers of unsmoked bacon

4 tablespoons olive oil, plus extra for cooking the partridge

1 large red onion, chopped

4 garlic cloves, chopped

4 canned wood-roasted peppers (see the Shopping Guide), sliced

3 celery sticks, chopped

6 fennel seeds

a large pinch of ground allspice

360g/12oz short grain Spanish rice

at least 1 litre/1¾ pints pheasant stock or other poultry stock

1 sachet of saffron powder

12 freshwater crayfish (see the Shopping Guide)

4 sprigs of flat-leaf parsley, roughly chopped

salt and freshly ground black pepper

Preheat the oven to 180°C/350°F/Gas Mark 4. Put a small knob of butter and some salt and pepper in the cavity of each partridge, then rub the skin with oil and place the pork fat or bacon on top. Place in a roasting tin and roast for 25–30 minutes, then leave in a warm place to rest.

Heat the olive oil in a large pan, add the onion, garlic, peppers and celery and cook until soft. Add the fennel seeds, allspice and rice and cover with the stock, throwing in the saffron powder at the same time. Bring to the boil, then cover the pan and cook over a very low heat for 30–40 minutes, until the rice has absorbed most of the liquid – add more stock if you need to. The rice should be just cooked, with a firm but not hard centre; be careful it doesn't become overcooked. Season to taste.

If the crayfish are raw, place them on top of the rice, cover and cook for another 4 minutes; otherwise place on top and warm through. Split the partridges in half and arrange on top. Scatter over the parsley and serve.

mallard (wild duck)

Mallard, or wild duck, is robust-flavoured meat that is elegant with fruit when hot, and makes an exotic salad, shredded with lime, toasted sesame seeds and peppery leaves. Wild duck also makes an elegant soup, to lace with brandy and pour over seasonal wild mushrooms and thinly sliced celery (see page 133).

roast mallard

You will need 1 bird per person. Preheat the oven to 190°C/375°F/Gas Mark 5. Put a little butter, salt and pepper in the cavity of each bird, rub the skin with oil and place a strip of pork fat or unsmoked bacon on top to baste. Roast for about 35 minutes for rare meat, 45 minutes for well done. Eat with fruit – or fruit jellies, such as quince, orange, rowanberry, or even sweet pepper jelly.

cold duck with mizuna, glass vegetables, lime and sesame

Mizuna is a peppery Japanese salad plant that grows easily in the UK – and much faster than rocket or baby spinach. You will see it, along with its relatives mibuna and mitzuna, in herb catalogues, and it is becoming more widely sold in shops. If you can't find mizuna use mibuna, watercress, young spinach leaves or small chard leaves instead.

There is nothing mysterious about glass vegetables, they are just grated raw turnip, celeriac and carrot. I find that using the fine grater on a food processor achieves a better result.

Serves 2 as a main course, 4 as a starter

1 turnip, peeled
¼ celeriac, peeled
1 carrot, peeled
juice of 1 lime
2 handfuls of mizuna leaves
about 180g/6oz leftover cold duck, shredded
2 tablespoons sesame seeds, toasted in a dry pan
4 sprigs of coriander, roughly chopped

For the dressing:
4 tablespoons soy sauce
1 tablespoon rice vinegar
1 tablespoon sesame oil

Grate the root vegetables and mix them with the lime juice to prevent discoloration. Mix roughly with the mizuna and divide between serving plates. Scatter the duck over, followed by the sesame seeds and coriander. Mix together all the dressing ingredients and pour it over the salad.

✳ kitchen note ✳

This salad is also good made with cold partridge, pheasant, beef or farmed duck.

part two

these chapters use the principle

of rolling food into more than one

meal, but they are chiefly about

changing perceptions. with more

information about fish, gluts of fruit and

vegetables, eggs and dairy foods, you

will learn to value them more and make

the most of the variety on offer,

including the overlooked foods that

contain a world of untapped potential.

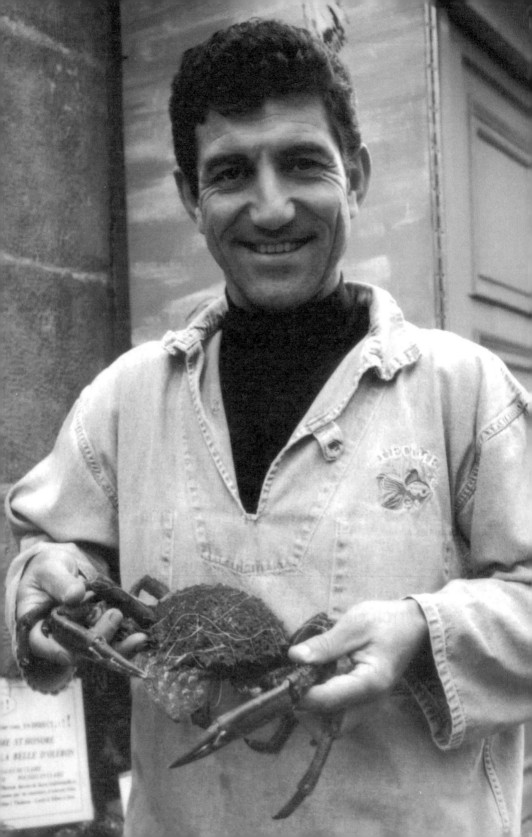

7
Fish and shellfish

Look at a supermarket fish counter and you will see heaps of what appears to be, give or take, just eight varieties of seafood. Cod, haddock, monkfish, salmon, tuna, trout, tiger prawns and squid usually feature, plus smoked versions of a few of the above and the occasional piece of warm-water exotica. Look at the counter again. Haven't many of these fish been in the news recently? Stocks are low, headlines warn; catch sizes are dwindling, and fish farms a pollutant. Soon jobs will go, warn the doomsayers, and the British fishing industry shut down for ever. It's all gloom. And yet here, courtesy of the bright and shiny superstore fish counter (the local fish shop closed down almost as soon as the supermarket opened) is a whopping great, gilt-edged invitation to buy these endangered species. The only clue that things might be changing is that the fish seems to have got rather more expensive lately. Confused? You haven't heard the half of it.

I want to show you how to take a broader approach to eating fish. This is not only necessary to conserve the remaining fish in the sea. It is also a chance to savour the extraordinary variety of fish on offer – some with firm meaty flesh for eating in robust soups and chowders; some with fragile, delicately flavoured fillets to which you wouldn't dare add anything more than lemon and butter. Once you learn how to buy truly fresh fish, you will notice an extraordinary improvement in flavour.

positive shopping

Shoppers have brought a certain amount of change to the meat industry, demanding improvement in animal feeding and welfare regimes because they threatened human health. Fish is different. The single greatest problem with eating wild fish is the damage it does to the marine environment. Not that the problem is small: every marine environment organisation is issuing dire warnings about the future of current favourite fish species. Stocks of certain species of fish in the North Sea have drastically dropped in number. A 2003 study by Globefish stated that worldwide the total cod catch has fallen by two-thirds in just three decades, and the number of breeding cod in the North Sea has shrunk by 90 per cent.

Shoppers may not be responsible for managing fish stocks, but if our habits don't alter, the problem will come back to us eventually. But it is possible to shop positively, with knowledge, care and imagination. The good news is that there is a choice. Responsibly harvested fish – even cod – is available. Currently it is at the niche end of fish selling, but if we demand it from our supermarket fish counter, we will send our powerful retailers a message they cannot ignore.

which fish?

Applying the pay-more, make-more philosophy to fish is trickier than adapting the idea to bread, eggs, meats or vegetables. Fish is delicate and highly perishable, and lends itself only to a few dishes that use up the remains of a previous meal. This chapter will show you how to make the most of the fish you buy, but it's really about the subsidiary aim of *The New English Kitchen*, and that is to show you how to be wise when buying your food.

new fish

In *The Good Fish Guide* (Second Edition, Marine Conservation Society, 2003) Bernadette Clarke warns, 'It is likely that more of the world's catch currently used for animal feed will be used for direct human consumption.' I'd like you to consider a new approach to how you eat fish. If it is to be a meaningful part of your plan to make the most of the food you buy and to understand its real value, you need to know more about it. That knowledge will help you to buy species of fish you did not even know existed, that are less expensive because they are still plentiful. These species are no less good than the usual suspects. Some will surprise you with their wonderful flavours. If you don't have a local fishmonger, you may have to persuade your local supermarket to stock them. And I will let you in on the secret, new and convenient way to buy the freshest, best-quality fish from expert fishmongers: home delivery (see the Shopping Guide). Nevertheless, it will always be necessary to see seafood as a delicacy – not an everyday dish, but a treat. Buy less and buy knowledgeably, and enjoy the adventure of tasting something new.

the great white fish disaster

'What would you say to a little fish?' said the waiter to Noël Coward.

'I should say, hello little fish.'

Will we be saying goodbye to the little fishes? I wondered, as I set off to find out how the whole damn fruit of the ocean thing ticks along. The quest to understand what is going wrong, and right, and why, in the fishing industry has been fascinating and is still, I admit, an ongoing job.

The story of cod perfectly illustrates the destructive love affair between man and fish. It was the whiteness of cod that appealed so much – those pearly flakes of flesh with their clean marine flavour. Moreover, cod were large fish with relatively few bones, ideal for salting to become a commodity with enormous value in economic and practical terms. It is hard to pinpoint the moment when the species entered what may turn out to be its terminal decline. Perhaps it was the moment the Basques tasted cod and fell for it, hook and line. Around AD1000 they expanded their cod markets to create an international trade in salt cod. By the fifteenth century cod was a highly profitable commodity in Europe, and the hunt was on for the best cod grounds to plunder. And each succeeding generation brings another avid market of cod eaters.

But when did the dramatic decline of the fish numbers begin? Summing it up as simply as possible, it was with the establishment of the Common Fisheries Policy (CFP). The concept of the CFP originated in 1957 with the Treaty of Rome, the agreement that created what is now known as the European Union. Central to the CFP's creation was the idea of equal access: in 1970 all member countries' waters were opened to fishermen from other member states. You can imagine what happened. The fishing fleets of the member states went on the rampage. Needless to say, the most and biggest boats were to be found where there had historically been the largest number of fish. In 1972 a much-needed alteration was made to the EU equal access policy, ruling that coastal waters up to a six-nautical-mile limit from the shore of a member country would be exclusive to that nation's fishermen. These inshore or coastal fisheries (a catch-all term for any style of fishing business) come under local regulation by sea fisheries committees, and tend to be well managed.

The local fleets that fish these waters live in the towns and work along the shore, so it is very much in their interest to co-operate and take a long view of the future. As a result inshore fisheries tend to be very well managed. Traditional fishing styles like hook and line and drift nets are used in place of high-tech catch methods. They often use day boats – small craft that go out and return within one day, bringing the freshest local fish to market.

Fish from inshore fisheries is the stuff to buy. Even species that are dwindling outside the six-nautical-mile limit are fine when caught in coastal waters using responsible methods. So you can have your cod, haddock, lobster, brown crab, halibut and monkfish . . . Much of the ultra-fresh, day-caught fish – around 60 per cent – is exported, so we know there is plenty available. Several inshore fisheries have set up direct delivery services with online ordering, so it is now possible to access the freshest, sustainable fish, no matter how far you live from the sea (see the Shopping Guide).

But there was little protection outside these coastal zones. The EU took action against overfishing in 1983. As a conservation measure the CFP came up with a total allowable catch (TAC) for popular species, to be reviewed every year. The TAC was then divided, and a portion or quota of it given to each member state. Their respective fisheries were then allotted a slice of the quota. The quota dictates exactly how much of each species can be taken in any one year, and is reviewed each December. When quota limits are reached, the fleet are not permitted to take any more of it. But these restrictions were not adequate.

Britain has a lot of coastline, and a lot of fish. Or rather, we *had* a lot of fish. Our fisheries moan about unscrupulous Spanish boats encroaching on their catch. This isn't an empty prejudice. The Spanish fishing fleet serves a population with the greatest per capita appetite for fish outside China and Japan, but despite having the Mediterranean on one side and the Atlantic on the other, Spanish waters do not yield a great deal of fish, so their fishermen must look for it far and wide. But they have not been the only ones to head for British waters. The Russians were crazy for mackerel and herring, and their eager exploitation of their historic fishing rights to our waters helped decimate British supplies of both species, but not without a little help from our own factory ships. And many British trawlermen sold their fishing quotas, in perpetuity, for large sums – although some have come to regret it.

management

Technology has played a major part in the problem of overfishing. The fault lies with the uninhibited use of purse seine nets, radars, Fish Aggregating Devices (FADs, which attract fish), sonars, dredgers, and beam trawlers with their giant nets – and of course the people who permitted the fishing fleets to use these technologies. Instead of netting a number that could be sustained after another season's breeding, entire shoals of fish were brought up in one net. And the most popular fish, such as the poor old cod, were bound to suffer sooner rather than later.

plenty more fish

If we have in the past overlooked our responsibilities, it's understandable – marine conservation is not a sexy subject. I can't see environmentalists making much headway protesting outside fish and chip shops. After all, fast food is all about *not* having to think about food. But even now, despite the well-publicised decline of fish stocks, popular demand for cod and other favourite species shows no sign of abating. People seem to expect the bureaucrats in some remote Whitehall or Brussels corridor to be taking care of the problem without any effort from us. But our habits need to change if the situation is to improve.

The oddest thing of all is that there are, as the cliché goes, plenty more fish in the sea. The EU's TAC system means that when fishermen bring up a mixed catch, they must throw back any fish whose quota has been exceeded for that particular season, or which are too small. Inevitably a high number of these unwanted fish die anyway, whether or not they make it back into the water. The inflexible nature of the system also means that unforeseen gluts of a species are often wasted. If a fishery catches an exceptional number of fish, above and beyond its quota, then it must move fast to get a dispensation from Defra (the Department for Environment, Food and Rural Affairs) or Brussels to avoid throwing thousands of often dying fish back into the sea, and with them, thousands of pounds.

It comes as no surprise that the EU's 1983 conservation measures are deeply unpopular with fishermen. They are thought plain ineffective by marine conservationists. We are locked into this wasteful system. The solution, says the oldest international marine science agency, the International Council for Exploration of the Sea (ICES), whom the EU, and you and I, pay handsomely for advice, is to close off areas of the ocean and allow the fish to spawn and develop a sustainable supply. But the EU also has its own scientific advisory board, the Scientific, Technical and Economic Committee for Fisheries (STEFC), which has the power to disregard the recommendations of ICES. The Common Fisheries Policy has changed little in recent years. However, fisheries have been advised to return to the hook-and-line method and a responsible fishmonger will seek line-caught fish of all types.

cheap cod is expensive

The troubles with cod are a perfect example of how ultimately the full price will always be paid for cheap food. The mysteries of fish are such that not even the scientists can accurately predict how to bring about the recovery of species. The Grand Banks fishing grounds off Newfoundland and Labrador were closed in 1981 due to overfishing and the drastic decline of cod stocks. Forty thousand jobs were lost. To date, over twenty years later, the cod have barely returned.

If our fish stocks continue to deteriorate, or even close, and thousands are left jobless, all of us will pay, one way or another. Cheap cod is very expensive.

the good news

But there remain reasons to be optimistic. One is that marine conservationists' criticism of the Common Fisheries Policy seems to be making an impact. It's now widely recognised that the CFP has contributed to the decline of fish stocks, and the politicians, the industry and conservationists have begun work on plans for sustainable fishing in the future. Thanks to advances in marine science we know more and more about the numbers of many types of fish. The Marine Stewardship Council (MSC), a worldwide organisation, is in the process of certifying the sustainable sources of certain species. These fisheries tend either to be inshore (operating within the EU imposed six-mile coastal zone), or to use traditional methods of catching fish such as hook and line or drift nets. MSC-approved sustainable fish is available in supermarkets or direct from the coastal fisheries (see the Shopping Guide). Look out for their blue-and-white logo.

Fish to eat less of

The following types of wild fish are classed, by the Marine Conservation Society, as overfished to the point that stocks are close to collapse:

Blue ling; brown crab; cod; dogfish; grouper; haddock; hake; halibut; ling; lobster; marlin; monkfish; orange roughy; plaice; wild warm-water prawn; ray; Atlantic salmon; wild and Chilean sea bass; shark; skate; snapper; swordfish; blue-fin tuna; yellow-fin tuna (see page 84); whiting.

Finding fish to eat more of

It sounds, I know, like all your favourite fish are off limits. But there are exceptions within the danger list. For example, Iceland manages its cod fishery well – although a row has erupted over the resumed whaling in its waters, which their fisheries say is to keep cod numbers up. There are sources of the above species which are sustainable – notably line or drift-net caught from coastal fisheries. In the case of shellfish, there are small well-managed fisheries. Line-caught yellow-fin tuna is also available. Numbers of certain species can also surge in certain areas, but it's hard to keep track. The best solution is to buy direct from small-scale fisheries, or a fishmonger you trust. It all comes back to a central theme of the *New English Kitchen* – buy food from a trusted source (see the Shopping Guide).

As with all other food, if you want to be confident about its origins, make friends with your supplier. They should be happy to answer your questions. Try to find out:

✳ What method was used to catch the fish – Handline-caught, troll-caught, drift net, creel or pot-caught and angler-caught is fine.

✳ Where was it caught and when – You want 'day-caught' fish, not fish from boats that are out at sea for a week. Day boats tend to belong to artisan-style fisheries, who use traditional forms of fishing, as per above point.

✳ If the fish has been previously frozen – You'd be surprised . . .

✳ Was the fish farmed? – Some 'wild' fish are not wild at all.

Good fishmongers will enthusiastically articulate all there is to know about everything they sell, even if there's a queue of twenty behind you. You should also be able to ask for the lesser-known types – many of which are normally shipped abroad due to lack of interest here. These are the alternative species; the ones that have not been overfished that are just waiting to be discovered by you.

The following species are at safe biological limits:

> Anchovy; brill; catfish (wolf-fish); cockles; spider crab; cuttlefish; dab; Dover sole; oysters (farmed); grey mullet; grey shrimp; gurnard; John Dory; langoustines; lemon sole; mackerel; megrims; mussels (farmed); octopus; North Atlantic prawn; redfish (ocean perch); red mullet; pilchards; sardines; scallops (diver-caught only); sea trout; skipjack tuna (see page 84); spider crab; sprat; British squid; turbot; weaver; witch.

The Marine Conservation Society publish regular updates about edible species on their website www.fishonline.org.

river clean-up

Recent improvement in rivers' water quality is due to the enforcement of laws to prevent the discharge of effluent from sewage treatment works and industry into British rivers. Water companies have spent over £4 billion improving rivers, and the work continues. Current stocks of wild freshwater fish, apart from a few species, are at healthy levels – improving in many places although there are still problematic rivers. Stocks of wild brown and rainbow trout are also thriving.

An angler friend, Mike McCarthy, brought me a huge brown trout one Sunday last year, fished out of the River Allen. We baked it in foil with branches of fennel that night. It had all the quality of that sadly endangered species, wild salmon.

british beach shellfish

Some of the best 'new' fish discoveries are to be made on our doorstep. Among the lesser-eaten delicacies, cockles, winkles and whelks, hand raked or tractor harvested from our beaches, are often overlooked in favour of more fashionable mussels and imported clams. But if you have a source of them, there is something unutterably homely about them. All are vulnerable to overfishing, so you should avoid irresponsibly harvested beach shellfish. Pollution is another threat.

Finding an acceptable source of beach shellfish is a matter of common sense. Buy from a trusted source, on the beach, or via mail order from a coastal fishery (see the Shopping Guide). If there is a real problem with the water's hygiene, there will almost certainly be a moratorium or ban on the fishery. In fact, quite often there is a moratorium where there's no problem, such is the scrupulous nature of our authorities.

farmed fish and shellfish

Since the 1980s there has been an alternative source to wild fish. Fish farming, or aquaculture, has been a *tour de force* in many ways. Anyone over the age of 30 may remember when salmon was a rare treat, mussels came from wild stock and oysters were seasonal and native. Now salmon can be cheap as broiler house chicken, mussels are abundant, oysters have Pacific parentage and – to hell with the need for an 'r' in the month – they can now be eaten all year round.

For a while everyone celebrated, then more and more bad news about the aquaculture of certain species began to emerge – of problems that affect the environment and human health. The scale of these problems has yet to be determined, but there is one undisputed fact about many types of farmed fish that I find hard to swallow: wild fish must be used to feed the carnivorous varieties such as salmon, trout and cod. It takes up to five kilos of wild fish to produce one kilo of farmed fish. Some of this wild fish is fit for human consumption, indeed some of it is delicious. This wasteful food production doesn't make sense to me either economically or environmentally. For these reasons I don't eat conventionally farmed salmon or trout, and look on their wild cousins as rare treats.

The standards of fish farming vary greatly, so inside information about individual farms is needed when choosing farmed salmon, trout, sea bass and prawns. As far I'm concerned, stocking density is a big issue: you'd be amazed at how many fish can be crammed into a cubic metre. Look out for those that operate a fallow system, moving the cages from one area of the sea loch to another, minimising pollution (see the Shopping Guide).

farming in tanks

The new way to farm fish such as halibut, Arctic char, cod, haddock and trout is not in lochs but tanks. This technology is in its early days, but the first cultivated cod have been produced this way and are on sale in certain supermarkets. It is too early to know if farming in tanks makes economic sense, or is an improvement on tidal water aquaculture. As it stands, the same problem comes to the fore: it will be necessary to plunder wild fish stocks to feed them.

ranching

How about this for a business idea: rearing young sea fish and shellfish then throwing them into the ocean. Hmm, not with my savings you don't. You might as well empty a suitcase of banknotes into the Solent. But there's a lot to be said for ranching seafood – there's a real chance it could boost wild ocean stocks. Early experiments with lobsters off the British coast have been encouraging, and the Marine Conservation Society believe marine ranching is the ocean's only hope of rebuilding its fish population. But who wants to invest in a scheme like that when there's a foreign fishing fleet, ready and waiting to scoop up your harvest, just six miles offshore?

global fish farming

Much of the sea bass and gilthead sea bream on supermarket fish counters is farmed. This should be stated on the label, but often it is not. The only wild sea bass that is sustainable is that caught with a rod and line. Sturgeon is farmed in Europe, for its caviar as well as its flesh, and Japanese fish farmers have found a means to ranch sushi-grade tuna (blue-fin and yellow-fin). They catch wild tuna at 150 kilos, then fatten them up to 180 kilos. This method is not judged as sustainable by marine conservationists.

good shellfish husbandry

Langoustines, prawns, clams and scallops can all be farmed, although standards vary as much as they do for salmon. Mussels are by far the most reliable farmed shellfish, because they cannot grow without high-quality water. There is also an emergence of individual shellfish farms who are looking for total sustainability, working hard to maintain the welfare of the animals and avoid damage to the environment (see the Shopping Guide).

the right farmed fish?

The best way to navigate the sometimes confusing array of options is to ask questions. Check labels for logos that advertise sustainability. And be suspicious of the words 'farm assured' and 'farm quality' – they are meaningless unless backed up with claims of sustainable farming. I know sustainable has an irritatingly worthy ring to it, but a future without fish would be dismal.

how to tell if fish is fresh

Maybe it is the legendary British politeness but I rarely see people examine fish as closely as they do in other European countries. In a French fish market you see customers bend down to the fish, looking, smelling, even touching them, and the fishmongers don't mind – they expect this behaviour. It is a bit like complaining – we're not too good at that, either. But don't be afraid to fuss. A fussy customer is never forgotten, although you may have to make frequent appearances at supermarkets really to get noticed. The freshness of the fish you're sold will improve the more noise you make.

When choosing fish, don't just ask if it is fresh: look at it, smell it and feel it. Be as inquisitive as you can, and don't buy unless it has:

* bright shiny eyes
* clear slime on the skin and a slippery feel
* redness under the gills
* flesh that resists finger pressure
* a clean smell with no hint of ammonia (which is literally a bathroom cleaner aroma)

where to buy fish

* Fishmongers – If you live near a fish shop that prides itself on the freshness of its fish, support it. These shops are very much under

threat from supermarkets. In ten years of living where I do, I have seen three good fish shops close and two supermarkets open.

✳ Markets – You can often buy excellent fish in markets in areas with a large ethnic community. Fish is highly valued, and if there is more than one market stall the competition will boost the quality of the fish on sale.

✳ Farmers' markets near the coast should have fish sellers. Ask for details about where the fish comes from.

✳ If you shop regularly at a market, ask about visits from a fish stall. If there is one, again, ask where they source their fish.

✳ Some coastal fisheries with fleets of day boats (fishermen return each day with the catch – supplying the freshest fish) can send fish, on ice, to your door overnight in sealed polystyrene boxes (see the Shopping Guide).

✳ Supermarkets pride themselves on having wet fish counters, but they are not the places to go to for the freshest fish: it may be at least a week old, having moved from market to processor to centralised cold storage to supermarket, a supply chain held together by long-distance lorry journeys. My local supermarkets have not trained their counter assistants to fillet fish correctly, or advise shoppers on how to use it. However, some supermarkets in coastal areas have adopted local buying policies and sell the catch of nearby fisheries. This should be made clear by labelling – they'd be mad not to do so. Ask your supermarket repeatedly for some of the more unusual species. Eventually you will be heard.

ways to cook fish

grilling fish over embers

Fish cooked slowly over embers has a slightly charred, woodsmoke flavour that does wonders for its skin, crisping it in an appetising way. If you can buy a double-sided mesh in a fish shape, it makes it easy to handle. Thai supermarkets sell banana leaves which, when wrapped around fish, offer protection from burning.

To cook fish perfectly over charcoal or a wood fire is a matter of judging the moment when the hot coals or wood have lost their burning heat but still have enough oomph to cook the fish through. Once the flames have died down and the embers are grey white, it's time to get the fish on to the grill. Cook whole fish or just their fillets. Brush them first with olive or sunflower oil, season with salt and pepper, adding herbs if you wish – thyme, oregano, rosemary – and lay the fish on a grill rack or in a wire mesh over the embers. Be patient. It should be cooked slowly – you do not want black stripes, which can ruin the flavour. Turn after a few minutes. When the fish feels firm to the touch, it is done.

Very fresh fish that has only recently come out of the water tastes truly remarkable when grilled over coals. I travelled to St Ives in 2004 with the food photographer, Jason Lowe, to cover a story for the *Telegraph* magazine about the alternative species of fish we never cook. He showed me how to get the fire to the right temperature, and I remember being impressed that he kept a barbecue in the boot of his car. We grilled large fillets of gurnard and weaver fish – the latter being the fish most people fear for their poisonous spines. They tasted so good, with their large, firm flakes of flesh, that they could have been the very freshest bass or monkfish. Jason decided to photograph them with no sauce, no lemon . . .

Fish suitable for grilling over embers include red gurnard, weaver fish (fillets only – avoid contact with the spines which can give a nasty sting), grey mullet and langoustines.

Frying Fish

Have ready a plate of plain flour or gram flour, seasoned with salt and pepper, and a bowl of water. Heat 2cm/¾ inch of groundnut oil in a large frying pan until it sizzles when a drop of water is thrown into it (at arm's length). Dip fish fillets or, say, a whole gutted, scaled red mullet, into the flour, then into the water (this removes excess flour and will give the fried fish a glimmering sheen when cooked). Gently lay the fish in the oil and cook until firm and crisp on both sides.

poaching fish

Some fish suit the simplicity of poaching – whole salmon, sea trout, brill, pollack and pouting among them. Poaching fish in a special stock, or court bouillon, is simple.

> 1 litre/1¾ pints water
>
> 2 carrots, roughly chopped
>
> 1 celery stick, roughly chopped
>
> 1 onion, roughly chopped
>
> 1 bay leaf
>
> 4 cloves
>
> 6 peppercorns
>
> 1 glass of white wine vinegar, or white wine

Bring all the ingredients to the boil in a wide pan and simmer for 30 minutes. Lower the fish into the simmering stock, cover the pan and turn off the heat. Even a 1kg/2¼lb fish will cook naturally in the cooling stock within about 20 minutes.

Eat poached fish hot or cold, with egg and herb sauce, Hollandaise Sauce, Mayonnaise, or butter and shallot sauce (see pages 395, 396, 393 and 288).

white fish pie

A rich fish pie is a good way to make fish go further. The first stage of this pie can be made well in advance.

Serves 6

1 onion, finely chopped

600g/1¼lb fillet of smoked pollack, line-caught cod or haddock
(see the Shopping Guide)

750ml/1¼ pints milk

1 bay leaf

a little grated nutmeg

6 semi-soft-boiled eggs, quartered (see pages 384–5)

60g/2oz butter

60g/2oz plain flour

300ml/½ pint double cream

freshly ground black pepper

For the topping:
1.4kg/3lb floury potatoes, peeled and cut into chunks

90g/3oz butter

1 egg

salt

Put the onion and fish in a pan and cover with the milk. Add the bay leaf, grate in a little nutmeg and add a few grinds of black pepper. Bring to the boil, then reduce the heat and simmer for 5 minutes. Remove from the heat and leave to cool. Drain the fish, reserving the milk. Pick the flesh of the fish away from the skin, remove any bones, and put it in a pie dish with the quartered eggs.

In a separate pan, melt the butter, then add the flour and stir to a paste. Remove from the heat and gradually whisk in the reserved milk. Return to the heat and bring to the boil, stirring all the time. Simmer for 1 minute, then add the cream and leave to cool. Pour this sauce over the fish and eggs and chill for 1 hour or until ready to cook.

Preheat the oven to 200°C/400°F/Gas Mark 6. Boil the potatoes in salted water until soft and drain well. Mash with the butter, then beat in the egg. Spread the mash evenly over the fish mixture. Scratch the surface with a fork and bake for 35–45 minutes, until the pie is bubbling and the surface is nicely browned.

any-fish stew

Every country has its fish stew but here is mine. Very flexible but all the elements are there. Choose pollack, megrim, red mullet and gurnard, and ask your fishmonger to fillet them and give you the heads and bones.

Serves 4–6

1kg/2¼lb mixed fish fillets, cut into 7.5cm/3 inch pieces, plus the heads and bones

1 litre/1¾ pints water

1 large glass of white wine

4 tablespoons olive oil

2 onions, finely chopped

5 garlic cloves, finely chopped

3 carrots, chopped

2 celery sticks, chopped

1 fennel bulb, chopped

10 tomatoes, skinned, deseeded and chopped

1 tablespoon crushed coriander seeds

a pinch of dried thyme

a good pinch of saffron strands

1kg/2¼lb cockles and mussels, cleaned (see pages 289 and 305)

a dash of Pernod

salt and freshly ground black pepper

To serve:

toasted bread, rubbed with oil

mixed grated lemon zest and chopped parsley, plus chopped garlic
if liked

Make a simple broth from the fish heads and bones: cover them with the water and wine, bring to the boil and simmer for half an hour, skimming off any foam. Strain, discarding the bones.

Heat the oil in a large pan and add the vegetables, coriander seeds, thyme, saffron and then the broth. Bring to the boil and simmer until the vegetables are soft. Add the fish and shellfish and cook, covered, for about 5 minutes or until the shellfish open. Finish with a dash of Pernod and season with salt and pepper. Serve over toasted bread rubbed with oil and scatter over the lemon and parsley mixture. It's also good with the Saffron and Chilli Mayonnaise on page 394.

stock

The heads and bones of all non-oily sea fish can be used to make the fish stock on page 123. If the fishmonger fillets fish for you, ask for the bones and heads to take home, and he will probably give you a few extra. But don't ask for salmon or freshwater fish heads – they make poor stock.

whole sea fish

The fish in this section's recipes have been chosen because there are still healthy numbers of them in the world's oceans. Look upon cooking the species that are new to you as an adventure. Be brave. Stun your guests with a magnificent pollack chowder.

the fish and shellfish to eat: an A to Z

brill

Viewed as a poor relation of the turbot, if only a few coins poorer. But the last brill I cooked arrived shiny and fresh first thing in the morning from a mail-order fish company. We baked and ate it with hot butter sauce and gasped at the quality of this underrated fish.

These flat fish can be huge, up to 75cm long, but usually measure 30cm and will feed three to four people. They are line caught or come as part of the by-catch of other species. There is a TAC for brill, which it shares with turbot, but there are no reports yet that it is overfished.

baked brill with butter and shallot sauce

The French call this sauce *beurre blanc*, and eat it with all fish. It is quicker and easier to make than hollandaise, and you can prepare it in advance and come back to it.

Serves 4

1 brill, weighing about 1kg/2¼lb (or 2 brill, weighing about
480g/1lb each), cleaned
a little olive oil
4 slices of lemon
salt and freshly ground black pepper

For the butter and shallot sauce:
2 shallots, finely chopped
250ml/8fl oz white wine
180g/6oz butter, diced

Preheat the oven to 190°C/375°F/Gas Mark 5. Lightly brush the brill with olive oil, then season it. Place it on a sheet of foil in a roasting dish. Put the lemon slices in the cavity and bake for about 15–20 minutes, until the flesh feels firm or flakes when parted with a knife.

Meanwhile, make the sauce. Put the shallots and wine in a small saucepan, bring to the boil and cook until the wine has reduced by half its volume. Over a medium heat, add the butter in degrees, whisking all the time; the mixture will emulsify into a shiny, pale yellow sauce (don't allow it to boil). Season to taste. If you are making it in advance, don't worry if it separates when it cools; you can always whisk it up again over the heat.

Serve the fish accompanied by the sauce.

✳ kitchen note ✳

I sometimes add chopped chervil to this butter sauce, or a mixture of chopped chives, chervil, basil and tarragon for a very fragrant, aromatic version to eat with all types of white fish, as well as stronger-flavoured fish such as red or grey mullet.

cockles

Cockles are bivalves with two matching shells and a single sweet-tasting, misshapen piece of meat inside. They can be used in the same way as clams; their flesh is very slightly saltier and a mite smaller. You rarely see live cockles in fishmonger's – but ask for them, because they are possible to get. Their season runs from September to April.

how to clean cockles

To clean cockles, check first that they are alive. If you tap a cockle on your work surface and it shuts tight, it is definitely active. With experience, you will be able to tell by rolling a few from one hand to another: the closed shells should feel heavy for their size and roll in a lively way (if you ever had jumping beans as a child, you will know what I mean). Cockles may contain sand. Run cold water gently over them for about 30 minutes to remove what you can. You can buy live cockles direct from fish delivery companies: they should be clean, having been soaked in sea water to remove any grit. The cockles you see in seaside fish stalls tend to be ready-cooked and dressed with vinegar, so do try to seek out live ones.

steamed cockles

Clean the cockles (see previous page) and put them in a large pan with a tablespoon of water or white wine and 1 finely chopped shallot. Cover with a lid and cook over a medium heat for about 3 minutes, until the cockles open wide. Serve with lemon juice, olive oil and parsley.

linguine with steamed cockles and red chilli

Serves 4

2 teaspoons salt

400g/14oz dried linguine (or another long pasta)

1 tablespoon olive oil

2 shallots, chopped

2 garlic cloves, chopped

1 teaspoon dried red chilli flakes

1kg/2¼lb cockles, cleaned (see page 289)

½ glass of white wine, shellfish stock or water

4 sprigs of flat-leaf parsley, chopped

Fill your largest pan with water and place over a high heat. When it boils, add the salt and pasta at the same time. Simmer until the pasta is cooked through but there is still some 'bite' (if you buy Italian branded pasta, the correct cooking time is usually printed on the packet).

Meanwhile, heat the oil in another large pan and add the shallots, garlic and chilli. Cook for 3 minutes, being careful the garlic doesn't burn, then add the cockles. Pour in the wine, stock or water, cover the pan and cook over a medium heat for about 3 minutes, until the cockles have opened wide.

Drain the pasta and mix with the cockles and parsley in a big bowl. Serve with lots of bread to wipe the plates clean.

brown crab

At the current rate of consumption, the brown crab will disappear unless fisheries start to restrict themselves to only the larger, mature crabs. The problem recapitulates the same old simple sum that adds up to lack of sustainability: the number of spawning crabs left in the ocean is less than it takes to supply demand.

But because the management of crab fisheries in England and Wales is decided locally, not all brown crab fisheries are on the way out. There are responsibly managed brown crab fisheries, notably the Cromer crab fishery off the Norfolk coast, and that of the southeast coast of the Isle of Wight.

Crab fishing is the lifeblood of Isle of Wight longshoremen, and they simply cannot afford to take more than a responsible number from the coastal waters. At Ventnor, Geoff and Cheryl Blake sell freshly caught crab from a hut on the beach. You can light-heartedly eat crab sandwiches on Ventnor beach until you can eat no more, and cheaply too, as all the longshoremen seem to be closely related to the publicans and café owners. Recently Defra and the local council paid for a small 'haven' harbour for the Ventnor fishery, to reward it for responsible management and protect their boats. A step in the right direction, and hopefully the future for these coastal fisheries.

how to cook and pick a brown crab

Always choose brown crabs with mature, well-worn shells, as they have the most meat inside. Brown crabs are often sold cooked, and it is possible to buy the meat freshly picked from the shell – at a price (see the Shopping Guide). If you buy live crabs, kill them kindly before cooking. Drowning a crab in fresh water as you bring it to the boil is inhumane, and putting one straight into boiling water will encourage it to shed its claws.

There are two ways to kill a crab. You can pierce it in one of two places on its underside with a spiked instrument or a Phillips screwdriver: behind the flap-like apron or behind its 'eyes'. Alternatively put the crab in the freezer for a couple of hours. It will become comatose, at which point you can cook it.

Heat a large pan of water to boiling point with at least a mugful of salt. Submerge the crab or crabs in the boiling water, bring back to the boil and simmer for 15 minutes. Remove from the water and leave to cool.

To remove the meat, pull off the legs and claws, break them open with a hammer or nutcrackers and pick out the white meat. Open up the crab body, pulling away the 'breastbone' from the main shell and revealing the grey-green gills, which should be pulled off and discarded. Pick up the main shell (carapace) and press the tab between the eyes; it will click and come away with the stomach, which should be thrown away. Spoon out any brown meat from the shell into a bowl. Chop the breastbone in half and use the handle of a teaspoon to scrape out as much white meat as you can from the recesses in the skeleton. Break it apart more if it helps you access the meat. A large crab will yield enough cooked meat for two to three people, about 240g/8oz.

Serve the crabmeat plain with brown bread and butter, in sandwiches, or beside a salad. Some home-made herb mayonnaise would be good, too (see page 383).

crab pasties

Mandy Caws is the fiancée of Jim, a crab fisherman at Steephill Cove, within walking distance of Ventnor on the Isle of Wight. She will become a member of the Wheeler family that has lived and worked at the cove for 400 years. Jim's father is the longshoreman. He cleans the beach, puts out deckchairs, helps push dinghies into the water and sticks a plaster on the occasional cut foot. For the trippers who walk down the steep steps to the beach, Mandy sells pasties stuffed with crab from her door. I prised her recipe, word for word, straight from her kitchen.

Makes 5

1 slice of wholemeal bread

240g/8oz crabmeat

120g/4oz leeks, chopped

2 teaspoons lemon juice

a walnut-sized piece of butter, melted

¼ teaspoon salt

a pinch of turmeric

480g/1lb bought puff pastry

a little milk

freshly ground black pepper

Preheat the oven to 200°C/400°F/Gas Mark 6. Chop the bread in a food processor, transfer to a bowl and stir in the crabmeat, leeks, lemon juice, melted butter, salt, turmeric and some pepper.

Roll out the puff pastry thinly and cut out 5 circles about 15cm/ 6 inches in diameter. Place a heap of the crab mixture in the centre of each one. Brush the edges with milk and then fold over and pinch them together to form a pasty. Brush the tops of the pasties with milk, place on a baking tray and bake for about 30 minutes, until golden. Serve straight from the oven, as does Mandy Caws. Otherwise, they will keep for about 3 days.

spider crab

The spider crab is a woefully neglected treasure of British seas that I would love to see more of on our menus, especially since the popular brown crab is overfished in some areas. In fish markets on the Cornish coast you can hear merchants on their mobile phones, flogging the spider crab catch to the Spanish, French and Italians who, in their wisdom, love these crabs to bits.

This clever creature sticks cuttings of sea plants to its spiny back with saliva, effectively to cultivate a small garden for camouflage against the seabed. Its legs are meanly thin – hence its name. There is some brown meat in the body shell, but it lacks the flavour of the rich brown meat in the brown crab. It is the white meat in the spider crab's legs that has the real value. It breaks into beautiful, clean strings when cooked. Available direct to your door from coastal fishery mail order between March and July, the crab mysteriously disappears in the intervening months (see the Shopping Guide).

how to cook and pick a spider crab

Fish merchants will sell you the crab ready cooked, or even the meat freshly picked from the legs. But should you buy or even catch a live one, you can kill it humanely by piercing it with a sharp tool or Phillips screwdriver under the flap-like apron on its belly side. Be warned: it will struggle. It is perhaps better to put it to sleep instead, by chilling it in the freezer for two hours before boiling it.

Fill a large pan with water and add a mugful of salt. When the water boils, lower the crab or crabs into the water, bring back to the boil and simmer for 12 minutes. Lift out from the water and allow the crab to cool naturally. Use a hammer or nutcrackers to break open the legs. They are quite tough and prickly, so wear rubber gloves if your hands are sensitive. Pick out all the white meat and break apart the chunks; they will separate into strings. Discard any cartilage – the transparent inner bones attached to the meat. A large spider crab will yield about 180g/6oz meat.

spider crab salad

Serves 2

the meat from 1 large, cooked spider crab, plus the roe if female
(reserve the shell)
3 tablespoons extra virgin olive oil
juice of 1 lemon
1 small fennel bulb, very thinly sliced
2 sprigs of soft fennel leaves, or bronze fennel (or flat-leaf parsley),
chopped
a pinch of freshly ground black pepper
a large pinch of sea salt

Mix all the ingredients together and pack the mixture back into the main body shell. Serve with toast.

✳ kitchen note ✳

Add the skinned kernels of fresh or frozen broad beans to the crabmeat, if you wish.

spider crab and prawn cakes with red chilli dressing

Makes 8

the meat from 2 large, cooked spider crabs (about 360g/12oz
in total)
4 tablespoons cooked peeled North Atlantic prawns, chopped
3 egg yolks
2 tablespoons milk
4 tablespoons breadcrumbs (see page 30), plus extra for coating
sunflower oil for frying
salt and freshly ground black pepper

For the red chilli dressing:
2 tablespoons pine nuts, crushed in a pestle and mortar
4 red chillies, deseeded and chopped
6 tablespoons extra virgin olive oil
4 sprigs of coriander, including the root if attached, chopped
1 teaspoon smoked paprika
1 teaspoon white wine vinegar or lemon juice

Mix all the dressing ingredients together in a bowl, season with salt and pepper and set aside.

Mix together all the ingredients for the crab cakes, season with a pinch of salt and some pepper and form into 8 patties. Roll each one in breadcrumbs. Heat 1cm/½ inch of sunflower oil in a frying pan over a medium heat and fry the crab cakes on both sides until golden brown. Serve with the chilli dressing.

grilled spider crabs with sherry and cream

There is something of the bistro, or the gentlemen's club, about this hot little gratin. Serve in a gratin dish, or make individual servings in ramekins, half scallop shells or even small spider crab shells if you have them.

Serves 4

the meat from 2 large, cooked spider crabs (about 360g/12oz in total)

3 tablespoons sherry

2 pinches of ground mace

8 tablespoons crème fraîche or double cream

2 egg yolks

4 tablespoons freshly grated Parmesan cheese or similar British cheese

a pinch of grated nutmeg

sea salt and freshly ground black pepper

Preheat the oven to 230°C/450°F/Gas Mark 8. Mix the crabmeat with the sherry and mace, then pack it into a gratin dish, seasoning it with salt and pepper. Put the remaining ingredients in a bowl – keeping back half the grated cheese – and mix well. Pour the mixture over the crabmeat. Scatter over the remaining cheese and bake for 10–15 minutes, until the surface is browned and the custard puffed. Serve straight from the oven, with brown bread and butter or a salad.

flatfish

If you take British restaurant menus as your guide, there is only one flatfish and that is Dover sole. This is insanity, because while numbers of Dover sole are holding up, there are plenty of similar fish in the sea. Due to lack of local demand, British catches of flatfish like megrim, lemon sole and dabs tend to be sold to Spain. But these fish are very good when fresh; historically, they have been put down by food writers who have not had access to the freshest supplies. Try buying them by mail order from Cornish fish merchants and your habits may change (see the Shopping Guide).

fried sole

Fry whole small fish in a mixture of butter and olive oil for a few minutes on each side, until they feel firm when pressed with a finger. Serve with melted butter, very finely chopped parsley and lemon juice.

✳ kitchen note ✳

Dab, another good flatfish that is fished in British waters but rarely eaten here, can be cooked in the same way. A dab usually measures just 20–25cm/8–10 inches in length. A perfect meal for one! The same goes for the larger witch flounder, also found in British waters, but when did you last see one in a supermarket? The flesh of the witch is truly excellent but again, make an effort to seek out a fresh supply.

hoki

Hoki is another white fish, with a similar texture to cod. The New Zealand hoki fishery has been certified sustainable by the MSC. Look for their MSC logo on boxes of frozen hoki in supermarkets, but avoid hoki without it.

paper-baked hoki with potatoes and tomato dressing

Serves 4

4 hoki steaks, thawed (they are sold frozen)
12 salad potatoes, boiled and sliced

olive oil

4 pinches of dried or fresh oregano

salt and freshly ground black pepper

For the tomato dressing:

4 tomatoes, skinned, deseeded and chopped

2 shallots, finely chopped

8 tablespoons olive oil

2 tablespoons sunblush tomatoes, drained of oil and finely chopped

1 tablespoon red wine vinegar

Preheat the oven to 200°C/400°F/Gas Mark 6. Cut out 4 large pieces of baking parchment and place a hoki steak on each one. Arrange a quarter of the potato slices on top of each steak, season and then shake over a little olive oil. Add a pinch of oregano to each, then wrap the fish in the paper, twisting the ends like a cracker. Bake for about 12 minutes; the fish should feel firm and resistant when pressed with a finger.

Combine all the dressing ingredients, season to taste and put them in a bowl on the table. Serve the fish straight from the paper, with new potatoes and the sauce spooned over.

john dory

This small spiky fish is marked out by a dark spot on its side, said to have been made by the touch of St Peter. It is a non-quota, non-protected species that is usually brought up as a by-catch. Its white flesh is delicious, parting into boneless flakes. If the fishmonger bones it for you, remember to ask for the carcass as it makes excellent stock.

john dory with fennel and sorrel sauce

The lemon flavour of the sorrel, with the anise of the fennel, matches John Dory perfectly.

Serves 2

2 John Dory fillets, about 180g/6oz each
flour for coating
30g/1oz butter
salt and freshly ground black pepper

For the fennel and sorrel sauce:
1 small fennel bulb, thinly sliced
juice of ½ lemon
125ml/4fl oz double cream
a handful of sorrel leaves, shredded

First make the sauce. Put the fennel in a pan, add enough water just to cover, then add the lemon juice and cook for about 15 minutes, until the fennel is very soft and about half the liquid has evaporated. Add the cream and sorrel and bring to the boil, then set to one side. Season to taste.

Pat the fillets dry and season. Roll them in a little flour. Heat the butter in a large frying pan, add the John Dory and fry for about 2 minutes on each side, until firm to the touch. Reheat the sauce and serve it in a pool on warmed plates, with the fillets of John Dory sitting on top.

kippers

Herring, the fish that becomes a kipper once smoked, is caught all year round. It is a lot less abundant than it was before the 1970s, when stocks collapsed after some horribly enthusiastic fishing around the British coast. Efforts to rebuild numbers are proving successful. One fishery – Thames Herring – has been awarded MSC certification for good management. Very fresh herring are good filleted, dipped in egg then medium oatmeal and shallow-fried in sunflower oil for one minute either side. Eat with the egg and herb sauce on page 395.

kipper butter

Serves 4

2 kippers
125ml/4fl oz milk or cream
120g/4oz softened butter
zest of ½ lemon
4 sprigs of flat-leaf parsley, chopped
freshly ground black pepper

Put the kippers in a pan and cover with the milk or cream. Bring to the boil, then turn the heat down and simmer for 3 minutes. Remove the fish from the pan, strain the milk or cream and reserve. Prise away all the kipper flesh, making sure you extract the bones. Beat the flakes of flesh with the milk or cream, butter, lemon zest, parsley and a little black pepper. Store in a container in the fridge and melt over a baked potato for a meal on your knee.

langoustines

Langoustines, scampi and Dublin Bay prawns are one and the same. Personally I love to call them by the unpretentious name of scampi; it is how I first knew them when they were chic on restaurant menus in the 1970s, but in today's cooking language they are langoustines, so that they must be to avoid confusion. Langoustines are overfished in southern Spanish waters and the Mediterranean, but their numbers in the North Sea remain inside safe limits. Buy the very largest raw langoustines you can find. You get more meat for your money and, crucially, these will have had a longer life. The price of fresh langoustines, and even finest grade frozen, tells you they are a luxury, but as the first line of this book says – when you buy a fresh langoustine, it gives you a present of its shell which you can use for stock.

north atlantic langoustines with rosemary

Cook these in a ridged grill pan, under the grill, or over the embers of a barbecue.

Serves 4

24 large, raw langoustines in their shells
8 small sticks of rosemary, with the leaves left on
olive oil
sea salt and freshly ground black pepper

To serve:
2 lemons, halved
melted butter
chopped parsley

First peel the langoustines. The prickles on the edge of these shellfish make pulling their shells away a painful business and you run the risk of tearing their raw flesh. You can avoid this by taking a pair of scissors and snipping down the edges of the underside, lifting away the 'belly' shell, then gently prising the meat from the cocoon of the hard, outer shell. The shells can be reserved for making stock (see page 122). Put them in a plastic bag and freeze, or keep them cool ready for use.

Thread 3 langoustines carefully on to each rosemary stick. Shake a little olive oil on to them and season with salt and pepper. Grill for 2–3 minutes on each side, then serve with the lemon halves, melted butter and chopped parsley.

broiled north atlantic langoustines with mayonnaise

This may seem an extravagance, but the discarded shells make stock in minutes (see page 122). It is possible to buy langoustines that have already been boiled. All you need to do is sit down to a plate of them and peel away, dipping their pink flesh in lots of home-made Mayonnaise (see page 393) as you do so. Raw langoustines need to be cooked in a boiling, wine-based broth for three to four minutes, depending on size (see Poaching Fish, page 284).

southwest mackerel

Mackerel are pelagic fish, which means they swim in the upper waters of the sea and are therefore easy to overfish. Trawlers sometimes bring up whole shoals.

The waters around Cornwall, Devon and along the south coast as far as the Isle of Wight have been dubbed the Southwest Mackerel Box. The Box was established in 1981 when mackerel numbers dropped to crisis levels.

Inside this area the only legal method to catch mackerel is by handline – gill nets are banned. The fishermen let a line down into the water, punctuated by hooks decorated with eye-catching coloured feathers.

The Marine Stewardship Council has certified the Southwest Mackerel Handline Fishery as sustainable, and it is a relief to be able to see their logo and buy a fish that you know is not endangered from a supermarket or fish shop. If you can't see the logo, you can always ask and stun the queue at the fish counter with the well-informed question 'Are these line-caught or netted fish?' A good shop will be able to answer you. Mackerel once had a poor reputation. Because they were frequently found near wrecks the myth had it that they contained the souls of the dead. The real reason mackerel were often bad was because they are oily fish and deteriorate quickly, so they must be eaten either very fresh, or smoked.

mackerel with rhubarb and chilli

This recipe transformed my opinion of both mackerel and rhubarb. Make it, if possible, with the bright-pink rhubarb from Yorkshire, sometimes sold as champagne rhubarb, that is available between December and April. It has been grown in the dark and has beautifully tender scarlet stalks. The look of this dish – silver mackerel, shocking-pink sauce – is nearly as good as the taste.

Serves 2

2 pink rhubarb stalks, cut into 1cm/½ inch pieces

1 tablespoon sugar

2 tablespoons lemon juice

1 mild red chilli, deseeded and chopped

1 tablespoon vegetable oil

the fillets from 2 fresh mackerel

salt and freshly ground black pepper

Put the rhubarb in a pan with the sugar and lemon juice and cook gently until just soft but still holding its shape. Add the chilli, stir once and leave to cool.

Heat the oil in a large, heavy-based frying pan. Season the mackerel, add it to the pan skin-side down and cook for approximately 2 minutes on each side, until firm to the touch. Serve the mackerel – skin-side up for looks – with a large spoonful of the rhubarb sauce on the side and a big watercress salad.

✳ kitchen note ✳

Grilled mackerel is also good with hot sauces such as mustard and horseradish.

red mullet

Red mullet have a slightly gamy flavour, and for that reason fit best with a tart companion. Baked red mullet are good with an orange sauce (try them in Paper-baked Fish with Seville Orange, page 343). But red mullet are also, along with other bony fish with strong, dark, good-flavoured flesh, ideal in fish stew. Good options include gurnard and rascas. Fish suppliers love to sell these last two. More than once I've been told there is usually 'no call for them'. Not so in the southern Mediterranean, where their flavours are valued as essential to the saffron-scented soups and stews.

mussels

My daughter Lara adores mussels and will get through buckets of them. They are one of the cheapest ways to consume a lot of fish. The obvious way to cook them, as well as the simplest and most pleasurable, is steamed in wine, but you can add other flavours too.

how to clean mussels

Given the time, I enjoy the ritual of cleaning mussels before steaming them. First check that the mussels are alive: they should close when handled or cold water is splashed on to them. Clean the outer shells under cold running water, using a small knife to scrape off any barnacles or dirt. (Dirty shells will taint the broth made during cooking.) Next, pull away the 'beard' fom the closed shell.

steamed mussels with wine and shallots

Serves 4

1 tablespoon butter

6 shallots, sliced

2 glasses of dry white wine

2kg/4½lb mussels – Scottish preferably, or French – cleaned

(see previous page)

Melt the butter in your biggest pan and cook the shallots in it until soft. Add the wine, bring to the boil, then add the mussels. Put the lid on the pan and cook over a fairly high heat, shaking every now and then to move the mussels so their shells can open wide: 2–3 minutes should be enough. Put the pan in the centre of the table, give everyone a bowl and a bowl for the empty shells, and get on with devouring them. Don't eat mussels whose shells remain closed.

more steamed mussels

* Add crushed lemongrass and chopped red chilli to the butter, replacing the wine with water or fish stock (see page 123).
* Use dry cider in place of wine and add 150ml/¼ pint crème fraîche at the end of cooking, stirring the mussels with a big spoon to coat them.
* Add a tablespoon of medium curry powder to the cream recipe above.
* Add 2 crushed garlic cloves to the butter with 4 skinned, deseeded and chopped tomatoes and a few sprigs of chopped basil.
* Follow the recipe for stuffed mussels on page 35.

octopus

Some Greek islands sell postcards showing octopus drying in the sun, like rubber shirts on a washing line beneath startling cobalt skies. These pictures are sadly out of date; the process was banned some years ago for logical reasons of hygiene.

After slow cooking, octopus becomes tender, but still nicely chewy. Its flesh is clean and white, the flavour lovely and delicate. When they were tiny, my children used to pick the octopus out of the fish *antipasti* in Italian pizzerias on holiday – loving its feel in their mouth, and its sweet taste after being marinated in lemon and olive oil. They recoil at their bravery now.

preparing octopus

Your fishmonger will prepare the octopus for you, removing the bony beak, eyes and ink sac. If you really want to do it yourself, use a knife to sever the legs from the head, then turn the head inside out. Discard the innards as you do so, cutting them away with the eyes. Then tackle the hard 'beak' – as you can imagine, this is macho stuff.

Your fishmonger will not remove the skin, which can be difficult, but if you plunge the prepared octopus meat in boiling water for two minutes, it will pull away easily.

Lastly, pound both sides of the flesh with the smooth face of a meat mallet to tenderise. You almost wish they'd bring back the old sun-drying method, which had the same effect.

octopus with lemon, oil and oregano

Prepare an octopus as described above and cut it into manageable strips. Score it with a knife on both sides to make a criss-cross pattern, then grill over a barbecue or on a ridged grill pan without oil for a few minutes, until the flesh turns from translucent to opaque and the edges are slightly charred. Slice into bite-sized pieces, put them on a plate and shake over some extra virgin olive oil with a big flavour and some lemon juice. Scatter a little dried oregano on top, season with sea salt and freshly milled black pepper and eat with bread or toast. This dish keeps well in the fridge for 3–4 days.

✳ kitchen note ✳

The same method works well for large squid.

a store of octopus

If you are going to go to the trouble of cooking an octopus, buy a large one, as they are not expensive. Once you have made the salad above, store it in a large jar in the fridge; the oil will preserve it. As long as it still smells good and sweet, it will last. You can pull it out of the fridge at any time to pile on to a hunk of fresh bread.

braised octopus with tomatoes

Eat this simple stew with boiled potatoes – you could add some mussels 10 minutes before the end of cooking. You could also use squid instead of octopus, but steer clear of baby octopus; they deserve to be left in the sea to grow to full size.

Serves 8

1 average-sized octopus (approximately 1kg/2¼lb)

6 tablespoons olive oil

2 garlic cloves, chopped

2 onions, chopped

1 fennel bulb or 2 celery sticks, chopped

a sprig of thyme

1 bay leaf

1 tablespoon ground coriander

1 can of tomatoes

about 400ml/14fl oz water or fish stock

Prepare the octopus and remove the skin as described on page 307, then slice it into 2cm/¾ inch chunks. Heat the oil in a large pan, add the garlic, vegetables and herbs and cook over a gentle heat until golden. Add the octopus and cook, stirring, for a minute, then add the coriander and tomatoes. Cook for a further 4 minutes or so, then add enough water or fish stock to cover. Bring to the boil, skimming off any impure foam that rises to the top, then turn the heat down to a simmer. Cover with a lid and cook for 1–2 hours. To check if it's done, just cut a piece open – don't expect the octopus to fall apart like stewed meat; it will stay firm but easy to eat.

pollack

Pollack is the latest answer to the cod problem, although I'm wary of over-promotion because a trend for it could devastate. It has white, good-quality flesh with not too many bones, and can be treated in the same way as cod. Pollack is a member of the cod family, and usually taken as a by-catch in trawler nets. Its fishing is restricted; there is a TAC in place aimed at protecting its future. The Handmade Fish Company in Shetland smoke pollack with great success (see the Shopping Guide).

Fried white fish with parsley and caper butter

Serves 4

4 pollack steaks, weighing about 150g/5oz each

1 bowl of maize meal (polenta), seasoned with salt and pepper

60g/2oz butter

2 tablespoons vegetable oil

For the parsley and caper butter:

90g/3oz softened unsalted butter

2 tablespoons parsley, finely chopped

1 tablespoon capers, rinsed, dried and chopped

Roll the pollack steaks in the maize meal. Melt the butter in a large frying pan and add the oil. When the butter foams, add the pollack steaks and fry over a medium heat until golden on both sides and firm to the touch.

Beat together all the butter ingredients. Serve each steak with a knob of butter melting on top.

✳ kitchen note ✳

Look out also for pouting, particularly if you are in Cornwall, where it is sometimes brought up on lines. Previously a sneered-at poor relation of cod, pouting has a good flavour and can reach the size of 40cm/16 inches.

pollack, spring onion and cream soup

Based on Jane Grigson's soul-warming New England chowder, this is a soup that is both comforting and beautiful. Grigson's recipe called for monkfish at a time when that firm-fleshed fish was not so popular, but the species is now exploited and the large female fish are very rare indeed. Male monkfish are small and often sold as individual tails. Their supply varies but the important thing is to restrict fishing the mature, egg-laying females. I now find myself avoiding monkfish in restaurants, and only buy the small tails of males occasionally. Gurnard works well as an alternative in this soup, and you could also use mussels, cockles and/or North Atlantic prawns.

Serves 6

30g/1oz butter
90g/3oz unsmoked back bacon, chopped
16 small new potatoes, scrubbed or scraped clean
1 litre/1¾ pints langoustine stock or other fish stock
200ml/7fl oz double cream or crème fraîche
1kg/2¼lb line-caught pollack fillet, skinned and cut into bite-sized chunks
8 spring onions, chopped
salt and freshly ground black pepper

Melt the butter in a large pan and add the bacon. Cook for 2 minutes, then add the potatoes and stock. Bring to the boil, then simmer for 20 minutes or until the potatoes are almost cooked. Abandon cooking at this stage until 10 minutes before you eat.

Add the cream to the soup and bring back to the boil. Add the fish and simmer for 5 minutes, then add the spring onions and cook for a further 5 minutes. Season to taste and serve with lots of good white crusty bread.

✳ **kitchen note** ✳

You can substitute pollack with fillets of weaver fish or large red gurnard fillets.

north atlantic prawns

Let's not be snobby about cold-water prawns from the North Atlantic: compared to the wild tiger prawn, the sea is positively crawling with them. Their flesh is juicy and their flavour is clean, faintly like salmon or sea trout, and more delicate than their warm water cousins', too. Their prime drawback is that they are always cooked straight after the catch, and then shrink drastically during the second cooking unless you just warm them through. They're responsibly fished, mostly using trawl nets that are fitted with exit doors for by-caught fish. Could we please, oh North Atlantic prawn fisheries, perhaps have a supply of frozen raw prawns for which we can no doubt find a thousand uses?

a pint of prawns with garlic and cayenne butter

A large bowl filled with pink prawns, accompanied by hot garlic butter or real mayonnaise, is the kind of dish I always hope to find in pubs but very rarely do. No matter, because I can always eat it at home; the sheer messiness of ripping off the shells is true, time-consuming pleasure. Those same shells also make a fine broth when toasted (see page 122).

Serves 2

enough cooked North Atlantic prawns to fill 2 large bowls

For the garlic and cayenne butter:
2 garlic cloves, crushed to a paste with a little salt
a pinch of cayenne pepper
90g/3oz butter

Put all the ingredients for the garlic and cayenne butter in a small pan and melt gently, without letting the butter boil. Pour into 2 warmed ramekins or dishes and put them on the table, together with the prawns. Don't forget to put a bin-bowl on the table for the shells, plus lots of paper napkins, and bowls containing hot water and a quarter of a lemon for finger-washing rituals at the end.

spiced prawns on fried flat bread

Inspired by the Indian takeaway favourite, *puri*, this is a recipe in which ready-cooked prawns do not suffer from being cooked again. If you do not own a pestle and mortar, I do recommend buying a small, tough ceramic or stone one. The spices in this dish will have a more interesting flavour if you toast them whole in a dry pan, then grind them freshly.

Serves 2

2 chapatis
1 tablespoon vegetable oil
30g/1oz butter
1 small onion, finely chopped
1 garlic clove, finely chopped

1cm/½ inch piece of fresh ginger, grated

1 green chilli, finely chopped

½ teaspoon turmeric

1 teaspoon ground cumin

1 teaspoon ground coriander

2 tomatoes, deseeded and chopped

2 large handfuls of cooked peeled North Atlantic prawns

leaves from 1 sprig of mint

yoghurt, to serve

Fry the chapatis, one at a time, in the oil and half the butter until golden on both sides. Wrap in foil to keep warm.

Heat the remaining butter in the same pan until it foams, then add the onion and garlic. Cook, stirring, for 2 minutes until golden. Add the ginger and chilli, then the spices, and stir-cook for another minute. Add the tomatoes and cook for 30 seconds. Finally add the prawns, warm them through, then tip the whole lot on to the chapatis. Scatter over the mint leaves and serve with a little cooling yoghurt on the side.

✳ kitchen note ✳

If you can't find chapatis, substitute naan or flour tortillas – or make the flat bread on page 22.

warm-water prawns

Warm-water prawns are normally identified as tiger prawns and are big favourites with the takeaway generation. But I would rather eat British scampi any day than warm-water tiger prawns from the seas around Asia and South America. Trawling for tiger prawns results in the need-less capture of other species – notably endangered turtles – although some fisheries are developing nets that let out the by-catch. Tiger prawn farming or aquaculture is big business in Southeast Asia. The impact of the prawn farming has been appalling damage to the Southeast Asian environment. According to the Marine Conservation Society, over 25 per cent of the world's mangrove forest has disappeared as a direct result of the industry. Setting aside damage to the environment, the need to use larvae from wild prawns means prawn aquaculture is not sustainable anyway.

salmon

Farming rights and wrongs

The west coast of Scotland is now peppered with salmon farms, most owned by just a handful of multinational companies. The yield from these farms stands at about 140,000 tonnes per year and is rising. Most fresh salmon in supermarkets come from Scottish fish farms, but the sashimi-loving Japanese also pay big money for it. Lately Scottish salmon has been getting a bad press, and the arguments rage on. There has been claim and counter-claim.

* Escaped fish damage the wild salmon population – The salmon farming industry blames the decline of wild salmon on other forces.
* The muck on sea and sea loch beds annihilates other marine life, damaging the ecosystem – The industry says it moves the fish cages regularly to avoid this and cleans up after itself.
* Farmed salmon is fatty due to the creature's sluggish lifestyle, and does not taste as good as wild – Emphatically not: it is delicious, says the industry.

The most damaging claim to have hit salmon farming is that there are toxins in the fat of farmed salmon, the very element of the fish that contains the essential Omega 3 fatty acids that are supposed to be so good for us. The fear is that farmed salmon contains, in its fat, toxins derived from the fishmeal that a salmon eats. Toxins are found because the manufacturers of fishmeal rely upon wild fish, some of which is trawled from deep waters all over the world – where toxic chemicals accumulate, having been dumped as waste. The contaminants in the fish feed – called PCB's – are known to cause cancer, hormonal disruption and neurological problems, and they accumulate in the fat of humans and animals that ingest them.

The salmon farming industry argues that levels of contaminants are not dangerous, but it has a way to go before it can convince the public – and the media – that farmed fish is as good for us all as it says it is. Intensive farming in general does not have the best track record, and public mistrust of farmed salmon is exacerbated by experience of past food scares. And now a new spectre looms: the development of salmon genetically modified to grow larger and faster, despite popular distaste for the idea.

Amid such confusion, it is difficult to know what is the sensible, responsible approach to farmed salmon. The Marine Conservation Society says that the environmental damage caused by salmon farms outweighs any environmental gain, but they admit not all fish farms are bad and recommend various sources as responsibly managed (see the Shopping Guide).

where to buy salmon

Organic salmon farming has taken off in the Orkneys and Northern Ireland. The fish from these farms is a good alternative to standard farmed salmon, with improved welfare and more natural feed. And it is available in supermarkets. All the same, even if this fish comes with Soil Association approval, I am uncomfortable with the use of the word 'organic' when the fish is reared in sea and lochs that cannot be shut off from outside influences.

organic feed for farmed trout and salmon

Between 60 and 70 per cent of feed given to organically farmed fish certified by the Soil Association is composed of fish oil and fishmeal. At least 50 per cent of the feed must be by-products of wild caught fish destined for human consumption – such as the bones, skin and heads of filleted fish. Any other fishmeal or oil in food must come from a guaranteed sustainable source. The remaining percentage of their diet is based on organically grown cereal with added vitamins and nutrients (see the Shopping Guide).

attitude to salmon

I don't wish to discourage you from eating salmon. Just approach it with respect. Feast on it, don't make it a dish for every day, and buy the best quality you can find. There are sources of sustainably caught wild salmon; notably that, during a brief summer season, from the estuaries on the south coast of the Irish Republic. For more regular doses of oily fish, look to sustainably caught skipjack tuna, mackerel, kippers and crab.

bay shrimps

All along the wide crescent of Morecambe Bay, on England's West Coast, witness the peculiar sight of tractors driving on the flats at low tide, dragging a rectangular wire net behind them. They are catching tiny shrimps that turn pinky-grey when cooked. Their flavour – gentle, salty and slightly earthy – is known to anyone who has eaten potted shrimps. In the past their diminutive size meant that the trouble taken to peel them alone accounted for their high price. More recently, an obsessed Dutch inventor came up with a machine which has thousands of tiny wire fingers that can undress the little grey shrimp in a nanosecond, reducing their exclusivity enough for Morecambe Bay potted shrimps to become available in some supermarkets. You can also buy them directly by mail order from the Morecambe Bay fisheries (see the Shopping Guide).

potted shrimps or prawns

I like these best when they are all together in a large, shallow dish, then carved out and put on plates with lots of toast to hand.

Serves 4

200g/7oz peeled grey shrimps or cold water prawns

a pinch of cayenne pepper

½ teaspoon ground mace

juice of ½ lemon

30g/1oz unsalted butter

2 sprigs of chervil, flat-leaf parsley or coriander

2 chives

Mix together the shrimps, spices and lemon juice, then pack them into a dish. Melt the butter gently and pour it over the shrimps. Pull the herb leaves from the stalks, chop the chives finely and drop them on to the butter. Use a spoon to submerge the herbs in the melted butter. Leave in the fridge to set.

squid

It is best to buy squid caught in British waters, where it tends to turn up in the nets as a by-catch of white fish and scampi, because there are various problems with the large dedicated squid fisheries in both the Atlantic and the Pacific. Buying British is not just an ethical choice. The freshness of locally caught squid is hard to beat. Choose medium-sized squid (about seven inches long) if you can.

preparing squid

Squid contain a single, easy-to-remove transparent bone and some jelly-like guts. Pull everything out of the white tube, then remove the hard eye. They are predators and it is not unusual to find a little fish inside, too. Then you can either slice the squid into rings or cut into squares for dipping in flour and frying in groundnut oil. Alternatively, for the barbecue or grill pan, slice down the length of the body, open them out flat and score the surface in a criss-cross pattern. Cut them into strips for the following recipe.

warm salad of squid with potatoes and shallots

There are two ways to cook squid and be sure it is tender – very fast or very slow. Anything in between will be indistinguishable from rubber.

Serves 4

12 new or waxy potatoes

2 tablespoons vegetable oil

2 medium squid, cleaned (see above), cut into strips and left on a towel to absorb water

soft sea salt and freshly ground black pepper

For the dressing:

2 shallots, finely chopped

4 tablespoons red wine vinegar

8 tablespoons olive oil

2 sprigs of parsley, chopped

Boil the potatoes in water with a pinch of salt until just tender. Drain, quarter them and set aside in a bowl. Mix together all the ingredients for the dressing in a bowl or mug.

Heat the vegetable oil in a wok or large frying pan and have ready a lid or mesh disc, because the oil is liable to spit when you cook the squid. Put the squid in the pan and cook over a high heat for 2–3 minutes, until they turn from translucent to opaque white. Lift them out of the pan with a slotted spoon and put them on top of the potatoes. Pour over the dressing, season with salt and pepper, and it is ready.

crispy squid with salt and pink peppercorns

A cooking method that gives you squid as crisp as that served in restaurants, but without using gallons of fat or deep-fat fryers. Frying it twice is the secret.

Serves 2

2 tablespoons plain flour
1 teaspoon soft sea salt, ground to a powder in a pestle and mortar with ½ teaspoon pink peppercorns
1 medium squid, cleaned (see page 319) and cut into strips
groundnut oil for frying

Mix together the flour, salt and pink peppercorns, then roll the squid pieces around in this mixture. Heat 2cm/¾ inch of groundnut oil in a wok until it sizzles when a drop of water is thrown in (at arm's length). Put on an apron because squid spit as they fry. Fry the squid for 1–2 minutes, then remove and allow to cool in a sieve or on a towel. Re-fry in the same oil for 2 minutes, until very crisp. Eat with a sweet chilli sauce.

trout

Trout farming shares some of the problems of salmon, but the farms are on rivers and the practice is being ever more tightly regulated and controlled to minimise damage. Organic trout farms are on the increase, and the fish are available in supermarkets. Trout farms produce rainbow and golden trout species. Both are delicious when fresh, but the wild brown trout will always taste superior. Trout can be substituted for sea trout and salmon in recipes, but you will need a large fish (1 kilo/2lb minimum) for the home-cured sea trout recipe.

home-cured sea trout

When I buy sea trout it is often in order to cure it in sugar and salt, then serve with a cucumber salad or on toast. It takes moments to prepare the fish and only 18 hours before it is ready to use. It will keep for about four days in the fridge.

> 2 fresh sea trout fillets, weighing about 360g/12oz each (taken from
> a 1.5kg/3¼lb fish)
> 1½ tablespoons sea salt
> 1 tablespoon golden caster sugar
> 1 teaspoon black peppercorns, crushed
> 5 sprigs of dill

Lay one of the sea trout fillets flesh-side up in an oval dish. Scatter the salt and sugar on top, then the pepper. Cover the fish with the dill sprigs and place the other fillet on top, skin-side up, to make a sandwich. Cover with cling film and a long piece of card. Weigh down with a few cans of food and refrigerate for at least 18 hours. Some liquid will seep out of the fish.

Uncover the fish and lift off the top fillet. Remove the pin bones with tweezers; you will find them running down one side of each fillet. Slice on the diagonal, working from the tail end towards the head end.

Arrange the slices on a plate and serve with Cucumber Salad with Mustard (see page 94).

✳ kitchen note ✳

The same method can be applied to other oily fish, such as herring and mackerel.

trout pâté

Serves 8

480g/1lb cooked trout, flaked and off the bone

120g/4oz Greek yoghurt or cream cheese

zest of 1 lemon

½ teaspoon crushed pink or black peppercorns

6 sprigs of dill, chopped

salt

Melba Toast, to serve (see page 30)

Combine the trout with the yoghurt or cream cheese, then stir in the lemon zest and pepper. Taste and add salt if necessary. Place in a container and chill for 1 hour. Serve the pâté decorated with the dill and accompanied by Melba toast. It will keep for about a week in the fridge.

sea trout and lentils

Lovely colours – grey-greens and pinks, with bright green leaves. No one will ever know this is leftovers.

Serves 4

120g/4oz Puy lentils

240g/8oz cooked sea trout

salt and freshly ground black pepper
For the dressing:
1 garlic clove, crushed
1cm/½ inch piece of fresh ginger, grated
1cm/½ inch piece of lemongrass, finely chopped
½–1 green chilli, finely chopped
1 tablespoon rice vinegar or lemon juice
4 tablespoons avocado oil
6 sprigs of coriander, chopped

Put the lentils in a pan, cover generously with water and bring to the boil. Simmer for about 30 minutes, until tender, then drain and leave to cool. Season to taste.

Break the sea trout into large flakes and mix it lightly with the lentils. Mix together all the ingredients for the dressing and pour it over the top.

✳ kitchen note ✳

This salad will also work with smoked white fish, very fresh grilled mackerel or trout, and even the flesh pulled from kippers.

whelks

These quirky sea snails, or gastropods, have their season in the summer, from April onwards. Fancifully I think of whelks as being both extravagant and benevolent old men. They live on a grand diet of oysters and scallops, then after death they donate their home, or shell, to the humble hermit crab. They are boiled after harvest, and their lovely chewy texture and gentle fishy flavour goes well with lemon juice, or the garlic-infused mayonnaise on page 394.

whelks with broken pasta, garlic butter and unwanted lettuce

Inspiration for this recipe came from a plate of ravioli that I ate in Dijon, home to the snail. The broken pasta is lasagne – while I get through pasta shells and tagliatelle in no time, I never seem to use that box of pasta sheets. Buy an Italian brand of egg lasagne and break it into pieces for this dish, which is also a useful vehicle for putting those unwanted outer leaves of floppy, oh-so-English lettuces to good use. Their pale hearts can be stored in the fridge for eating raw.

Serves 2

120g/4oz unsalted butter
2 garlic cloves, crushed to a paste with a pinch of salt
8 sheets of egg lasagne
20 cooked whelks, prised out of their shells with a long pin
outer leaves from 2 round lettuces
salt and freshly ground black pepper

Bring a large pan of water to the boil. Meanwhile, melt the butter in a separate pan and add the garlic. When the water boils, add 2 teaspoons of salt and the lasagne. Boil until the pasta is just tender, then drain, keeping back a little of the cooking liquid. Put the pasta back in the pan, with the small amount of cooking liquid to keep it from turning rubbery.

Add the whelks to the pan containing the melted butter and garlic. Cook over a low heat for half a minute, then add the lettuce and season with salt and pepper. Cook until the lettuce collapses. Throw in the pasta, mix it all together in a big bowl and put it on the table.

winkles

Winkles are basically gastropods with a muscly texture and a delicate, slightly salty flavour. Their season runs from September to April. Fishermen boil them immediately after harvest, so they are best eaten dipped in red wine vinegar and chopped shallot, with Mayonnaise (see page 393) or with a little Tabasco sauce.

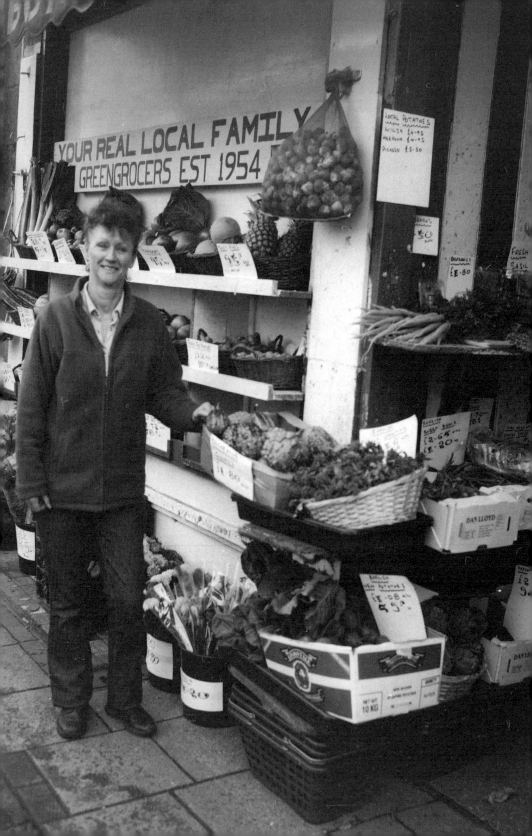

8

gluts of fruit and vegetables

The glee I feel when a favourite fruit or vegetable arrives in season comes not only from the welcome you would give any friend you haven't seen in a year. There is also the excitement of knowing that an hour or two's work is going to fill the kitchen with useful food. And that work will be repaid several times over during subsequent days and weeks. It's an investment that gives you the leverage to indulge yourself – with whatever you like. You can use the money saved for meals out, or spend it on something completely different from food. Isn't that what we all want?

Every month of the year brings a gift. And the gift is twofold, because a week or so after a fruit or vegetable's first appearance, when its season gets in swing, the price drops, but the quality is at its best. These periods, when shops and markets are suddenly flooded with certain varieties of produce, are my gluts.

This is not a book where you will find a recipe for every vegetable, every fruit. Those included are personal favourites, and all lend themselves very well to the philosophy of taking time out to get ahead. Buy into gluts when prices are low and prepare them for storage, or feast on them at once, capitalising on the advantages of eating in tune with the seasons. Either way you win. It's successful kitchen commodity trading: you are buying futures in food.

what one hour of cooking gives you

A large quantity of tomato sauce made from a glut will take approximately half a very relaxed hour to prepare and one hour to cook to the sweetness you want (it may need longer if the tomatoes are not ripe enough). You are left with a number of potential meals halfway to cooked. What's more, you have cooked at a time to suit you and the food is good quality and made from ingredients sold at their correct value.

Squirrelling away food cuts the cost of living while increasing the quality of life. The time saved frees you up to put in some extra work, go shopping, catch up on the post, or help with children's homework. You might prefer to have a rest. Hopefully it will be time for pure fun too. And you will not have to resort to expensive ready-made meals.

tomato economics

A five-kilo box of tomatoes bought late in the day from a chartered market should set you back around £5. Depending on the level of ripeness and the type of tomato, this should yield you around four litres of sauce. Allowing £1 for the cost of oil, energy, onion and garlic, this batch will yield 33 helpings of 120g/4oz, each serving costing 18 pence.

the right price

The price of a food goes up the moment it comes into season and drops after a week. Buying smart is a matter of knowing when to strike. As soon as a particular food is abundant in markets and groceries you will get it at the right value. Out-of-season food can be two to four times as expensive as it is in season, and it never tastes quite so good.

Seasonal gluts don't impact on supermarkets to the same extent. As Joanna Blythman has written in *Shopped* (Fourth Estate, 2004), the supermarkets' perpetual summer means that seasonal factors are less obvious. Indeed, they will carry on selling Spanish asparagus alongside English, even if we're heaving with the native crop.

producing the produce

Barely a day passes without the airing of one anxiety or another about produce. Sometimes I feel rather like the person in the old painkiller advert: there are so many alarm bells ringing you want to cover your ears with your hands. First the government wags its finger: you must eat five portions of fruit and vegetables a day! Then the organic lobby chimes in, saying your healthy five-a-day have been sprayed with poison. And then the environmentalists tell you the contents of a mixed salad have clocked up 20,000 food miles between them. To round things off, the cookery sections in Sunday newspapers encourage you to turn the lot into an exciting new pasta dish. Aaghh!

where on earth

Once confronted with the facts, most shoppers loathe the idea of others being exploited for their gain. This has been known since the Fairtrade Foundation was established to buy directly from farmers in the developing world and bypass the commodity exchanges that can have such a devastating impact when prices fall. Since 1986 we have been able to identify Fairtrade goods by their logo, but in general we are pretty powerless to do much about the exploitative nature of much food production. We are locked into a system that favours the West and creates poverty elsewhere, and with the production processes so far out of sight, it is easy to put them out of mind.

Food miles – how far the carrot, potato or apple flew, aided by fossil fuel, in order to sit on your plate – are a big issue for environmentalists. There are those who say that we should never eat foods that have been air-freighted or shipped to our shops. I'm not one of them. It isn't that I have no sympathy with the environmentalists' concerns: bringing in parsnips from New Zealand does not make sense when our own farmers could grow them themselves, were they minded to. But there is a lot of rot talked about the solution to the food miles problem. Why is it that an environmentalist can happily wear a pair of pants made in China, but disapproves of Caribbean bananas? Is it all right for one person to have a job stitching knickers, but not for another who picks and packs green beans?

unfair trade

I could write an entire chapter about the failure of the European Union's Common Agricultural Policy, protectionism, and the power of the food corporations. But the nub of it is this: for 50 years shoppers in Europe, and the USA and Japan for that matter, have been promised low-cost food. In Western Europe farmers are subsidised to produce certain crops, which keeps prices artificially low. Meanwhile, high levies protect the market from imports from poorer countries. So Western food production is protected and entrepreneurship is inhibited in the places that most need it.

The answer is not to stop buying imported food, but to try and buy more sensitively: by that I mean, try to buy British produce when it's in season, and, when you're able, to choose imported produce from a source you know is benefiting the people who are growing it. Britain could be self-sufficient in many vegetables and fruits if the supermarkets were prepared to pay a fair price for them (yes, there are poor farmers in Britain, too). Being less reliant on imported food would reduce fossil fuel usage, which would be a start. Were British farmers' favourite grain crops not subsidised, and more farmers diversified into growing vegetables for no subsidy, the reward for them, and us, would be great. I'm prepared to pay more for produce and that is a choice I am happy to make, because I am lucky to know how to make higher-priced food stretch further.

supply chains

While being by all accounts good employers, major retailers, with their vast buying power, enjoy something of an appalling reputation generally when it comes to dealing fairly with growers. They are known to pressurise food suppliers to cut their prices and many producers, who wish to remain anonymous, have complained to me that supermarkets squeeze their prices down to the point where they cannot profit. With costs of farming and food production in Britain constantly rising, the majority of suppliers face two grim choices: go out of business or break even. If they want to keep going, they cannot complain, out of fear that the supermarket buyers will simply take their business elsewhere.

In its report on supermarkets in 2000, the Competition Commission identified some situations in which competition is distorted and works against the public interest. A code of practice was proposed to stop the abuse of buying power, which had created a 'climate of apprehension' among food producers. The Commission concluded this code should be legally binding for those chains with 8 per cent or more of the British market. But the code drawn up the following year by the Office of Fair Trading was only voluntary. And the 'climate of apprehension' still dominates the relationship between supermarket buyers and food producers.

It's not all gloom. Smaller chains of supermarkets build long-term relationships with farmers. For example, some support watercress growers in the South, and Yorkshire rhubarb growers are well supported. Others encourage farmers to grow specialist vegetables such as squash, 'wild' mushrooms, violet pearl aubergines, and spiny artichokes. Waitrose are particularly good for potato varieties: it's fair to describe Alan Wilson, their agronomist, as a spud fanatic (he has revived numerous old favourites). Reports about Marks & Spencer and the northern supermarket chain, Booths, are also good, and Sainsbury's are frequently praised by the Soil Association for their commitment to British organic produce.

solutions

Variety and your good judgement can help change the British food market for the better. If UK farmers and food producers grew a greater variety of crops, they would live less under the threat of abandonment by supermarket buyers. Increasing numbers are already finding alternative ways of selling food through mail order, markets and independent shops. And if shoppers become more circumspect about buying and avoiding certain foods, supermarkets will prick up their ears and listen.

In the meantime, here is my five-point guide to choosing fresh vegetables and fruit:

buy british in season

✳ Never feel guilty about buying imported produce that does not grow in Britain.
✳ Try your best to buy from shops who will supply information on an import's country of origin and proof of fair trade and responsible farming methods.
✳ Pay more for better-quality, responsibly sourced food.

where to buy glut food

✳ Greengrocers – Greengrocers are fast vanishing from the British high street. During the last seven years the three fruit and veg shops nearest my home have closed down. They couldn't compete on price or footfall with the new high-street 'local' stores operated by Sainsbury's and Tesco, which started opening once planning permission for superstores began to dry up in the late 1990s.

I miss our local fruit and veg shops. They were run by enthusiasts who called everything 'lovely' and always had a box of slightly overripe odds and ends that you could snap up cheaply to use that day. If you have a local greengrocer's, support it. They buy their produce straight from the traditional wholesale markets, who buy straight from the grower. This simple supply chain means you can buy vegetables that were picked the previous afternoon, and you will taste their freshness. So encourage your green-grocer to sell the produce you want at the time of year that you want it.

✳ Box schemes – A good source of fruit and veg in season. Box schemes are run by market gardens, who on payment of a subscription will send you a selection of seasonal vegetables once a week. You get the freshest produce for an excellent price. This is a great way of buying organic vegetables. What's more, you are buying direct from the producer (see the Shopping Guide).

✳ Farmers' markets – These have sprung up all over the country in recent years. There you will find growers selling the pick of their crop.

✳ Pick-your-own market gardens (PYOs) – For me, PYOs are a particular favourite. I enjoy the peaceful pastime of selecting my produce, alone to do some quiet thinking, or with a friend to chat and catch up. It's a high-quality way to spend an hour, ending with a car boot full of food bought at a price that hasn't been inflated by middle men. All of these options allow you to buy food for its true value.

✳ Chartered vegetable markets – Since the arrival of farmers' markets, traditional chartered markets have become the targets of food snobs, who criticise their lack of organic produce or just plain imagination. It's true that stalls selling little more than apples, oranges, potatoes and cabbages are dull compared to a farmers' market trestle piled high with courgette blooms or lovely duck-egg blue, crown prince squash. But the chartered markets have begun to improve. The last five years have seen a definite surge towards greater diversity. Many sell herbs, Southeast Asian ingredients, bunches of young vegetables, flavourful tomatoes, and good-quality salad leaves.

On Saturday mornings, if I am in Dorset, I go armed with a £20 note to see Pete on Blandford's marketplace. This is usually enough to buy all the fruit and vegetables I need for the week – in fact, it's enough to feed a small family of gorillas. The cost hasn't risen in three years, but the increasing variety has been remarkable to witness. I can buy purple sprouting broccoli, sprout tops, calabrese, sweet bunches of carrots, and great bags of Jersey Royals. There is, of course, the ever-useful box of tomatoes, and perhaps a tray of bargain peaches or a box of black figs. Pete also supplies Blandford's Indian restaurants, and always has a spare bunch of coriander and a few ripe limes. We chat, he gives the children Victoria plums, I stop by with the car later on to pick everything up. I know few more enjoyable ways to shop.

✳ Privately grown fruit and vegetables – Screeching to a halt when you see blackboards on the roadside has its risks, not least for the car behind, but the rewards can be enormous. Honesty box sales have always been a great source of summer vegetables and fruit. Look out for the sign, the box of home-grown produce and the jam jar waiting for your payment. When I can, I even buy honey and eggs this way. Such produce is likely to have been grown in a leisurely way, with a low use of chemical pesticides, if any at all. No shop front and no middle man means no mark-up, so you and the grower both come out well.

✳ Supermarket fruit and vegetables – When a food is in season it will certainly be cheaper at the grower's end, but there may well be a big mark-up by the time it reaches the supermarket shelf. Each of the Big Four supermarket chains occasionally boasts of their loyalty to British produce. But as yet none has broken the habit of selling cheaper imported apples when British grown are on the shelf. If you ask supermarkets to sell the produce you want them to sell, when you want them to sell it, they will start to respond as demand grows. So insist!

wild foods

Anyone who likes to walk can help themselves from the public larder. Even municipal parks have blackberries, and the odd giant puffball grows on playing fields: look out for them in the morning before everyone else gets there. Wild foods are not necessarily organic; the land they grow on can be subject to the same chemical treatment as farmland. So wherever you find it, wash wild fruit thoroughly when you get home.

be a food pirate

I loathe the notion of typically English food. People drone on snobbishly about pork pies, roast beef and Marmite, but I really don't want to rediscover the great bland dishes of England, the cow-heel pies or suet puddings. I'd rather see fields of artichokes growing in Lancashire, and twisted, sweet peppers in Cornish greenhouses. I love to find herbs and chillies in my food, and the new fascination with ingredients fills me with optimism for the future development of our cooking.

Many talk about our new food as borrowed from the Mediterranean, Asian and so on, but in fact this is another chance, like so many we have had in the past, to expand the repertoire of English cookery. A delicious curry is now authentic English food.

Remember the British have a history of being terrific food pirates. Living on a small island breeds a natural curiosity for what is eaten on other shores. Much of our very English diet is based on the foods brought to Europe by the early explorers. Thanks to the likes of Columbus, Vasco da Gama, Ralegh, Marco Polo, maize, chocolate, turkeys, coffee, potatoes, strawberries and tomatoes came to us from the Americas. And where would we be without our favourite spices?

the season tells you what to eat

When a fruit or vegetable comes into season there is nothing wrong in eating it every day, even twice a day. There are certain things I cannot leave alone once they are 'in': asparagus, so expensive at other times of year; forced rhubarb; purple sprouting broccoli; strawberries; corn on the cob.

As the year unfolds various foods will come and go. By all means buy into gluts of imported foods when you see them, but the following sections are arranged according to when different gluts occur through the British seasons, beginning in January, the month traditionally reserved for hibernations and a withdrawal from richness. The food it yields reflects that.

winter

forced rhubarb

I know that the post-Christmas weeks are no one's favourite unless they have flown off in search of sun, but I still like them. It's time to get back to work and take time off from the rich food you have tired of during the holidays. I tend to eat a lot of citrus-scented coconut curries, using up cold meat, and to hunt around for something fresh and colourful.

Forced rhubarb has its glut moment from January to the end of February and has everything I want to cheer up these dark months. It's shocking pink, even brighter when cooked. Last year I bought a box of it at market, ate some that week, chopped, bagged and froze some more, and gave a bunch instead of flowers as a thank-you present to friends.

candlelit harvests

Chance discoveries punctuate culinary history. There is the legend of the chef who burnt the sugar in anger when the kitchen boy dropped a tray of nuts, then mixed the two together and came up with praline. It was another accident in the nineteenth century that brought about the unorthodox growing technique for rhubarb. The story goes that a Yorkshire farmer threw a rhubarb root on to a compost heap one autumn and forgot all about it. A few weeks later he found the rhubarb had sprouted wan, pink stalks in the warmth of the rotting heap. Rhubarb at that time was eaten for its purgative qualities, but an exploratory sample revealed that these rogue stalks were infinitely nicer to eat than the tough stuff he'd grown that summer.

When cultivated in the dark, rhubarb hunts for light and grows at three times its natural speed. In the low, unlit sheds that are still scattered around Wakefield, it takes one week for the unfurling stalk that audibly pops from the corm to reach two foot in length. It's still harvested in candlelight (brighter light will stop the plants from growing). Forced rhubarb's proudest moment came during the Second World War, when a train left Lofthouse every day of the winter months for London, a snaking twenty carriages filled to the hilt with the long boxes of highly nutritious stalks.

The best thing of all about rhubarb is that the season begins in mid-November and ends in March. It is not a fruit, despite its good marriage with sugar, but a wonderful native British vegetable perfectly designed to lift winter kitchens out of their gloom. I like to eat it with my favourite winter store fruit, frozen raspberries, brewed into a compote and lightly sweetened. It sits in the fridge for a week or so, ready to be stirred into yoghurt or eaten with ice cream. But there are more fascinating ways to eat rhubarb. Be brave and try the next recipe. It's wonderful with rice, a few unsalted pistachios and a sprig or two of dill.

beef braised with rhubarb

This is adapted from Claudia Roden's recipe for *khoresh* in *A New Book of Middle Eastern Food* (Penguin, 1986).

Serves 4

60g/2oz butter

1 onion, finely chopped

480g/1lb lean beef steak, cut into 1cm/½ inch cubes

beef stock or water, to cover

1 teaspoon ground allspice

480g/1lb forced rhubarb, cut into 2cm/¾ inch lengths

juice of ½ lemon

4 sprigs of dill, chopped

1 tablespoon shelled unsalted pistachio nuts, chopped

salt and freshly ground black pepper

Heat half the butter in a large casserole, add the onion and cook until pale gold. Add the meat and stir-fry until browned on all sides. Cover with beef stock or water and add the allspice. Bring to the boil, skimming off any rising foam. Turn down to a simmer and cook slowly, partly covered, for 1–1½ hours, until the meat is tender.

Heat the remaining butter in a separate pan, add the rhubarb and cook for a few minutes, until just tender. Squeeze over the lemon juice, then stir into the simmering meat sauce. Cook for another 10 minutes, then season to taste. Serve over plain boiled white rice with the dill and pistachio nuts scattered over the top.

rhubarb fool

Serves 4

480g/1lb rhubarb, cut into 2cm/¾ inch pieces
150g/5oz golden caster sugar (or you could substitute Apple Jelly –
see page 365)
300ml/½ pint whipping cream

To serve:
demerara sugar, or multi-coloured sugar crystals (see the Shopping
Guide) and Moroccan dried rose petals

Put the rhubarb in a pan with the sugar and a splash of water, then cover and cook gently until soft. Allow to cool, then refrigerate. Whip the cream until it holds its shape and fold it in to the rhubarb. Spoon into a glass bowl or individual glass dishes and dust with a little demerara sugar or a few coloured sugar crystals and Moroccan rose petals.

purple sprouting broccoli

Just as Christmas is over, in comes purple sprouting broccoli, the finest flavoured of all the cabbage family. It's slightly citrus, with slim fibrous stalks and unopened flower heads. Buy it at about six inches long, and always inspect it first to make sure it's young, firm and sweet smelling. Good purple sprouting broccoli is as great a vegetable as asparagus and can be treated in similar ways.

warm purple sprouting broccoli with lemon and oil

This is my favourite way of eating purple sprouting broccoli, and useful too, because timing vegetables to arrive hot at the table is one of my least favourite aspects of entertaining. Fiammetta Rocco, who is Kenyan–Italian and a wonderful natural cook, made it for me one winter lunchtime and I have been hooked ever since. She cooked it quite a while before we ate and served it in an unworried way at room temperature with the roast lamb. As long as you drain the water fully out of the broccoli, it keeps its freshly cooked texture.

Serves 4

480g/1lb purple sprouting broccoli

olive oil

juice of ¼ lemon

salt and freshly ground black pepper

Strip off the leaves from the broccoli, leaving the flower heads, and peel away any tough skin on the stalk using a potato peeler. Bring 4cm/1½ inches of salted water to the boil in a large pan and lower in the broccoli. Cook until just tender, then lift out with a slotted spoon and leave to drain on a dry cloth.

Put the broccoli in a bowl and shake over some olive oil. Squeeze over the lemon juice and season with salt and pepper.

more ways with purple sprouting broccoli

✳ Eat hot as a starter, with Hollandaise Sauce (see page 396) or Egg and Herb Sauce (see page 395).

✳ Pare hard ewe's milk cheese over the broccoli at room temperature, or grate a little bottarga (dried pressed grey mullet or tuna eggs, available from Italian delis) on to it.

✳ Cut thick slices of a creamy soft-rind cheese, such as Flower Marie, Durras, Chabis or Camembert, and place in the oven to make a natural gratin.

sprout tops

Sprout tops are exactly that – the head of the Brussels sprout plant. For a long time they were ignored while we munched our way through millions of sulphurous mini cabbages each Christmas. The British Sprout Growers' Association – there is such a thing – decided something must be done about the image of everyone's least favourite vegetable and, with the help of a Dutch horticulturalist, Dr Hans Van Doorn, spent 10 years perfecting a sweetish sprout. Two years ago, when I heard sprout tops were the latest thing on restaurant menus, I was wary. But trying them dressed with crème fraîche, lemon and rosemary was a revelation. Incidentally, there is a point to those sprout 'trees' you see for sale around Christmas: sprouts stay sweeter longer if left on the stalk.

sprout tops with cream, lemon and rosemary

Serves 4

2 whole sprout tops, quartered

300ml/½ pint crème fraîche (or whipping cream)

leaves from 1 sprig of rosemary

½ lemon

salt and freshly ground black pepper

Bring a large pan of water to the boil, add a little salt, then the sprout tops, and cook for 8 minutes, until just tender. Lift out and drain on a dry cloth.

Heat the cream in a small pan with the rosemary leaves, add the lemon juice and season with salt and black pepper. Put the sprout tops in a dish and pour over the flavoured cream. Eat while hot.

seville and blood oranges

The merest hint that winter will end comes with the arrival of Seville and blood oranges, the former bitterly sour, the latter with glorious ruby flesh and a sweet, rounded flavour. The monotony of year-round oranges makes Seville and blood oranges seem all the more exotic, and the glut in the third week of January makes a bulk box a steal.

January is a happy month of blood oranges juiced for breakfast and six o'clock cocktails mixed with prosecco, the northern Italian sparkling wine. Seville oranges can of course be turned into marmalade, but they are also good used in Cumberland Sauce (see page 219) with cold roasted game birds and roasted ham. The juice, which can be frozen, makes the most delicious sour-sweet sponge-capped pudding imaginable.

blood orange and shallot salad

In Sicily the cold winter nights followed by mellow days develop the anthocyanin in these unique oranges – the pigment that gives them their colour. Try to find very mild, sweet shallots for this salad, which is lovely served with cold duck leftovers.

Serves 4

4 blood oranges
4 sweet pink shallots
2 tablespoons olive oil
salt and freshly ground black pepper

Peel and slice the oranges, removing any pips, and put them in a dish. Peel the shallots and slice them as thinly as you can. Mix with the oranges, then shake the oil on top. Throw over a little sea salt and season with freshly ground black pepper.

blood orange water ice

Serve in glass tumblers for pudding, with a plate of fresh cheeses and oatcakes.

Serves 4

240g/8oz golden granulated sugar
750ml/1¼ pints freshly squeezed blood orange juice
2 egg whites
dried rose petals (optional) and mint leaves, to decorate

Put the sugar in a small pan with 250ml/8fl oz of the juice. Bring to the boil slowly, stirring until the sugar has dissolved, then raise the heat and boil fast until it has become syrupy and reduced by half its volume. Leave to cool completely, then stir in the remaining juice. Freeze in a plastic box until soft crystals have formed. Whisk the egg whites until slightly foamy, then whisk them into the semi-frozen mixture. Freeze again until solid.

Remove the water ice from the freezer 15 minutes before you want to eat it, spoon it into glasses and throw a very few rose petals and mint leaves on top.

✳ kitchen note ✳

This recipe can be made in an ice-cream maker and you can also use other citrus juices – lemon, pink grapefruit, orange – with lovely results.

paper-baked fish with seville orange

When baking strongly flavoured fish such as red mullet or pilchards in paper, place a few triangles of Seville orange flesh inside and outside the whole fish. Shake over a small quantity of olive oil with a little pinch of sea salt and ground pink peppercorns. Wrap each fish into a cracker of baking parchment and bake in an oven preheated to 200°C/400°F/Gas Mark 6 until it feels firm, with no 'give' when pressed through the paper. Open at the table – the aromas are so appetising.

seville orange pudding

There are lots of versions of this ingenious pudding. It's a mixture of milk, citrus juice, eggs and sugar baked in a soufflé and it never fails to surprise me that it doesn't curdle. Instead it cooks to a sublime cream, and the surface becomes a cap of light sponge. This is my favourite version, made with Seville oranges; substitute lemons when their season is over.

Serves 6

2 Seville oranges
60g/2oz butter
90g/3oz golden caster sugar
2 eggs, separated
15g/½oz plain flour
300ml/½ pint whole milk

Preheat the oven to 180°C/350°F/Gas Mark 4. Pare the zest of 1 Seville orange (keep the other for beef stews) and chop it finely. Squeeze the juice from both oranges – you will need 2 tablespoons. Beat the butter with the zest and sugar until soft and pale, then beat in the egg yolks. Fold in the flour, then mix in the milk by degrees. Add 2 tablespoons of the juice.

In a separate bowl, whisk the egg whites until stiff. Fold them into the mixture, which will be disconcertingly sloppy. Pour into 6 small ramekin dishes and bake for 20 minutes, until the surface is golden brown. Serve immediately, with a little double cream.

spring

jersey royal and cornish potatoes

I love the moment when Jersey Royals become plentiful. Grown near the sea and flavoured with the seaweed that is used to fertilise them, Jersey Royals are particularly fine, although similar potatoes grown in Cornwall arrive at the same time and can be just as good.

After a winter of floury spuds and tasteless, undersized waxy salad potatoes, the distinctive lemony flavour of these new potatoes is so welcome. (A true new potato's skin will rub off with your fingers, so don't be misled by imposters.) The season begins in late February but takes off in late March, ending in June or mid-July, depending on the weather. I once travelled to Jersey to watch the potato harvest. In so doing, I discovered the secret that keeps Jersey's potato producers strong in the face of widespread pressures to lower prices: co-operation.

The Jersey Royal is a particular variety of potato grown in special conditions by a growers' co-operative in Jersey. The head of the group grades each farmer's potatoes as they arrive at the depot and the finer the quality, the more the farmer is permitted to sell through the group. The head of the group then handles the sale of the potatoes to wholesale markets and supermarkets (they can also be bought online – see the Shopping Guide). This mini-monopoly leaves supermarkets and wholesalers no choice but to buy through the co-operative or to do without, and it keeps prices at a reasonable level for the producer. In my opinion the empowerment of farmers through co-operatives is the way forward. Farmers in continental Europe tend to work together this way, but British farmers have been slow to stop seeing each other as competitors.

cooking new potatoes

Scrub the potatoes, or better still scrape away their weakly clinging skins with a knife. Boil for up to 20 minutes, until just tender, then drain and serve simply with butter and mint. Alternatively, serve with olive oil and dill, or sliced with canned anchovies and hard-boiled eggs, or mixed with shallots, parsley and soft goat's cheese.

✳ kitchen note ✳

Cook more potatoes than you need and store them in containers. You can then quickly fry them up to go with sausages, make them into a salad or cube them and eat in a soup with herb oil (see page 91).

stinging nettles

It was a sign of the times when the 2003 Chelsea Flower Show had stinging nettles on display. Perhaps soon we can expect to see a show of ground elder.

It's good to learn to love the stinging nettle, and not just for the butterflies that visit it. In early spring, when about 10 inches tall, it is deliciously eatable, and it loses its sting when cooked. Carefully snip off the top five inches – gardening gloves are necessary – and use it as you would spinach. I add it to rice dishes, pastas and vegetable curries.

wild garlic

In March and April you can smell wild garlic in woodland all over the UK. Don't walk by. If in doubt, wild garlic can be recognised by its white globe-shaped flower and leaves as long as the hyacinth's, and the same deep green. Always leave the bulb in the ground so that more will grow next year, but harvest the leaves sensibly and you will do no harm. They are edible raw, but the intense garlic taste can repeat unpleasantly so I prefer to eat them wilted: they keep their colour, while their power is subtle. They are delicious stirred into rice or pasta dishes, or cooked in a frittata (see page 397).

asparagus

The glut everyone looks forward to. I confess to eating Spanish asparagus while I wait for the English to arrive in May, but then I'll eat nothing
but home grown. Always sniff asparagus tips before you buy, avoiding
any that have a compost aroma or with open 'flowers'. It should smell
of asparagus and nothing else.

cooking asparagus

I don't bother with fussy kettles. Just bring a large pan of salted water
to the boil and lower in the asparagus. Test after five minutes: it is
cooked when just tender. Lift it out of the water using tongs or a slotted
spoon and drain on a tea towel to absorb all the water. Then eat with
melted butter, Hollandaise Sauce (see page 395) or egg and herb sauce
(see page 396). You can also fry young asparagus in a pan with olive oil
and eat it with Parmesan, Pecorino or parings of good British ewe's milk
cheese (see page 426).

elderflower

There's a three-week glut of elderflowers between the last week of May
and the second week of June. They grow everywhere: in hedgerows, on
the edge of woodland and in public parks. Don't be afraid to help yourself in a public place, but you should not have a problem seeking
consent to cut the flowers of this weed from bushes on private land. The
blooms are sprays of tiny white flowers with a centre dusty with pollen.
Eaten raw they are said to stave off colds, but most elderflower lovers
use them to make cordial.

elderflower cordial

Citric or tartaric acid is necessary to stop mould growing in this cordial. Buy it from Asian shops, if possible; it is very expensive bought from the chemist.

Makes about 4 litres/7 pints

5 lemons, halved

5 oranges, halved

1.9kg/4lb golden granulated sugar

4 litres/7 pints water

25 very large elderflower heads

60g/2oz citric acid

Put the fruit and sugar in a large pan and cover with the water. Bring to the boil, stirring occasionally to dissolve the sugar, then add the elder-flower heads. Turn off the heat and leave to cool completely. Add the citric acid, strain through a cloth into very clean bottles and cork. Drink diluted with water.

summer

garden peas and beans

Once garden peas are picked they immediately begin to lose their sweet-ness. This failing explains the success of frozen peas, which are garden peas (called that even though grown in fields) that have been podded then blast-frosted directly after the harvest. Nevertheless, there is a heady moment, usually in late June, when English garden peas suddenly appear in greengrocer's and farmers' markets. If their skins are a juicy bright green, the peas inside should be sweet enough to add raw to salads. Open one and taste before you buy. Freshness is the big issue, and size does not necessarily matter – a pea does not have to be the size of petits pois to be good (incidentally, petits pois are a variety, not extra-small peas). Even mature, fat peas picked before they have burst inside will be delicious.

At roughly the same time of year, in come the beans. French beans are the tender, much-prized, soft fine beans. Bobby beans are plumper and coarse – good to add to Thai curries in place of the authentic Southeast Asian yard bean, which is, as its name suggests, a very long bean with a toughish texture.

pea stock

A carrier bag full of fresh peas in their pods gives you more than something good to eat with lamb. The pale green stock that simmered pea pods yield makes the best springtime rice dishes and pea and herb soups with extra peaness.

Makes enough for 6 helpings of soup or risotto

the pods from ½ carrier bag of peas
1 onion, halved
1 celery stick, chopped
2 litres/3½ pints water

Wash the pea pods and put them in a large pan with the onion and celery. Cover with the water and bring to the boil. Turn down to a slow bubble and simmer for 20 minutes. Strain the stock, discarding the vegetables, and leave to cool. Bag up and store in the freezer.

peas and beans with rice

We made this on a Sunday night, returning with vegetables from a market. I used the only rice I had, pudding rice, and it was perfectly fine.

Serves 4–6

30g/1oz butter

1 onion, finely chopped

240g/8oz short grain rice

480g/1lb fresh peas, podded and the pods made into stock
(see page 349)

300g/10oz French beans

750g/1lb 10oz fresh broad beans, podded

120g/4oz hard ewe's milk cheese, such as Malvern, Somerset
Rambler, Lord of the Hundreds or pecorino

salt and freshly ground black pepper

Melt the butter in a pan, add the onion and cook gently until soft. Add the rice and cook, stirring, for a minute or so. Over a medium heat, stir in the pea stock a ladleful at a time, allowing each ladleful to be absorbed by the simmering rice before adding more (you will need about 1 litre/1¾ pints of stock). The rice will take about half an hour to cook.

Meanwhile, cook the French beans in a large pan of boiling water for 3 minutes, then add the peas and boil for 1 minute. Finally add the broad beans, which need only boil for 1 minute. Drain in a colander and then spread out on a dry cloth. If the broad beans are large, pop the green centres out using your thumb and forefinger, discarding the skins.

Stir the vegetables into the rice and add salt and pepper to taste. Using a potato peeler, pare 1 tablespoon of the cheese into the rice and stir. Eat the rice in bowls, with more cheese scraped over the top.

pea soup

Follow the recipe for Smooth Vegetable Soup on page 128, using peas and substituting Pea Stock for the chicken stock. Scatter dill on top before serving.

french beans with shallots and olive oil

The French love the gentle, savoury taste of shallots with dwarf beans. Why mess with something that good? Eat these with roast poultry, a salty ewe's milk cheese like feta or with a tomato salad. To get the full flavour eat them at room temperature.

Serves 4

480g/1lb dwarf French beans
large pinch of salt
2 shallots, peeled, halved and sliced very thin
5 tablespoons extra virgin olive oil
black pepper

Snip off stalk ends of the beans. I leave the pointed ends on – I like their appearance.

Bring a large pan of water to the boil and add the salt. Add the beans and cook for about 4 minutes until tender – they should still be a bright green but not squeak when you bite them. Drain, then toss the beans in a bowl with the shallots, oil and a twist or two of black pepper and take them to the table.

great garden salad

There are no limits in a salad, although I err on the side of keeping it largely green, allowing tomatoes to have their own salad and avoiding spring onions and raw peppers altogether because they overpower. I mix herbs with the leaves, and add runner beans, cucumber and anything from the pea family. For substance, I add small cubes of cooked waxy potatoes, green pumpkin seeds and/or pine nuts.

¾ of a large salad bowl filled with mixed salad leaves, such as
Cos lettuce, spinach, curly lettuce, mizuna (see Kitchen Note
overleaf) and rocket
8 sprigs of dill, chopped
10 chives, chopped
4 sprigs of coriander, chopped
leaves from 4 sprigs of mint
6 new potatoes, cooked and cut into 1cm/½ inch cubes
2 tablespoons green pumpkin seeds or pine nuts, dry-toasted
(optional)

Plus any or all of the following vegetables:
4 runner beans, cut into diamond shapes
a small bundle of French beans
a handful of broad beans and fresh garden peas

For the dressing:
6 tablespoons olive oil
2 tablespoons red wine vinegar
1 tablespoon Dijon mustard
1 teaspoon golden caster sugar
½ teaspoon soft crystal sea salt

2 tablespoons water

½ shallot, finely chopped

freshly ground black pepper

Put the leaves in the bowl with the herbs. Bring a large pan of water to the bowl and blanch all the green vegetables in it for 1–2 minutes. Drain and splash with cold water, then drain again on a dry cloth. Leave to cool, then add to the salad bowl with the potatoes and the seeds, if you are using them.

Put the dressing ingredients in a jar and shake. Strain on to the salad 15 minutes before you eat and toss well.

✳ kitchen note ✳

Mizuna is a fast-growing salad leaf that does very well in the UK. Plant it straight into pots or beds, cover with garden fleece (available by the metre from garden centres) and three weeks later you have a crop. Cut the taller leaves with scissors, leaving the immature ones and, provided you keep it damp, it will keep coming.

samphire

This succulent dark green weed grows on beaches in the summer and is lovely with seafood. It's available in greengrocer's, fishmonger's and specialist food shops from June, and free on the beach. When you buy it make sure the plants are small – four inches is ideal – and not woody. To cook, bring a pan of salted water to the boil, add the samphire, simmer for three minutes, drain and serve hot with butter, or cold and dressed with olive oil. It's also delicious with egg and herb sauce (see page 395).

indian runner beans

I have recently learned to love the vegetable that has had so much abuse. Remember the grey-green soggy strips that kept coming out of the freezer, right up until Christmas?

The Indian runner bean is, to my mind, a vegetable best eaten fresh when it's in season, which begins in July and reaches its glut moment in August (although, unsurprisingly, supermarkets are beginning to tap into an out-of-season source from abroad). Seasonal eating means using the best, not too large beans. Try them in the Great Garden Salad (page 352), or in Peas and Beans with Rice (page 350), or boil and mix them with another green vegetable, such as young leeks or French beans. And of course they're delicious hot, alone, with butter.

They are a common honesty box sale. Keep an eye out for them when you're driving through the countryside. Always buy firm beans that have not been allowed to grow so large that the beans inside are bulgy and hard. To prepare, top and tail them and cut diagonally for good-looking diamond shapes. Plunge them in boiling salted water for a minute or two – not a moment more! After cooking they should remain green and crisp. Drain and splash them with cold water to set the colour.

soft orchard fruit and berries

Summer means banks of apricots, peaches and plums. In truth I am not one of those people who can set aside a day to make twenty pots of jam from the fruit that pours into markets from June onwards. Instead I tend to buy trays of peaches, apricots or plums from Pete in Blandford market to eat fresh. But if it looks like they are going to be wasted, or the fruit flies start to attack, I have simple methods to put them to good use. The following recipe for 15-minute Jam can actually be made while you snatch a quick bite.

15-minute jam

Suitable for all types of plums, apricots, peaches, berries and cherries, this is a fresh jam to make the moment you notice that soft fruit has had its day. It is particularly good for slightly bruised apricots or raspberries that are too soft to serve.

It will never set textbook style, and does not have the long keeping qualities of conventional jams. Make it in small quantities and store in the fridge. You will need 480g/1lb preserving sugar for every 480g/1lb fruit. Add the sugar to the fruit, then leave it until you have 15 minutes to cook the jam.

Remove any stones from the fruit, put it in a stainless steel pan and cover with the sugar. Leave for several hours or overnight. The sugar should have virtually dissolved. Bring to the boil and allow to bubble quite fast for 15 minutes – the heat should not be so high that the mixture sticks to the pan. Pour into sterilised jars (see Kitchen Note below), then seal and store in the fridge. The jam will keep for about 1 month.

✳ kitchen note ✳

✳ To sterilise jam jars, wash them well, rinse in hot water, then place in a low oven to dry.

✳ Without jam jars, such a small amount of jam can be put in plastic containers with lids and kept in the fridge.

pickled fruit

This recipe works with peaches, pears and firm plums or greengages. Pickled fruit with cold leftover meat and game, or braised or baked ham, makes a bright Saturday lunch that yields extras to add to Sunday supper pilaffs.

480g/1lb peaches or other soft fruit

240g/8oz golden granulated sugar

a pinch each of ground cinnamon, allspice, coriander and cloves

4 cardamom pods

250ml/8fl oz white wine vinegar

Halve the fruit and remove the stones or pips. Put all the ingredients except the fruit in a pan and bring slowly to the boil, allowing the sugar to dissolve. Add the fruit and simmer for 3 minutes. Lift it out with a slotted spoon and pack it into sterilised jars (see previous page). Boil the pickling liquid fast to reduce it until thick, then pour it over the fruit and seal the jars.

✳ kitchen note ✳

Pickles can be eaten almost immediately. Don't make too much; they are best eaten within 5 months of being made.

pickled gooseberries

Follow the recipe on previous page but put raw gooseberries into jars and pour the pickling liquid over them. Seal and store.

mustard-pickled fruit

Follow the recipe on previous page but add 1 teaspoon of mustard oil (available from Asian shops) and 1 teaspoon of yellow mustard seeds with the sugar and vinegar. We eat this with poached salt tongue or beef.

corn on the cob

There's a cottage garden close to a hairpin bend on the Blandford–Shaftesbury road that sells perfect vegetables in high summer: tender Indian runner beans, carrots, beetroot and the youngest, sweetest corn on the cob.

We almost always eat the corn that day, boiled in water with a little salt for seven to eight minutes, then covered with butter. Sometimes I boil it for half that time and put it on to the cooling embers of a barbecue until it takes on a bit of colour (I even like it burnt). The browned kernels taste like caramel. Utterly irresistible.

using surplus corn

When you have more corn than you can eat, parboil the cobs for four minutes and then use a knife to pare off the kernels. Store them in the freezer in small bags, ready to be shaken around in a frying pan with a nut of butter, or made into fritters.

✳ kitchen note ✳

Sweetcorn keeps for up to four weeks in the freezer and is just as good cooked direct from frozen.

corn fritters

From Constance Spry. These were the little fritters we ate as children, with fried chicken drumsticks and bananas.

Makes 8

2 eggs, separated
200g/7oz frozen or sugar-free canned sweetcorn
a small pinch of sea salt
1 teaspoon baking powder
about 90g/3oz fresh breadcrumbs
corn oil for shallow-frying

Put the egg yolks in a bowl and add the sweetcorn and a small pinch of sea salt. Whisk the egg whites until stiff, then fold them into the corn mixture with the baking powder. Carefully stir in enough breadcrumbs to make the mixture just thick enough to handle, then form into little cakes.

Heat a thin layer of corn oil in a large frying pan and shallow-fry the fritters for about 2 minutes, until they are golden underneath and a few bubbles appear on the surface. Turn and cook the other side.

overripe tomatoes

A whole box of sweet, overripe tomatoes, bought for a song in August, becomes a large pan of sauce, cooked down with onions and oil until deliciously sweet. I don't add basil if I'm cooking for storage, because I can use this sauce instead of fresh tomatoes in a whole host of different recipes. Now I can have the base for a coconut-infused curry of lamb or mutton. A ladleful will brighten the taste and add texture to the juices of a braise. Add a pinch of brown sugar, a dash of vinegar, and you have the makings of a heartening sausage and bean stew. But you needn't do so much. Liquidised with creamy milk it is a delightful, foamy soup into which you can throw a sizzling piece of fried Spanish sausage and toasted day-old bread. Thinned with stock, it can be poured over beans or pasta and scattered with cheese for a substantial broth. I add basil or fresh oregano when I use it on pizzas, or in the most simple way of all, with a bowl of pasta.

tomato sauce

I buy boxes of tomatoes from street markets at the end of the day when the traders are packing up, or from market gardens in summer. It doesn't matter if the tomatoes are too soft – the sweeter they are the better. The essential tool, though, is a mouli-légumes (food mill). It takes just a few minutes to push through the cooked tomatoes, leaving behind their skins and hard pips, and you are left with a full-bodied purée.

> 250ml/8fl oz olive oil
>
> 8 onions, roughly chopped
>
> 5 garlic cloves, roughly chopped
>
> 3–4kg/7–9lb overripe tomatoes (cherry or standard)
>
> sugar (only if necessary to remedy sourness)
>
> salt and freshly ground black pepper

Heat the oil in a pan large enough to accommodate all the tomatoes – you can use more than one pan, evenly dividing the ingredients as you go. Add the onions and garlic and cook until soft but not browned. Add the tomatoes and cook, partially covered, over a fairly low heat until soft, then simmer for at least an hour. Some of the liquid will evaporate; this is no bad thing, especially when you use British tomatoes, which tend not to have the fibrous texture of tomatoes from Mediterranean countries. Turn an occasional eye to your bubbling pans, making sure the mixture is not sticking to the bottom. After an hour, taste the sauce; it should be sweet and cooked down. Season with salt and pepper, then judge whether you want to add sugar. Outside the summer season, the bitterness in tomatoes can be inescapable and there is nothing wrong with adding sugar as a remedy. I also tend to add an extra 2 onions to a sauce made in winter, for sweetening *and* thickening.

Put the tomatoes through a mouli-légumes. Feed the wasted pips to the birds. I haven't put them in the compost since the year tomato plants began to sprout all around the garden and in the pots, sapping all the energy from the pelargoniums.

✳ kitchen note ✳

Fresh tomato sauce will keep for up to 5 days in the fridge or for several months in the freezer. Freeze it in small quantities, in strong freezer bags; their odd shape will help them squash in among the other food and the smaller quantity will enable them to be defrosted quickly, straight into a pan over a low heat, if you wish.

tomato sauce with herbs

Add fresh torn basil leaves, 300 ml/½ pint *passata* and a further 3 tablespoons olive oil to 600ml/1 pint of the above tomato sauce for a classic *salsa pomodoro*. Use dried oregano in the absence of basil. Cook for a further 30 minutes. The sauce will become paler in colour as it stews with the added oil.

Spread this sauce on your pizza dough (see page 25). As well as pasta, I eat it for lunch with rice, or poured over pasta wheat or cooked barley.

tomato soup

A heartening, foamy hot soup to take on winter picnics in flasks.

Serves 4

1 litre/1¾ pints Tomato Sauce (see page 358)
500ml/16fl oz creamy milk (you could substitute double cream for some of the milk)
salt and freshly ground black pepper

Liquidise the sauce with the milk, then heat to just below boiling point and season to taste. Pour into bowls, or warmed flasks for a picnic.

For guests, drop a spoonful of crème fraîche into the centre of the soup, or perhaps make it bigger still with coriander leaves and fried slices of chorizo sausage.

curry

Everyone should be able to make a curry from stores – with lamb, poultry, vegetables or canned chick peas. Serve with basmati rice and relishes made from cubed bananas in lime juice with mint or coriander leaves, and yoghurt with grated cucumber or chopped tomatoes and black onion seeds (nigella).

Serves 3–4

2 tablespoons ghee or butter
2 garlic cloves, crushed to a paste with a little salt
2cm/¾ inch piece of fresh ginger, grated

1 onion, finely chopped

1 tablespoon medium Madras curry paste

250ml/8fl oz Tomato Sauce (see page 358)

250ml/8fl oz coconut milk

salt

Plus any one of the following:

480g/1lb raw chicken, rabbit or pheasant meat

480g/1lb lamb shoulder, diced

480g/1lb mixed vegetables, cut into chunks

2 cans of chick peas, drained

Melt the fat in a pan, add the garlic, ginger and onion and cook until soft, allowing them to brown very slightly. Add the curry paste and cook for a minute. Add the main ingredient and stir it into the hot, spiced oil, then pour over the tomato sauce and coconut milk. Simmer for 5 minutes for chicken, rabbit or pheasant, 20–30 minutes for lamb or vegetables. If the sauce becomes too thick, add a little water. Taste for salt, then serve.

❊ kitchen note ❊

Instead of using bought curry paste, you could make your own by grinding together 1 teaspoon each of dried red chillies, fennel seeds, cardamom, fenugreek, cumin seeds, coriander seeds and turmeric, then binding the mixture to a paste with a little vegetable oil.

tomato and grain soup

This is a soup I make from stores for my working lunches. I suffer from sleepiness in the afternoon and find this soup has a slow energy-release effect. I like to serve it with a few slices of Lord of the Hundreds or Malvern cheese scraped over the top. These are British cheeses you could liken to the hard ewe's milk cheeses of Italy and Spain (see page 426).

Serves 2

150g/5oz whole wheat (sometimes sold as Ebly) or pearl barley
250ml/8fl oz Tomato Sauce (see page 358)
250ml/8fl oz chicken or other stock
salt and freshly ground black pepper

To serve:
a little hard ewe's milk cheese
chilli oil and/or parsley oil (see pages 91 and 212)

Fill a large pan with water and bring to the boil. Add salt, then the wheat or barley. Cook for 15 minutes (20–25 minutes for pearl barley), then drain. Meanwhile, heat together the tomato sauce and stock and season with salt and pepper to taste. Add the cooked grains, then reheat to boiling point. Pour the soup into bowls, scrape over a few parings of hard cheese with a potato peeler and put on to the table with one or both of the oils.

giant puffballs

I am hopeless at finding wild mushrooms, not to mention wary ever since I read a report in an Italian newspaper of an entire family wiped out after a mushroom-hunting expedition. But even I can spot a giant puffball if I get lucky, from late August on. They are exactly as their name suggests: a big pure white ball that can grow up to the size of a watermelon. To be sure of identification, check your find against a reputable mushroom guide (see the Shopping Guide). It's well worth the effort of looking. Their meaty white flesh is a true treasure among wild mushrooms. To cook one, dip in beaten egg then breadcrumbs, slice into one-inch rounds and fry on either side in a mixture of butter and olive oil until pale gold. Eat sprinkled with parsley.

autumn

apples

After a hot summer the apple harvest will be early, but the glut usually comes in September. It's a very enjoyable glut too, with dozens of fascinating apples every shade of red and green, or the charming rusty hues of russets. Flavours range, too, from sourly tangy to fragrantly sweet. Look out for traditional varieties in local markets and groceries where they will be cheapest.

To make a store of cooked apple, buy a whole box of them. An hour or two of admittedly hard work, peeling and coring, will produce several containers of fresh-tasting cooked apple to use in puddings and sorbets, or eat with juicy roast pork.

stewed apple

4kg/9lb eating apples – if you use Bramleys you will need to add
more sugar
water
juice of 1 lemon
golden granulated sugar

Peel, core and slice the apples. Put them in a large pan with a teacup of water and the lemon juice. Place over a low heat and cook, stirring occasionally. When the apples are tender – about 20–40 minutes depending on the type – taste and add some sugar if they are too sour. Store your apple sauce in jars, or plastic freezer bags. It will keep for a week in the fridge, or six months in the freezer.

how to use apple sauce

✳ Unsweetened, as a sauce for roast pork
✳ Warmed, seasoned with cinnamon and nutmeg, with hot fresh custard

✳ In a pie – sweeten with sugar to taste and put in a pie dish. Place sweet shortcrust pastry rolled to 0.5cm thick over the top, cut slightly larger than the dish. Brush with milk and bake until golden. Scatter caster sugar on top as it comes out of the oven.

✳ As a sorbet – purée 600ml/1 pint apple sauce, season with half a teaspoon ground cinnamon, add sugar to your taste. Beat well with two egg whites and freeze until solid, stirring once when the mixture is half frozen.

apple snow

An easy, whisked-up pudding that shows off the glorious flavours of the old apple breeds that appear in shops after the September harvest. Serve this pudding in glass tumblers with sweet biscuits. Any remainder can be frozen to make an easy sorbet.

Serves 4

2 egg whites

120g/4oz golden caster sugar

375ml/12fl oz unsweetened apple sauce, puréed

1 pinch cinnamon

4 teaspoons golden muscovado sugar

Whisk the egg whites until stiff and fold in the sugar, whisk again until shiny and smooth. Mix the apple with the cinnamon and then fold into the egg white mixture. Divide the mixture among the glasses and sprinkle muscovado sugar on top of each.

windfalls

Apples found lying on the ground are not always in a perfect state for eating, but will make a failsafe jelly that lasts for years. I find it even more useful than frozen apple purée.

apple jelly

A gentle task for a September weekend. Add a few sloes or blackberries to this recipe, if you wish. Red chilli added to one jar only makes a good sauce for sausages.

> 3kg/7lb windfall apples, roughly cut into quarters (stalks, pips, cores and all)
>
> golden granulated sugar

Put the apples in a large, heavy-based pan and cook, partly covered, over the lowest possible heat until they become a thick, reddish pulp. Stir occasionally and check that they are not burning or sticking to the bottom of the pan; you may find you need a heat diffusion mat under the pan (traditionally the cooking was done in earthernware crocks placed over boiling water and left all day).

Turn a chair or stool upside down and suspend a jelly bag or baby muslin between the 4 legs – alternatively a hook from which you can hang the bag is perfect. Place a bowl under the bag, then spoon all the apple pulp into the bag. Allow it to drain into the bowl naturally; do not push or force it in any way or the jelly will not set. Leave overnight and the bowl will fill with a slightly cloudy, rusty pink liquid. Measure the liquid and for every 500ml/16fl oz add 480g/1lb golden granulated sugar. Put in a clean pan and bring to the boil – the liquid will become clear. Simmer for about 15 minutes or until setting point is reached (see Kitchen Note below). Pour the jelly into sterilised jars (see page 355) and seal.

Eat with meat or spread on toast; dilute with water to make a cordial; add to gravies; melt to glaze tarts; or put in blue cheese sandwiches for picnics.

✳ kitchen note ✳

To test for setting point, put a teaspoonful of the jelly on to a saucer and leave to cool, then push it gently with your finger; if it wrinkles, setting point has been reached.

blackberries

Pick them and store in small quantities in the freezer, where they will sit happily for six months. Just 100g, mixed with 500g of apples, makes a perfect compote. Add a few to the apple jelly recipe, on the previous page, or put some inside a game bird with butter to infuse the juices with fruit.

sloes

Sloes are best used in sloe gin, although a few can be added to the windfall apple jelly recipe, to eat with cold duck and game. Sloe gin is a wonderful dry winter shot for afternoon walks or before Christmas lunch. Put the sloes you pick in the freezer and leave them overnight. They will split when defrosting, helping the maceration process move quickly. Remove a third of the gin from an ordinary bottle and push the sloes in one by one. Add a split vanilla pod, seal the bottle and leave for 12 weeks. Taste and add golden caster sugar if you want to sweeten it, but I do find the vanilla takes the sourness off the sloes. Use the same method for small wild plums (bullaces) and damsons.

quince

Quince is a wonderful, fragrant fruit that lost credit in Britain during the twentieth century. It has been here for centuries, although it is native to western Asia. The fruit is similar in appearance to pear and apple, but larger, harder and slightly sour. I have a quince tree that yields over 150 huge fruits a year. We barter them with a local hotel restaurant, the Castleman, and receive in return pots of versatile Quince Cheese. (You can make fruit cheese from apples and pears too.) It forms a firm fruit purée when cooled, and if left to dry wrapped in a muslin cloth for 48 hours in a warm place, like an airing cupboard, it becomes very firm and darkens in colour like the Spanish delicacy, membrillo.

You can buy quinces between September and December from southern Mediterranean and Middle Eastern shops. They are heavy to carry and can seem expensive, but you can use everything but the stalk and pips. Don't buy fruit with any rust-coloured spotting on the skin; it's a sign of age and the flesh inside will be brown and tasteless.

The sweet-sourness of quince lends it both to meat and cheese dishes as well as the stickiest puddings. Eat Quince Cheese sliced with hot or cold roasted pork belly, and Lord of the Hundreds cheese, which is similar to Manchego. Barbara Garnsworthy of the Castleman makes an extraordinary Quince Frangipane Tart, with nice thin pastry, not-too-sweet Quince Cheese, and a melting almond sponge on top.

quince cheese

8 quinces

juice of 1 lemon

preserving sugar

Wash the fruit and chop it roughly. Put it in a heavy-based pan and add the lemon juice, plus enough water barely to cover. Partly cover the pan and cook the quince to a pulp over a very low heat – this may take some time. Pass the mixture through a mouli-légumes. Alternatively you can push the pulp through a metal sieve, scraping at it with a spatula to get the most out of it.

Weigh the pulp and for every 480g/1lb add 360g/12oz preserving sugar. Return to the pan and stir over a low heat until the sugar has dissolved. Simmer for about 15 minutes, until the mixture leaves a clean channel across the base of the pan when you draw a wooden spoon through it. Pot in sterilised jars (see page 355), seal and store.

✳ kitchen note ✳

Simmering the quince and sugar mixture for longer will produce a much firmer paste, which when cold can be sliced to eat with fresh cheeses. Be careful not to burn the quince pulp as you cook it down.

quince frangipane tart

From Barbara Garnsworthy's kitchen in Chettle, Dorset. Barbara uses a lot of local food. She also runs a terrific store cupboard full of fruit jellies and cheeses, which she uses in her cooking.

Serves 10

240g/8oz unsalted butter

240g/8oz golden caster sugar

240g/8oz ground almonds

3 eggs, lightly beaten

4 tablespoons Quince Cheese (see page 367)

flaked almonds

For the sweet pastry:

60g/2oz icing sugar

270g/9oz plain flour

a pinch of salt

135g/4½oz softened unsalted butter

1 large egg yolk

1–1½ tablespoons double cream

You can make sweet pastry using a light, cool touch with your fingers, but it is quicker and even better made in a food processor. Put the icing sugar, flour and salt in the processor and whiz for a few seconds. Add the butter with the egg yolk and enough double cream to form a paste when the mixture is whizzed briefly. Do not overwork the paste. Remove from the food processor, place on a well-floured board and lightly work into a ball, then roll out to about 5mm/¼ inch thick. The pastry will be very soft. Lift it by wrapping it around the rolling pin, then use to line a 28cm/11 inch tart tin. Don't worry if it tears; just patch it up with spare pieces of pastry. Chill for half an hour.

Preheat the oven to 200°C/400°F/Gas Mark 6. Prick the base of the pastry randomly with a fork, cover with greaseproof paper and fill with dry rice or beans (this will prevent the pastry bubbling up). Bake for about 15–20 minutes, until the edges are crisp and the base of the pastry dry. You may want to lift away the paper and beans for the last 5 minutes of cooking so the base can dry out.

Remove the pastry case from the oven and leave to cool. Meanwhile, make the frangipane. Melt the butter and sugar together over a low heat, stirring with a spoon or whisk, and then cook for 2–3 minutes, until the mixture has a golden fudge consistency. Remove from the heat, add the ground almonds and the beaten eggs and stir until well combined.

Turn the oven down to 190°C/375°F/Gas Mark 5. Spread the Quince Cheese over the base of the tart and pour the almond mixture on top. Scatter a few flaked almonds over the surface and bake for 15–20 minutes, until the frangipane is just firm and slightly puffed. Eat hot or cold.

the squash family

Pumpkins and squashes of every shape and colour are now readily available in markets. The more unusual ones have their season in late September, and home-grown pumpkins are not usually in shops until mid-October, but you can buy butternut squash and orange-skinned Caribbean pumpkins all year round.

Creamy squash soup is lovely with a few pieces of crisp bacon or fried slices of peppered sausage (see page 128 for a basic soup recipe). Sometimes pumpkin soup can be unpleasantly sweet. Counteract this with extra garlic and onion.

roasting squash and pumpkin

Peel and slice into 2cm wedges, season with salt and rub with sunflower or olive oil. Bake in a roasting tin at 220°C/425°F/Gas Mark 7 for 20–30 minutes until golden on the outside. Scatter with coriander leaves and serve with sour cream on the side.

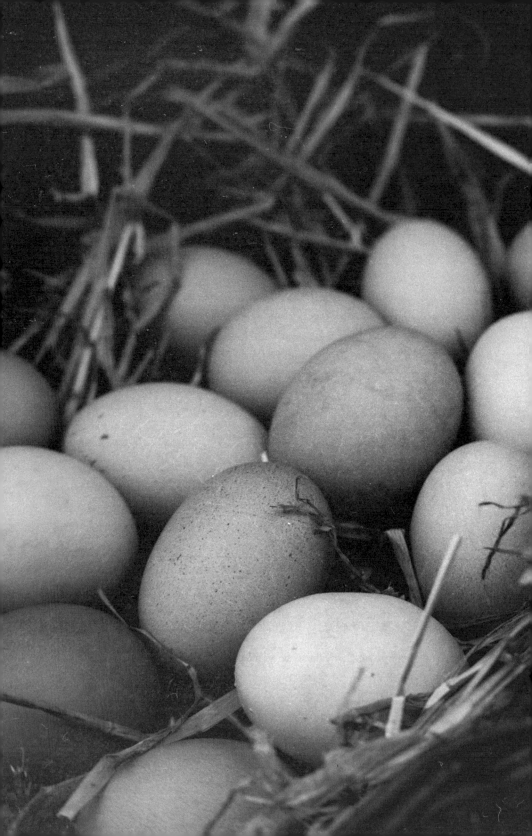

9
eggs

I always think of the egg as food's conjurer. It can use its bag of tricks to perform extraordinary feats in recipes – to trap great air bubbles in a choux pastry bun, gel a light fresh cheesecake, or to lift a buttery sponge. In soufflés egg white transforms a heavy blend of yolks, butter, flour and cheese into a high, airy mousse. Beaten into sauces the yolks disperse into a million droplets and hold on to fat, making velvety mayonnaise or a rich hollandaise. And even in its purest form, boiled or poached, a good egg from a well-bred, well-fed hen is impossibly delicious.

But a good egg can be hard to find. Who in the Western world was not shown, at some point in their childhood, an illustrated tale set in a farmyard? If all you had to go on was the storybook, you would imagine that every farmer keeps black and white cows in wooden barns, jolly pink pigs, white sheep, with brown hens running about in his bright green meadow. I was seven years old in 1969, the year that not one single commercial free-range egg farm existed in the UK. As far as I was concerned Old MacDonald had a farm and on that farm he had some hens. *Some* hens? The farm that produced my egg in its Peter Rabbit eggcup would have had several thousand of them, immobile and caged in a shed. Oh, and as for Peter Rabbit, I was always on Mr McGregor's side in that one. We grew vegetables in our garden.

It was only in the 1990s that free-range egg farming took off again on a commercial scale. At the time of writing, just 3 per cent of British egg farms allow their hens to roam totally free. Standard free-range eggs make up 27 per cent of the market. Welfare for standard free-range hens is a great improvement on those kept in cages, though their conditions are still a far cry from those in storybooks. Battery eggs now make up 60 per cent of the market (10 per cent are imported), and the remaining 10 per cent are barn eggs – that is, from hens that are kept loose indoors, although their welfare is debatable as they can be very densely stocked.

But still the educators are peddling fantasies. My children are taken on school trips to city farms where they see little wooden hutches housing a handful of well-exercised rare-breed birds. Imagine if they were shown the places where the majority of eggs come from. Would it be kind? No, but at least it would be accurate. Viewed another way, if a method of farming is so revolting that you cannot show it to children, should it exist at all? I don't think so, but that's because I know that a good egg laid in natural circumstances is valuable, in the same way that meat from naturally reared livestock is valuable.

hens

When I think of eggs, I always think how much I like hens. Given the chance, I could spend hours watching these almost prehistoric creatures strutting and pecking about.

They are decorative, noisy and fascinating, and will nobly continue to lay even after each egg is taken from them.

The relationship between humans and hens goes back more than 4000 years. They were the hunter-gatherer's perfect food provider, supplying regular gifts of protein encased in a hygienic wrapping. It's no wonder that humans have made eggs symbols of birth and renewal in religion and art – no wonder the great jeweller, Fabergé, immortalised their form and covered them with diamonds and rubies.

Look at the way we care for our hens now. Most are kept in battery egg farms. There they spend short, miserable lives captive in a cage with floor space no larger than a sheet of A4 paper – just 550 square centimetres. Left to their own devices hens lay between 60 and 180 eggs each year, but selective breeding and special techniques in battery farms – such as 24-hour lighting, to create a perpetual day – have seen hens laying 280 eggs each year. They lay egg after egg after egg until they are worn out – usually within 17 months. It is as if hens, once a prized farmyard beast, have become no more than machines, to be disposed of once worn out, and replaced with ease.

For a hen to be happy she must be able to perch whenever she feels vulnerable, forage for food, preen her feathers and take dust baths. She should also be able to build a nest. This totally natural behaviour is denied to the caged hen. Her feet can become caught in the wire floor of the cage, preventing her from reaching her water and food supply. Hens kept this way become aggressive, attacking each other through the mesh of their cages. To prevent hens from harming each other, battery farmers use a hot blade to cut off the sharp point of their beaks. On commercial egg farms, both battery and free-range, hens live on average for just 72 weeks. Premature death and slaughter when egg laying slows are given as reasons for this shortened lifespan.

To cheer myself up, I think of the following experience of a dairy farmer friend, John Sansom. Walking into a barn one day, he noticed something moving in the corner. It was a hen, barely feathered and shivering, with each foot encased in thick boots of chicken muck. It turned out that the lorry that transported the waste from a nearby battery egg farm had passed through the village. Somehow this hen, which had been scooped up with the muck at the farm, had managed to jump off the lorry. Sansom spent hours washing the mess from her feet, then let her loose with the motley collection of chickens, guinea fowl and geese that roamed his garden. Henny grew a magnificent set of feathers and rewarded the Sansoms by out-laying all her companions. She came to a sad end when a fox broke into the chicken pen one night and took her, but it made a lot more sense than being swept out with the battery farm's sewage.

the cost of half a dozen eggs

The cost of an egg varies hugely. At the time of writing prices are as follows:

Battery eggs (British)	61 pence
Battery eggs (imported)	59 pence
Standard free-range eggs	81 pence
Totally free-range eggs	£1.20
Organic totally free-range eggs	£1.50
Eggs sold at the farm gate/food co-operative (see the Shopping Guide).	80 pence

But it can be difficult to know what you are paying for.

cheap eggs are expensive

Battery farming is a consequence of the post-war drive to produce cheap food, and plenty of it. After the Second World War and years of rationing factory farming was seen to be food's way forward. Hen cages were invented in the 1930s but not widely used until the early 1960s. The automated egg battery came after 1956, when drugs were developed that prevented hens kept in high densities from developing the disease coccidiosis. As a result eggs became cheap, and they still are.

People who support battery egg farming say it provides budget protein to those who cannot afford better. But there's more than one way to eat inexpensive protein. What about peanut butter, hummus and dal? I would argue that cheap eggs are expensive. The former Health Minister Edwina Currie was not wrong when she told the country in 1988 that British egg farming was infested with salmonella bacteria. It was there, and it was the consequence of packing too many birds into a small space. Salmonella poisoning, and the ensuing clean-up, cost the taxpayer millions.

The association of salmonella with eggs continues in many people's minds, so it is worth knowing that 80 per cent of British hens are now vaccinated against it, and instances of food poisoning have come down dramatically. Eggs from vaccinated hens carry the Red Lion stamp on their shells and boxes. But bear in mind that disease in egg farming is a clear symptom of poor husbandry, namely overcrowding. Buying non-vaccinated eggs from a responsible farmer who gives his hens plenty of room to move is a salmonella-safe, positive choice.

If shoppers come to decide that battery farming is unacceptable, in any form, then eggs must become a food that we pay more for, and eat less of. Eggs laid by totally free-range hens, with spacious night shelter and drug-free supplementary feed, are valuable; a food to respect as much as it would have been by the earliest civilisations. I am happy to eat a good egg in place of meat, and happy to pay for the privilege. A good egg from a hen that is farmed totally naturally may cost significantly more than the factory farmed alternative, but it also has a firmer, thicker yolk and tastes so much better. Cooking with eggs this good takes on greater meaning: even a boiled egg is a luxurious indulgence. So vote for good eggs with your money, because the supermarkets will take note.

good eggs?

So how do you find a good egg? An alternative to battery farms is offered by the free-range system of egg farming. Yet on investigation the level of welfare varies hugely. They can be kept indoors and out. Space for each bird can differ. The legal minimum is 1000 hens per hectare outdoors (395 per acre), or 11 hens per square metre in barns, which is not much. At the other end of the scale is the free-range hen kept in a vast field where it's free to peck about, eating an assortment of grasses, wild plants and seeds, and pulling those all-important grubs from the ground, which give eggs their flavour.

There are seven separate bodies that issue organic certification in the UK. Of these, the Soil Association is recognised as the main independent body, with the most demanding criteria, particularly for animal welfare. Organic egg farms with Soil Association approval do not have more than six hens per square metre when they are in the hen houses, which is why they are so much more expensive.

the eggs to buy

If I did not live in a city I would keep hens. I often look at my copy of Ray Feltwell's *Small-scale Poultry Keeping* (Faber and Faber, 1980) and just wish and wish. Hens eat your leftover vegetables, and the reward in taste is great. When, in later life, my mother took to keeping her own hens, she fed them all her vegetable peelings, and you could actually taste the celery, pumpkin or spring greens in their eggs. A little band of Welsummers would be perfect for me – they do indeed lay the brownest eggs (although Maran owners would go to war over the question). But sadly the dream will have to wait.

If you want a boiled egg, look for the best you can find: you will taste the quality with every bite. Fortunately the variety of options is growing all the time. When commercial free-range farming was revived in the 1990s, farmers found the battery breeds too inactive and aggressive to be let loose. They had been bred to have shorter legs, found walking exhausting, and turned cannibal when left free to roam with other birds. As naturally produced eggs become more popular, old breeds are being revived or cross-bred to produce traditional-looking and -tasting eggs from rather more efficient, docile and leggy hens.

Now there are blue, olive and pink eggs from Cotswold Legbars, a Gloucestershire breed derived from a hen brought back from Patagonia in 1927 by the botanist Clarence Elliott. Stonegate Farms created the Columbian Blacktail, a mix of Rhode Island Red and Light Sussex, which is an outdoor-loving bird that will continue to lay throughout winter (traditional breeds tended to work to rule in cooler months).

Once again there are freckled eggs in eggcups, laid by a new cross of the old farmyard friend, the Speckled hen. Even eggs from old-style seasonal layers are popping up as well. I am looking forward to the revival of the Wodehousian Buff Orpington, or perhaps the notoriously inefficient layer, the Chilean Araucana. Now *that* would be an expensive egg.

When driving through the countryside I will often call in on a farm that advertises eggs on the roadside. If the hens are there to see, are healthy and having a good time, I buy. When I buy eggs in shops and supermarkets the words 'free range' are no longer enough. I follow the maxim that a responsible farmer will trumpet his good husbandry all over the box, or on signs in the shop where he sells his eggs. I am happy to read a positive litany of good news on packaging to know what I'm paying for.

the future of hens – and eggs

The present caging system in battery egg farms is due to be phased out. By 2012 batteries will be made illegal in the European Union's member states. The old A4-sized hutch will be replaced by a larger, intriguingly named 'enriched' cage, with a nesting space, a scratching spot and a perch. Several hens will share the enriched cage, however, so they must compete for access to the nesting space. Compassion in World Farming says the perch is too near the floor to make a satisfactory roosting place. Such an enriched cage represents the barest improvement, a bit like having an extra foot of leg room in a train carriage, but not being allowed to leave your seat: there won't be enough space to allow for stretching and wing flapping, and the birds will still get little exercise. While the cage will allow hens to be more sociable, this will itself create disturbance for laying hens. There are calls to scrap cages in Britain altogether, but in any event, the price of eggs in the EU will rise. Countries which over-produce eggs in the old factory-farming style will no doubt benefit.

It's harder to check the welfare and hygiene standards in overseas egg farms, and well-managed British egg farms need consumer support

– that means demanding British and paying more. Our gradually increasing standards of welfare and hygiene should be a comfort to shoppers.

New laws now require each egg to be stamped with its place of origin, so, if I can say so, read your eggs. At the time of writing 10 per cent of eggs eaten in Britain are imported, many in liquid form, from as far away as India, the USA and the Ukraine. These eggs 'hide' in ready-made or restaurant food. It seems a shame, when Britain has the capacity to be egg self-sufficient.

alternative eggs

Much as I love hen's eggs, there are other delicious eggs to choose from.

* Duck eggs – You will often see duck eggs for sale on the roadside because people love to keep these prolific layers as pets. They produce lovely eggs that can be substituted for hen's eggs; indeed, all the recipes in this chapter are suitable for duck eggs too. They taste the same as hen's, only richer, and best come into their own in a cake or soufflé, but are also wonderful hard-boiled. As duck eggs weigh more than hen's, you should increase their cooking time by a quarter when boiling them and use approximately one third less in recipes (see Shopping Guide).

* Goose eggs – They're very large and very rich, but many people love them, including my son, Jack. He went through a phase of eating one of these giants, soft-boiled with toast, for tea (see the Shopping Guide). 'Just how big is a goose egg?' a curious visitor once asked. Jack, who was five at the time, replied, 'Fucking big.' Quite.

* Gull's eggs – They have a rich, reddish-yellow yolk and pretty, blue speckled shells, and their flavour is sublime – delicate and rare as wild salmon. They are wild and only available – where you can find them – for about four weeks of the year, between mid-May and mid-June. Gull's egg gatherers hold licences to gather eggs in certain places, in a government-regulated scheme to prevent

plunder from any unsustainable source. As a consequence, they're extremely expensive, averaging at £2 each, but if, like me, you take the view that every delicacy must be tried once, do so when the opportunity arises. Licensed game dealers sometimes sell gull's eggs, as do some old-fashioned fishmongers because the eggs are often sold by wholesalers at Billingsgate fish market (see the Shopping Guide). Usually they are sold ready boiled, but should you find a raw supply, to cook them, prick each egg with a pin on its rounded end, and plunge into boiling water for seven minutes – they should be firm. Peel away their shells, and eat with celery salt mixed with soft sea salt and a few specks of cayenne pepper.

✳ Quail's eggs – Do not be fooled by their wild appearance. Most quail's eggs come from housed birds. Commercial free-range quail farming is struggling to get off the ground because these birds are unpredictable layers if they don't have the right habitat. As with the re-emergence of free-range chicken farms, successful free-range farming of quails may come with new breeds. But just occasionally free-range quail's eggs pop up in farm shops or farmers' markets (see the Shopping Guide). Seize them when you see them. The creamy, savoury flavour of quail's eggs sprinkled with sea salt is incomparable. Incidentally, treating them like hen's eggs and frying or poaching them is a gimmick: just not worth the bother.

storing eggs

All types of raw egg have a long shelf life. As long as it's stored at a constant temperature, an egg will keep for a month. You can keep them in or out of the fridge, but in summer the fridge is best. Make sure they're clean, and if you buy them from the farm gate, wash off any dirt. Always keep them away from unwrapped raw meat or dairy products.

Hard- and semi-soft-boiled eggs keep for about a week, refrigerated and unshelled. They're precious for sandwiches, and you can also separate whites and yolks and chop them very finely or mimosa them, that is, push them through a sieve to scatter over salads or vegetables. Hard-boiled egg yolks make a delicious egg and herb sauce (see page 395).

Raw egg yolks do not freeze well, but will keep for four days in a sealed container in the fridge. Add half a teaspoon of water to stop them drying out. After two days or more, only use them in recipes where they will be cooked. Raw egg whites last far longer: up to two weeks in a sealed container in the fridge. They can also be frozen for up to six weeks. I use a system whereby I keep adding them to a container in the freezer, then defrost the whole lot to make, say, a lot of meringues or macaroons for a party. A medium egg white weighs 30g/1oz and the yolk weighs 20g/⅔oz.

plain boiled eggs

Even the best eggs crack sometimes when they are put in boiling water. To prevent this, prick the rounded end of the shell with a pin; this provides a vent for the air to escape from a cold egg when it is added to the water.

cooking times for medium-sized hen's eggs

> Lightly boiled (soft yolk, soft white): add to boiling water and
> cook for 3 minutes
> Soft boiled (soft yolk, firm white): add to boiling water and
> cook for 4½ minutes
> Semi-soft boiled (semi-soft yolk, hard white): add to cold
> water, bring to the boil, then cook for 5 minutes
> Hard boiled (hard yolks, hard whites): add to cold water, bring
> to the boil, then cook for 7 minutes

I add salt to the water when boiling eggs. If anything 'escapes' during boiling, the salt keeps it to a minimum. Remove the eggs from the pan after cooking. I always tap them on the pointed end to prevent further cooking.

While very fresh eggs are best for frying, poaching and making omelettes, eggs that are at least a week old are best for hard boiling, as they peel easily. If you boil an egg that has been laid that day, the white will stick to the shell.

soft-boiled eggs with purple sprouting broccoli

A good-quality soft-boiled egg in a cup acts as a sauce for seasonal green vegetables. The broccoli is boiled for just a few minutes so it keeps its crunch. On a rainy day, however, toast soldiers are the alternative.

Serves 4

16 spears of purple sprouting broccoli
4 medium eggs
soft sea salt crystals and freshly ground black pepper

Bring some water to the boil in a large pan, add a pinch of salt and boil the broccoli for about 4 minutes. Remove one spear and cut through the lower part of the stalk to test; it should be just tender, not soft. Drain and set aside on a cloth or kitchen paper.

Soft-boil the eggs (see page 380), then drain and put each into an eggcup. Take the tops off the eggs using a knife – a quick tap on the shell and cut through, an action that brings mothers to mind. Serve on a plate, the broccoli piled to one side, salt and pepper nearby.

✳ kitchen note ✳

You could use goose eggs for the same purpose, as an offering with drinks. Prick the eggs and boil them for 10 minutes. Season the yolks with a little celery salt and cayenne pepper to cut the richness.

the boiled egg store

This is a way to save time or use up leftover hard-boiled eggs from other meals. Boiling a few eggs to the semi-soft or hard stage at the beginning of the week will be a useful squirrel store that you can dip into for quick lunches, work picnics and starters for dinner. Unshelled boiled eggs keep for five days in the fridge. The following recipes are for semi-soft and hard-boiled eggs.

open egg sandwiches

A lunch and summer supper dish – or, forgive stating the obvious, stick a second slice of bread on top and it will travel.

Serves 2

2 eggs

butter

2 thin slices of wholemeal bread

1 punnet of mustard and cress, or a few stalks of watercress

or rocket

cayenne pepper

salt and freshly ground black pepper

Boil the eggs until semi-soft or hard (see page 380), whatever you prefer. Drain and leave to cool. Butter the bread and put it on plates. Pile up the cress on each slice. Peel and chop the eggs and put them on top. Twist pepper and throw salt on to the egg, with a few grains of cayenne pepper.

cold boiled eggs with herb mayonnaise

Bright, shiny green sauce on the white of an egg, with the fresh flavour of herbs. I eat these beside cold roast beef with a watercress salad.

Serves 6

6 eggs

For the herb mayonnaise:
2 egg yolks
1 tablespoon capers, chopped
leaves from 4 sprigs of tarragon, torn
leaves from 4 sprigs of basil, torn
about 10 chives, chopped
150ml/¼ pint sunflower or olive oil
salt

Boil the eggs until semi-soft (see page 380), cool them under the tap and peel them. Cut them in half lengthways and put them on a plate.

To make the mayonnaise, put the egg yolks in a small ceramic or glass bowl (metal bowls can discolour the sauce), add the capers and herbs, then a few drops of the oil. Stir with a wooden spoon until well blended, then add a few drops more. Continue until the oil is used up – you will find as you go that you can add it slightly quicker and the sauce will not split or curdle.

Add a little salt, taste the sauce, then put a teaspoonful on to each half egg.

✳ **kitchen note** ✳

Keep the raw egg whites. You can use them for making meringues (see page 404), or whisk them through boiling stock to remove impurities – the method for clarifying stock (see page 117).

semi-soft-boiled eggs and lettuce hearts

Simplicity and beauty on a plate. You will need 1 egg and 1 small lettuce heart per person. The outer leaves of the lettuce can be used for soup (see page 129).

Serves 4

4 eggs

4 romaine or Cos lettuce hearts, quartered

For the dressing:

1 tablespoon Dijon mustard

1 tablespoon white wine vinegar

3 tablespoons olive or sunflower oil

2 tablespoons water

a pinch of salt

a pinch of sugar

freshly ground black pepper.

Boil the eggs until semi-soft (see page 380), then drain and cool under the tap. Peel and cut into quarters lengthways.

Whisk together all the dressing ingredients. Put the lettuce in a deep bowl and pour over the dressing. Stir or toss thoroughly. Put the quartered eggs on top and eat with bread.

You could add bacon, fried over a low heat for 10 minutes until crisp, if you wish.

boiled eggs mimosa with summer vegetables

You have to rid your mind of the image of a boiled egg in salad that came too close to the beetroot and got a nasty pink stain, then drowned in a pool of watery cucumber. Think instead of a mixture of blanched summer vegetables – broad beans, runner beans, dwarf French beans, mangetout – with finely chopped egg whites and mimosa yolks strewn on top. Mimosa is the culinary term that describes an easy yet grand way to chop hard-boiled egg yolks by pushing them through a sieve.

Serves 4

3 eggs
about 700g/1½lb mixed green vegetables – broad beans, runner
beans, dwarf French beans, mangetout (or use purple sprouting
broccoli in winter/early spring)
5 tablespoons extra virgin olive oil
juice of 1 lemon
salt and freshly ground black pepper

Hard-boil the eggs (see page 380), then drain and cool. Bring a large pan of water to the boil, add a pinch of salt, then the vegetables, and blanch them for 1 minute. Drain and splash with cold water to set the green colour. Toss with the olive oil and lemon juice and season with salt and pepper.

Peel the eggs and separate the whites from the yolks. Chop the whites finely and scatter them over the salad. Push the hard yolks through a metal or nylon sieve, allowing them to drop on to the vegetables, then serve.

roasted pepper mimosa on baked bread

Cooked egg yolk and roasted peppers are a wonderful combination. I buy canned wood-roasted peppers from Spanish shops for this (see the Shopping Guide). They are cheaper and better than Dutch peppers, which you will have to spend ages roasting and peeling.

Serves 4

4 slices of stale white bread

virgin olive oil

2 eggs

8 pieces of canned wood-roasted red peppers

a few parsley leaves

soft sea salt and freshly ground black pepper

Preheat the oven to 220°C/425°F/Gas Mark 7. Brush each slice of bread on both sides with oil and bake until crisp and lightly browned. Leave to cool to room temperature. Hard-boil the eggs (see page 380), then drain and cool.

Put the bread on 4 plates, lay 2 pieces of pepper on each and shake a small amount of oil over them. Peel the eggs and separate the whites from the yolks. Chop the whites finely and scatter them over the peppers. Push the yolks through a metal or nylon sieve, allowing them to drop on to the peppers, then season with salt and pepper and scatter the parsley leaves on top.

poached eggs

Poaching eggs is easy when they are very fresh, but if you do not know how old the eggs are it is incredibly frustrating cracking them into simmering water only to see the whites completely detach themselves from the yolks and dash off to the other side of the pan. The result is a terrible mess, with strings of white all over the place and a separate, waterlogged yellow ball.

Treat poached eggs, then, as something of a luxury. When you come across some eggs that you know have been laid within the week, make a note to poach them. Never use vinegar to bind the egg white, as it leaves an unpleasant flavour.

To poach eggs, bring about 5cm/2 inches of water to the boil in a wide, shallow pan and add a large pinch of salt. Crack an egg into a small bowl or a cup, hold it close to the gently simmering water and carefully tip it in. Allow it to cook slowly – it will take 3–4 minutes – until the white is firm and there is an opaque film over the yolk. Lift out with a slotted spoon or a fish slice and drain on kitchen paper or a clean cloth.

✳ kitchen note ✳

If your eggs are not very fresh, line a ramekin with cling film, crack in an egg and twist the cling film over the top to seal. Then lower into the water and poach as above. Drain and unwrap.

baked eggs

I can't write a book without including these hot little Sunday supper eggs. Butter, cream and eggs – but in such a small quantity you could almost allow yourself two. Sometimes I put sliced, canned wood-roasted peppers (see the Shopping Guide) in the bottom of the ramekins, for piquancy.

Serves 2

butter

2 large eggs

4 tablespoons double cream

leaves from one small sprig of tarragon, if available

salt and freshly ground black pepper

Preheat the oven to 220°C/425°F/Gas Mark 7. Butter 2 ramekins, crack an egg into each and season with salt and pepper. Add the tarragon, pour the cream on top, then place the ramekins in a roasting tin containing 2cm/¾ inch of boiling water. Place in the oven and cook for about 10–12 minutes, more if you like your eggs hard.

baked eggs and bacon

This is a supper I remember from childhood and remains something to come home to on a dark winter afternoon. It needs a small, shallow pan that can be used on the hob as well as in the oven, but investing in one is well worth it. The best are the French, Le Creuset-type enamelled pans measuring about 15cm/6 inches across. Hob and oven cooking gives the eggs and bacon a rustic edge – as if they have been cooked in a wood-fired oven.

Preheat the oven to 220°C/425°F/Gas Mark 7. Put 3 or more rashers of green or smoked back bacon in the pan with a tablespoon of lard and fry gently over a medium heat until the bacon is cooked on one side. Turn the bacon, crack in 2 or 3 large eggs, then transfer to the oven and bake until the whites are set.

baked eggs with sweet red peppers and tomatoes

The Tunisians call this *chakchouka*; it is a pepper and tomato casserole with eggs cooked in it. You could use fresh peppers and tomatoes but I see this as a store dish that can be thrown together, providing you keep the basic ingredients in the kitchen. Make it in a casserole pot with a lid.

Serves 4

2 tablespoons lard or olive oil

2 large onions, finely chopped

3 garlic cloves, chopped

2 canned wood-roasted peppers (see the Shopping Guide)

400ml/14fl oz Tomato Sauce (see page 358)

4 eggs

leaves from 4 sprigs of coriander or parsley

salt and freshly ground black pepper

Heat the fat in a flameproof casserole, add the onions and garlic and cook until soft but not brown. Add the peppers and tomato sauce, then bring to the boil and simmer for 5 minutes. Remove from the heat and season to taste. Make 4 wells in the stew with the base of a ladle and crack an egg into each one. Place over the heat, cover with a lid and cook until the whites are set. Scatter the herbs on top.

cooled scrambled egg on thin toasts

I serve these to line tummies when drinking before dinner. Made with good-quality eggs, they are perfect eaten on their own, but you can add a few chopped herbs (chervil, chives or dill) or mix in a little smoked trout or eel or sautéed black pudding. Alternatively try grating over a little bottarga (air-dried grey mullet roe). If you are in a hurry, pile the egg on to ordinary toast. Duck eggs make beautiful, deep-yellow scrambled eggs.

Serves 6–8

6 eggs

60g/2oz butter

2 tablespoons cream

sea salt

For the toasts:

6 slices of white bread (old bread is best)

60g/2oz melted butter, or 4 tablespoons olive oil

Toast the bread and cut off the crusts. Run a sharp serrated knife between the toasted sides of each slice until it separates into 2 very thin slices. Cut each one in half. Brush the uncooked side with melted butter or olive oil and place in a dry frying pan over a medium heat until it is crisp underneath. Set to one side.

Lightly beat the eggs and add a generous pinch of sea salt. Melt the butter in a non-stick pan over a low heat and add the eggs. Stir slowly, incorporating back into the scramble any egg that sets on the bottom of the pan. Keep going until the eggs are thick but still slightly runny, then immediately stir in the cream (at this stage you have traditional hot scrambled eggs). Set them to one side to cool.

Spoon a little heap of scrambled egg on to each toast and serve.

✳ kitchen note ✳

Use any remaining scrambled egg to make an open sandwich (see page 382).

soufflé

An overly scientific approach to cookery can take all the joy out of it. You can end up a slave to cookery books and measuring equipment. However, there are times when it helps to know not just how to cook something, but why ingredients behave in the way they do. And best of all, why soufflés rise.

The reason few people get into baking is because they have one disaster and decide there and then never to be humiliated again. If you are an occasional baker, it does help to have an understanding of the science behind pastry and bread, and it is worth knowing for a soufflé, too, because it is food too good *not* to be able to cook confidently. A soufflé provides a great opportunity to use up any soft or hard cheese. Once you know what you are about, try adding other things. Hard to believe, I know, but you can make the soufflé mixture in advance, right up to the point where it is ready to be put in the oven. Just freeze it until you need to use it. It will last for two weeks.

a few things you should know about making soufflé

✳ The oven must be the correct temperature, 200°C/400°F/Gas Mark 6 for a large dish. Individual dishes cook at the same temperature but you must reduce the cooking time.

✳ The egg whites should be beaten to a really stiff foam in a metal or ceramic bowl. Plastic bowls often have a slight grease on them, which softens the whites.

✳ A good, stiff foam will hold the bubbles of air, which expand during cooking, making the soufflé rise. If the foam is not really stiff, the bubbles will break, and the soufflé will not rise fully.

✳ Allow the base mixture to reach room temperature before folding in the whites. If any fat in the soufflé is warm, it will weigh down the whites.

✳ If you use cheese, do not let it melt in the base mixture before you bake the soufflé.

✳ Pour the mixture into the dish cleanly, because drips on the side of the dish can prevent the soufflé from rising evenly.

cheese soufflé

If you use a hard cheese, choose one with a nutty flavour, such as Gruyère. There is no British or Irish alternative to Gruyère or Emmental but I like to make soufflés with Coolea or Gubbeen, or a washed-rind cheese such as Bishop Kennedy.

Serves 4 as a starter, 2 as a main course

35g/1¼oz butter

30g/1oz plain flour

300ml/½ pint milk

a pinch of grated nutmeg

4 large eggs, separated

120g/4oz hard cheese, grated, or semi-soft cheese, finely chopped

1 teaspoon finely grated strong cheese, such as Parmesan

salt and freshly ground black pepper

Preheat the oven to 200°C/400°F/Gas Mark 6 – it must be hot for the soufflé to rise to its fullest – then butter a soufflé dish, about 20cm/8 inches in diameter. (You can cook your soufflé in individual dishes – my favourite size is 10cm/4 inches in diameter, 5cm/2 inches deep – cook at the same temperature but reduce the cooking time by 12–15 minutes.) Tie a piece of baking parchment around the outside of the dish to prevent an overflow.

Melt the butter in a saucepan and add the flour. Cook for a minute, until the mixture becomes gritty in texture. Gradually add the milk, stirring all the time. Bring to the boil, still stirring, and let it simmer for 3 minutes. Season with the nutmeg and some black pepper. Let the mixture cool to room temperature, then beat in the egg yolks and cheese (but not the Parmesan).

Whisk the egg whites with a pinch of salt until very stiff. Stir a heaped tablespoonful into the cheese mixture to loosen it, then gently fold in the remaining whites. Pour carefully into the soufflé dish and run a wet finger around the edge of the mixture to help the soufflé rise neatly. Dust the top with the finely grated Parmesan. Bake for 20–25 minutes, until the soufflé is well risen and still slightly wobbly. When you take it out, cut the string to remove the paper and take it straight to the table. Eat immediately.

egg sauces

There is a rightness to eating clean-tasting green vegetables with a rich yellow sauce made with eggs. The colours alone seem to say it's a perfect balance of all that is good. Picture a late-summer globe artichoke with a bowl of chopped egg and herbs, bound with olive oil, or a plate of asparagus with hollandaise poured across its spears. And then there is mayonnaise, either the strong-flavoured, green-tinged type made with virgin olive oil to eat with raw veg, or the paler mayonnaise that comes from lighter oil. The latter is the base for garlic or saffron and chilli mayonnaise.

mayonnaise

Always use a ceramic, stainless steel or glass bowl and a wooden spoon for making mayonnaise, or it may discolour.

Makes about 300ml/½ pint

3 egg yolks
2 teaspoons Dijon mustard
250ml/8fl oz ordinary olive oil, or ½ olive and ½ sunflower oil
juice of ½ lemon
sea salt and ground white pepper

Put the egg yolks and mustard in a small bowl and slowly add the oil, beating with a wooden spoon. Begin adding the oil drop by drop, but you can increase the flow as you go. The mixture will gradually get paler and heavier and should be a smooth emulsion.

When you have finished adding the oil, season with a squeeze of lemon juice and a little salt and pepper. Taste and add more if you think it needs it. Mayonnaise will keep in a sealed plastic container in the fridge for 4 days. Before use, bring to room temperature and give it a stir.

✳ kitchen notes ✳

✳ For economy, buy olive oil in large cans from home delivery companies or delis.

✳ Use leftover mayonnaise to make Potato Salad (see page 79). Alternatively, add it to mashed squash, parsnip or celeriac – it will be beautifully rich.

garlic mayonnaise

Known in the South of France as *aïoli*, this sauce is used for dipping raw vegetables or spooning over soup or *bourride*, a white fish stew.

Crush 2 garlic cloves with a pinch of sea salt (if there are green shoots in their centres, remove them), then follow the recipe for mayonnaise above, adding the garlic to the egg yolks instead of the mustard. Serve with sautéed squid or grilled fish, or with quartered lettuce hearts, whole baby carrots and radishes. Leave the leaves on so you have something to hold on to when dipping.

saffron and chilli mayonnaise

This is the sauce, known in France as *rouille*, for a fish broth made with the rough-and-ready oddities that are so often overlooked (see page 286). *Rouille* comes from the South of France but its ingredients bow to the land across the water – North Africa.

Put a large pinch of saffron strands into a small bowl and pour over a tablespoon of boiling water. Leave to steep for about 15 minutes.

Meanwhile, follow the recipe for mayonnaise above, adding 1 crushed garlic clove and about 1 tablespoon of finely chopped deseeded red chilli with the egg yolks. Strain the saffron water and add it to the mayonnaise after you have incorporated about half the oil.

✳ kitchen note ✳

You can use saffron powder for *rouille*. Available from Italian shops, it does not have such a strong flavour as pure saffron strands, but it saves a little time because you don't need to steep it.

an egg and herb sauce for summer vegetables

When there are gluts of asparagus, artichokes or leeks (especially early in the year when English leeks are small), serving them with this sauce will make them into a meal.

In the winter, use watercress to make the sauce, or even chopped spinach or chard leaves that have been plunged into boiling water for 30 seconds, then drained well. In the summer, use chopped parsley, chives, chervil, basil and tarragon.

Serves 4

4 eggs
chopped herbs or leaves, roughly the same volume as the eggs
150ml/¼ pint olive oil
1 teaspoon white wine vinegar or lemon juice
sea salt and freshly ground black pepper

Boil the eggs until semi-soft (see page 380), then drain and cool. Peel the eggs and chop them finely, but not to a mush. Mix in the herbs, then stir in the oil. Season with salt and pepper and stir in the vinegar or lemon juice.

hollandaise sauce

I make hollandaise in a food processor and no other way. I have no patience with volatile ingredients in double boilers, and the food processor makes a beautiful shiny sauce. Use the plastic blade, if there is one.

Serves 4

240g/8oz unsalted butter

4 egg yolks

lemon juice

sea salt

Gently melt the butter in a pan without letting it boil. Put the egg yolks into a food processor and switch it on so it runs continuously. Begin adding the melted butter through the feed tube a few drops at a time, then in a thin stream until it is all incorporated. Stop the machine, squeeze the juice of approximately ½ lemon into the sauce, then add a good pinch of sea salt. Whiz once more, and it is ready to serve with green vegetables or fish.

✳ kitchen notes ✳

✳ If you are not going to use the hollandaise sauce immediately, keep it in a Thermos flask for up to half an hour, because it must stay at the same temperature and is not easy to reheat.

✳ To make a citrus-flavoured hollandaise, add a handful of finely chopped sorrel leaves at the end. This is delicious with asparagus.

✳ Don't worry if leftover hollandaise splits when it cools; the basic ingredients are still valuable. Mix it with leftover mashed potato or other root vegetables and either bake it till golden, fry it in little patties or spoon it over fish in cream to make an instant fish pie.

duck egg omelette with spring vegetables

I specify using duck eggs for this picnic omelette because they have a nice habit of sticking to the vegetables. Using very fresh eggs will lighten the omelette. Include only one or two vegetables, in order to keep the flavours simple. Spring vegetables are good in omelettes – little broad beans or the green centres of large ones, asparagus, artichoke hearts, or Jersey or Cornish potatoes. In winter use cooked potatoes, squash, purple sprouting broccoli, canned artichoke hearts (in brine, not oil), frozen peas or the green centres of frozen broad beans that have been boiled for 1 minute.

Serves 4

2–3 tablespoons olive oil

5 eggs, beaten

700g/1½lb cooked vegetables (see above)

grated hard cheese, such as Saval, Somerset Rambler or

Pecorino, for dusting

salt and freshly ground black pepper

Heat the oil in a medium-sized frying pan – use one that you know will not stick. Season the beaten eggs and pour them into the pan. When the edges begin to cook, add the vegetables. Cook over a low to medium heat until the surface of the omelette is almost set, then place a plate upside down over the pan. Put your hand on top and quickly invert the pan and plate together so that the omelette falls on to the plate. Lift away the pan, turn it the right way up and slide the omelette back into it. Carry on cooking for 1–2 minutes, so it sets underneath, then slide the omelette on to a clean plate. Allow to cool, then dust with grated cheese and serve.

pancakes

Pancakes make a traditional pocket in which to recycle cold meat and vegetables left over from other meals. If everyone valued eggs highly, the number finding their way into pancake batter would be a matter of acute awareness. You would have to go back a long way to find a time when eggs were so precious that giving them up for Lent – along with all animal fats and meat – was still thought a great sacrifice. Then, what remained of the eggs, butter and cream were thrown into a batter for a pancake blowout. These days fasts are more likely to exclude chocolate, alcohol and cigarettes than humble eggs.

Perhaps it is no bad thing that pancakes' suitability as a fasting food is now less meaningful – it gives us an excuse to eat them more often.

pancakes

Makes 8–10

150g/5oz plain white flour (replace 1 tablespoon of the flour with buckwheat flour, if you wish)

1 egg

1 egg yolk

1 tablespoon sherry

1 tablespoon melted butter or vegetable oil

300ml/½ pint milk

a little butter or lard for frying

Sift the flour into a bowl, make a well in the centre and add the egg, egg yolk, sherry and melted butter or oil. Add about a quarter of the milk and whisk, drawing in the flour. When the paste is too thick to whisk, add more milk and whisk again. Gradually add all the milk in the same way – the whole point is to make a smooth, lump-free batter (you can always make it in a food processor). Leave it to rest for about half an hour.

Melt a little butter or lard in a 25cm/10 inch frying pan and pour in enough pancake mixture to cover the base thinly. Quickly tilt the pan so the mixture runs all over the surface, then cook over a medium-high heat until set. Lift the lacy edge of the pancake with a palette knife, then flip it over – practised cooks can toss them with the flick of a wrist – and cook for about 1 minute longer. Store pancakes, one on top of the other, in the fridge for up to 5 days or in the freezer for up to 4 weeks.

things to put inside pancakes

cauliflower and fresh goat's cheese

These pancakes are a lighter take on cauliflower cheese, and make use of cooked cauliflower, perhaps left over from another meal. Look for a soft British goat's cheese with a fresh aroma, such as Chabis or Golden Cross. The goat's cheeses sold in small cartons in supermarkets are fine. Alternatively, try the soft British ewe's milk cheese, Flower Marie. These cheeses will not heat to a runny melt but to a nice, soft, cakey texture.

You could also substitute chopped field mushrooms, sautéed in a little oil, for the cauliflower.

Serves 4

240g/8oz fresh goat's cheese

4 egg yolks

a pinch of grated nutmeg

2 egg whites

4 pancakes (see previous page)

240g/8oz cooked cauliflower, broken into florets

15g/½oz hard cheese, such as Saval, Somerset Rambler,

Cheddar or Pecorino, grated

soft sea salt and freshly ground black pepper

Preheat the oven to 190°C/375°F/Gas Mark 5 and butter an ovenproof dish that will accommodate 4 rolled pancakes. Mix together the cheese and egg yolks and season with the nutmeg and some pepper. Whisk the egg whites with a pinch of salt until stiff and fold them into the cheese mixture. Fill each pancake first with the cauliflower and then with the cheese mixture, roll them up loosely and place in the baking dish side by side. Sprinkle the grated cheese on top and bake for 20 minutes. They will puff up, browning on the surface. Serve immediately, a green salad to one side.

chicken, broad bean and tarragon

Very rich stuffed pancakes, for a supper dish.

Serves 4

30g/1oz butter

30g/1oz plain flour

150ml/¼ pint chicken stock

a pinch of grated nutmeg

150ml/¼ pint double cream

4 sprigs of tarragon, chopped

2 egg yolks

240g/8oz roast chicken (or pheasant), cut into bite-sized pieces

8 heaped tablespoons frozen broad beans, the green centres only
(see page 80)

4 pancakes (see page 398)

15g/½oz hard cheese, such as Saval, Somerset Rambler or
Pecorino, grated

salt and freshly ground black pepper

Preheat the oven to 190°C/375°F/Gas Mark 5 and butter an ovenproof dish that will accommodate 4 rolled pancakes. Melt the butter in a small saucepan and add the flour. Cook for 1 minute, until the texture is gritty, then remove from the heat and slowly add the stock, stirring or whisking all the time so the sauce is lump free. Season with nutmeg and black pepper, bring to the boil, stirring, and simmer for 3 minutes to 'cook out' the flour. Add the cream and tarragon, whisk in the egg yolks and taste for seasoning.

Divide the meat and beans between the pancakes, pour over some of the sauce and roll them up. Place side by side in the baking dish and pour over the remaining sauce. Dust with the grated cheese and bake for about 20 minutes, until browned on top.

pancakes for pudding

Use the recipe above to make pancakes for puddings or teatime. A cheat's version of *crêpe Suzette* follows. Make a butter cream – equal quantities of sieved icing sugar and unsalted butter – and work the zest of an orange or lemon into it. Place a blob in the centre of one quarter of an open pancake. Fold into a fan shape. Repeat with 6 pancakes. Squeeze the juice from the orange, put in a large frying pan with 30g/1oz butter and melt together over a medium heat. When it bubbles, fry each pancake on either side for 1 minute. The edges should crisp as the butter cream melts inside. Remove to a warm plate and repeat with the other pancakes. You should be able to fit more than one pancake in the pan at a time. Eat the pancakes with crème fraîche or vanilla ice cream.

puddings made with eggs

custard

The happiness scale of custard memories is a good way to judge the generosity of the cooks in your childhood. Cornflour is a useful stabiliser if you want the custard to keep. I make custard and store it in the fridge for children's meals and for making ice cream.

Makes about 600ml/1 pint

600ml/1 pint whole milk

1 teaspoon vanilla extract

1 tablespoon cornflour

6 egg yolks

1–2 tablespoons golden caster sugar

Put the milk and vanilla in a pan and heat to boiling point. In a bowl, whisk together the cornflour, egg yolks and sugar until smooth. Slowly pour in the hot milk, whisking all the time. Return the mixture to the pan and reheat, stirring, until it thickens. Pour into a container, cover with greaseproof paper and leave to cool. Store in the fridge for 3 days.

✳ kitchen note ✳

Bird's custard is one of the few sauce mixes I use, partly because the addition of a little cream and vanilla sugar works magic, but also because its inventor, Alfred Bird, created it in 1837 out of love for his wife, who was unable to eat eggs. Irresistible.

making ice cream

Once you have your store of custard, making a rich ice cream is simple. Stir melted chocolate into custard until you have the richness you want and freeze until solid. Alternatively mash mango, banana or passion fruit flesh, mix with the custard and freeze. You can do the same with raspberries, loganberries and strawberries; orange flesh and zest; or Lemon Curd (see page 405) mixed with whipped double cream and broken meringues (see page 404).

baked pear custard

An easy pudding that uses up ripe or unripe pears.

Serves 4

4 eggs

120g/4 oz caster sugar

20g/¾oz plain flour

small pinch salt

100ml/3½fl oz whole milk

150ml/5floz single cream

half teaspoon vanilla extract

4 pears, peeled, cored and quartered

15g/½oz butter

icing sugar for dusting

Preheat the oven to 200°C/400°F/Gas Mark 6. Whisk the eggs and sugar together until pale and fluffy; then beat in the flour with the salt. You should have a smooth batter. Add the milk, cream and vanilla, whisking constantly. Butter a shallow rectangular baking tin and lightly dust it with flour.

Arrange the pears in the dish, pour over the custard mixture and bake for about 25 minutes, until it is just set, puffed up and golden. Remove from the oven, allow to cool, then dust with a little icing sugar.

✳ kitchen note ✳

If you have dregs of brandy, Calvados or pear liqueur in the drink store, marinate the quartered pears in a tablespoon or two for a grown-up pudding.

meringues

If you have a store of egg whites, you can put it to good use by making meringues. Rather than attempt to remember how many are in the container, write the number on the side. If you forget you could always weigh the whites. Put a bowl on the weighing scales and then add the egg whites. A medium egg white weighs about 30g/1oz. It is easier to work in grams – just divide your total weight by three, and subtract a nought. You will then know how many whites you have. Incidentally, egg yolks weigh about 20g/⅔oz.

easy meringue

So called because there is no need to fold the sugar into the meringue halfway through and risk losing those stiff peaks. I have used this recipe for years, adding unsalted pistachio nuts, dried fruit, cocoa powder or even raspberries, and believe it to be indestructible. It cooks faster, too – meringue within an hour.

> 4 egg whites
>
> 270g/9oz golden icing sugar

Preheat the oven to 150°C/300°F/Gas Mark 2. Put the egg whites and sugar in a clean, dry bowl (don't use a plastic one, as they can be greasy) and beat with the whisk attachment of an electric food mixer or hand-held electric beater until the mixture is foamy and stiff. This will take about 10 minutes, so don't even try to use a hand whisk.

Spoon the meringue on to baking trays lined with baking parchment, either in small dollops for individual meringues or 2 large discs for a cake. Remember that it will spread as it cooks, so leave room between individual meringues. Cook for 35–45 minutes, until crisp, then remove from the oven and leave to cool. Eat with cream or ice cream, or fresh fruit (save broken meringues for lemon meringue ice cream, see page 402).

✳ **kitchen note** ✳

Freestanding electric mixers are wonderful machines for committed cooks who want to invest, but a handheld electric beater is a good, economical starter tool that can be stored in a cupboard.

lemon curd

Lemon curd made at home with the best eggs is twice as good as shop bought. You can make it with whole eggs or use up egg yolks. It is lovely spread on fresh bread or English muffins, and is also a useful store cupboard item – a vital ingredient of lemon meringue ice cream (see page 402).

Makes 2 pots

4 lemons
360g/12oz golden granulated sugar
120g/4oz unsalted butter, diced
4 eggs or 8 egg yolks, beaten

Scrub the lemons, grate the zest very finely and mix it with the sugar. Squeeze the juice from the lemons. Place a bowl over a pan of simmering water, making sure the water is not touching the base of the bowl. Tip in the sugar and zest, plus the butter, lemon juice and eggs. Stir slowly with a wooden spoon until the mixture is thick enough to coat the back of the spoon. Strain through a sieve, pour into sterilised jars and seal.

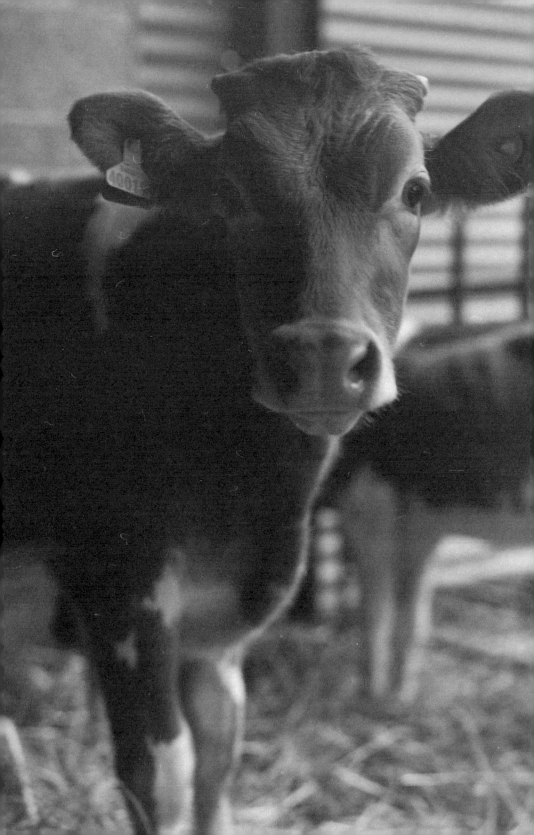

10
dairy

If much of this book is about getting more from the better-quality food you buy, this chapter is about voting power – the clout contained in the shopper's wallet. We can't avoid knowing there are problems in the food chain: the media constantly tell us so, in increasingly alarmist language. There has been gradual improvement in certain areas, but we could wait all century for politicians, big food businesses and supermarkets to bring about any more radical change. However, the simple act of walking into a shop and asking for the food you want, made the way you want it, will make an enormous difference.

This approach is especially relevant to dairy foods because, not to put too fine a point on it, dairy is one of the most disturbing areas of the food chain. Milk is no longer a whole food but a processed drink. And this impacts on all dairy products, because before there can be tangy cheese, silky yoghurt, cream or even veal, there must be milk. So it makes sense to find out why milk production has altered so much over the last fifty years.

Almost all milk sold in the UK has been pasteurised, that is, heat-treated to kill harmful bacteria, and in the main for very good reason. But before it even reaches that stage nearly every bottle of milk sold in Britain, even whole milk, is skimmed to a standard level of fat, then homogenised – that is, whizzed in a centrifuge so that the fat that once sat on the top of the milk is dispersed throughout it, before being pasteurised. To do all this, then pack and deliver the milk to supermarket, costs the milk processor five to six pence per litre.

Farmers do not benefit from this elaborate process. The price they are paid for their milk is dismal. On average one litre of milk costs the consumer 50 pence, a fair price were it not for the fact that the farmer typically receives little more than a third of it. Depending on the season, they receive an average of 18 pence per litre, when the cost of producing it runs at between 21 and 22 pence, which makes a loss of 3 to 4 pence per litre.

Many dairy farmers, particularly the little guys, are going out of business, selling their herds to larger farms. They can then produce more milk and just about survive on the margins. It is predicted that without an improvement in the price paid for milk all but the largest dairy farms will eventually give up.

It was not ever thus. In 2003 the Farmers' Union of Wales calculated that farmers need to produce three times as much milk to buy a tractor in this decade as they did in the 1950s. It's hard for farmers to negotiate a better deal when the buying power is concentrated in the hands of four dairy giants, and the business seems to be consolidating all the time. The dairy giants blame the supermarkets for the low prices farmers get paid, while the supermarkets blame the dairies.

It's frustrating to witness how popular Fairtrade bananas, coffee and tea have become with shoppers and supermarkets while plenty of unfair trade goes on, largely unnoticed, in our own back yard.

animal welfare

It is fair to say that small dairy farms are the most welfare friendly (there are, of course, a few exceptions). On smaller farms the farmer or herdsman can look after each cow personally. He will know what kind of milker she is, be familiar with her behaviour in the herd, and know how to get the best out of her. In general, the bigger the herd, the more mechanised is the milking process – and the less the herdsmen are hands-on. As the old farmer's saying goes: you can 'shepherd' 250 sheep, 'look to' 500 and 'look at' 750.

milk across the pond

There are other powerful reasons why we do not want milk and other dairy foods to become the exclusive domain of big dairy business. In the United States dairy farms are very big indeed and milk is cheap. These farms are profitable because it is common practice to add protein-rich grains and a bovine growth hormone (rBGH) to cows' feed, boosting milk production by one third. Increased lactation can tire the cow and cause repeated attacks of the infection mastitis. These cows can be milked up to four times a day and live an average of five years when, with natural methods of husbandry, they could survive into their teens. The EU has resisted the introduction of rBGH into the European dairy industry – so far. Further consolidation of the dairy industry in Europe will threaten this resistance.

raw milk

You're lucky if you can find a source of raw, unpasteurised milk. It is by law only available at the farm gate, and the farmer must pay for regular tests against harmful bacteria if it is to be sold as green top. Bottles of raw milk carry health warnings akin to those found on packets of cigarettes, and successive governments of all political persuasions have attempted to ban the sale of it. But records of illness caused by bacteria in milk show that there is no greater threat from raw milk than pasteurised. And without raw milk, we would not have over a third of the exciting new British artisan cheeses. Incidentally, because heat treatment damages the protein structure, pasteurised milk goes off quicker than raw milk, which keeps for up to ten days in my fridge.

renaissance cheese

During the Second World War cheese-making on British farms was banned to satisfy the need for milk powder to feed the forces. Before the war Britain could boast 1,500 farmhouse cheesemakers. By 1945 only 126 remained. The ban was lifted after the war ended, but by then, a shortage of experienced cheesemakers meant that much of the precise, slow art of artisan cheese-making had fallen from use.

In the early 1980s there was a renewed interest in British cheeses. The hard work of gurus, especially the exceptional Randolph Hodgson of Neal's Yard Dairy, has helped to bring about a revival. Twenty years ago he tracked down the few farmers that still made cheese and encouraged them to keep going, offering them a market in London. He sold their cheese in his now-famous shop in Covent Garden. Then enterprising dairy farmers noticed that these cheese-makers could not meet the growing demand and set about learning how to make cheese. There are now over 220 artisan cheesemakers at work in Britain producing 450 different cheeses, 170 of which are made with raw milk. Many of these are set to become classics. I list some of the best in the cheese section below.

These cheeses are a revelation eaten alone. Why cook when you can eat a good piece of cheese with bread or a salad? But then some of them melt extremely well, too. Recipe books habitually use Continental cheeses, but we now have cheeses that eat and cook just as well as Gruyère and Vacherin, Pecorino and Manchego, and Fontina. It begs the question why do we need to buy cheese that has travelled a thousand miles? Encouraging, with the vote in your wallet, supermarkets and shops to sell more British cheese, and in turn, inspiring beleaguered dairy farmers to make more cheese, will help dig British dairy farmers out of their post-war grave.

butter

While few things can be nicer for breakfast than fresh butter spread on to good bread, the greatest pleasure to be had from butter is in cooking. Even in small quantities it gives a sublime, savoury flavour to hot food. Think baked or waxy new potatoes, asparagus and shellfish. The basic ingredient of butter is ripened cream that has been skimmed off the milk. The cream is churned until the fat inside it begins to amalgamate, at the same time blending with the water that naturally occurs in the cream. But as with all dairy foods, butter varies. The same principles apply when buying the best butter as for any other dairy product. Butter made on the farm, using milk from cows that feed naturally on pasture, silage or hay, will always have the finest flavour. Obviously butter of this quality is not always easily available. I have a particular weakness for the beautiful creamy butters of France, but farm-made British butter is a good choice too. While on the subject of imports, be careful when reading labels to check for the words 'blended butter' or 'produce of more than one country'. There is no telling where the butter in these packs comes from, nor can you be sure about the welfare and feed of the animals that have produced it.

cream

Cream is a changed food. Once it was skimmed or separated from the milk, then left to ripen before refrigeration, developing a flavour not unlike the crème fraîche so popular today. Contemporary fears about food safety put an end to that and the modern process sees it chilled through every stage of production. By the way, the tang in modern crème fraîche comes from added cultures – not natural ripening – nevertheless, I like to use it in cooking and eat it fresh with berries.

As with milk, the quality of single and double cream varies widely, from the mainstream, bland white stuff with its uniform thickness to the yellow mass – part-liquid, part-solid – made by artisan producers. The former is perfectly fine to use in cooking or as a pouring cream, but try the latter and, just as with other beautifully made dairy foods, you will find not flavour but flavours that conjure up green pastures in spring. And that is before dipping into a pot of clotted cream, a food worth buying for its importance to the dairy economies of Devon and Cornwall alone.

Incidentally, unlike raw milk, raw, non-pasteurised cream can be sold away from the farm gate. Very occasionally I come across it in village shops or specialist food shops.

yoghurt

Like cream, yoghurt has two personalities. One is the whole milk, home-style yoghurt that is creamy enough to use in a savoury sauce (see page 422), the other skimmed of almost all fat with added thickeners that never quite improve its grainy texture. Yoghurt is milk fermented with live cultures. It is a simple enough, living food – so why do manufacturers muck about with it to the extent they do? Much of the space allocated for yoghurt in supermarkets is taken up with weird plastic containers that have separate compartments filled with either industrially made jam, chocolate or fizzy sherbet balls to tip into the bland white slime in the other half. A little locally produced real yoghurt in supermarkets would be very welcome. Yoghurt is meant, after all, to be a health food.

alternative milks

While cow's milk forms the greater percentage of the milk we drink, there are alternative natural milks produced in Britain to drink or use fresh in cooking. Goat's and ewe's milk are used in some great artisan cheeses and yoghurt, and butter made from goat's milk has a pleasing ripe flavour. I have not had as much success cooking with goat's milk as its distinctive taste can overwhelm other ingredients, but the natural creaminess of ewe's milk makes it a good base for savoury gratins, filled with sliced potato and seasoned with garlic, and there are some delicious hard ewe's milk cheeses. As with cow's milk, there is more pleasure in buying fresh goat's and ewe's milk from small farms that take pride in their high welfare standards, some of which have home delivery services.

Water buffalo are reared mainly for the purpose of making cheeses although it is possible to buy cream made from buffalo milk and the milk. Buffalo milk has a creamy taste and a ripeness that will take regular drinkers of standardised cow's milk by surprise. This ripeness is merely flavour, so don't be put off. I have also tried buffalo milk ice cream, a great delicacy for milk lovers; if you can tap into a source of it try using it in the recipe on page 420.

where to buy milk and other dairy foods

✳ If you are touched by the plight of the farmers, aim to buy milk from retailers who publish mission statements about the fair price they pay for it.

✳ There are a few dairy co-operatives run by groups of farmers fed up with the meagre prices they were getting. They either operate milk rounds or sell into local shops and sometimes garages (see the Shopping Guide).

✳ Raw or untreated milk is available only at the farm gate. Organic dairies can be traced through the Soil Association directory (see the Shopping Guide).

✳ Non-homogenised milk is available in supermarkets and from small dairy co-operatives (see the Shopping Guide).

✳ It is possible to buy cream and butter direct from farms via mail order (see the Shopping Guide).

✳ Artisan cheeses are becoming more widely available. Specialist cheese shops are mushrooming in cities and market towns, but if you live too far away from one there is always home delivery or mail order (see the Shopping Guide).

✳ Supermarkets sell some artisan cheeses, but have a tendency to keep them at temperatures that hinder ripening, or wrap them incorrectly. It is vital you feed back to them any comments, negative or positive, about the standards of the cheese they sell if you want to encourage the best practice.

✳ Goat's, ewe's and buffalo milk are available fresh in health-food shops and supermarkets, as well as direct from the producer (see the Shopping Guide).

veal

The famously unpleasant rearing conditions of much veal have dented its popularity with British shoppers. But we seem to have forgotten that veal is an inevitable by-product of all dairy foods. Veal belongs in this chapter, but let me say immediately that I am talking about British veal, not the veal of ill-repute – the cruelly crated type from Europe. British farmers are subject to strict rules on the welfare of veal calves. Our veal farming methods are no more cruel than those used for naturally rearing beef steers. Even farming experts at the RSPCA approve.

Buying British veal is another way to bring about positive change in the world of dairies as farmers look for ways to diversify and make their products more profitable. New regulations, implemented in 2003, have seen an increasing amount of veal farmed in Britain. If you love dairy foods, it's time to learn to love veal again and dust off some delicious recipes.

Dairy farmers are no longer permitted to destroy their unwanted dairy calves – those often forgotten calves which must be born to enable cows to make milk. This vile slaughter went on for years because farmers were permitted to bury dead livestock on their land. So it was simple and cheap to take those dairy bull calves and any dairy heifers not destined to join the herd, then shoot and bury them. This amounted, in 2001, to 350,000 unnecessarily slaughtered three-day-old calves. It's enough to make any milk drinker with a conscience spit out their Rice Krispies.

But the game, as they say, is up. The practice has been banned for reasons of hygiene, protection of the underground water supply and so on. And while some farmers are whingeing away – 'There are so few livestock markets left', 'We'd have to pay to transport the calves elsewhere' – my, there are plenty of farmers I'd happily throw bricks at – others have actually taken their hands out of their pockets and begun to rear these calves on their mothers' milk, or bought-in, reconstituted feed made from whey powder and vegetable fat. These calves have a lifespan of about six months before they are ready to slaughter, by which time they are a small cow weighing 130kg.

The new welfare rules say they must be reared loose in small groups in large barns, on a bed of straw. They behave naturally, frolicking and playing as young animals should. They have a life. 'A life well-lived is better than no life at all,' a veal farmer told me when I visited her farm.

cooking with milk

It is strange to feel so strongly about a food that I cannot take in its raw form. While I'm happy to discuss the politics of milk all day, I couldn't swallow a glass of the stuff. But I love to cook with it.

Treat good milk as you would great meat. Don't marginalise it as a breakfast food but show it off. It is a great source of calcium and protein, and useful in delightful recipes for main courses and puddings. Hindus braise chicken in cardamom-scented sauces; pork cooked in milk, as the Italians do, is a star turn. Versatile and enriching, milk harmonises foods in cooking, most significantly by smoothing their texture. Vegetables simmered to a soup with milk, blended until velvety, are filling little meals for a non-meat day with the foamy lightness of a cappuccino. Milk-based puddings have all the allure of cream without being too rich.

Rice puddings, flavoured lightly with spices and eaten with figs, are a surprisingly weightless way to end a meal. The same is true of ice cream made with plain good milk and the best eggs you can find.

watercress soup

I make most smooth vegetable soups with meat or vegetable stock as the primary liquid and milk or a dab of cream coming secondary. But you can also make some soups with mainly whole milk. Using vegetables such as watercress, squash, mushrooms or frozen peas, I liquidise the soup until it is very smooth, and a foam forms on top. This is soup to eat in small quantities. It makes a lovely starter or a filling lunch. You can garnish it with ground pink peppercorns, which are very good with vegetables, or add finely chopped crisp bacon. For the richest soup of all, drop a whole peeled semi-soft-boiled egg (see page 380) into the watercress version.

Serves 4

1 tablespoon unsalted butter

2 white onions, roughly chopped

2 potatoes, peeled and roughly chopped

1 litre/1¾ pints whole milk

250ml/8fl oz stock – veal, beef, chicken or vegetable

4 bunches of watercress, finely chopped

sea salt and white pepper

Melt the butter in a large pan, add the onions and cook until soft. Add the potatoes, milk and stock, bring to the boil and simmer for about 15 minutes, until the potatoes are tender. Add the watercress and bring back to the boil. Simmer for 1 minute, then remove from the heat and leave to cool.

Liquidise the soup until very smooth. It is well worth passing it through a mouli-légumes (food mill) as well to remove any threads of watercress stalk, but not absolutely necessary. Reheat without letting it boil, adding 2 pinches of white pepper and sea salt to taste.

chicken cooked in cardamom and milk

Eat this delicate chicken curry, based on the milk cookery of the Hindus in India, with flat bread or rice, and dishes of flaked almonds and diced banana in lime juice on the side.

Serves 4–6

30g/1oz butter

1 red chilli, sliced

2 garlic cloves, chopped

2 onions, chopped

12 cardamom pods

12 fennel seeds

1 teaspoon turmeric

1 teaspoon ground fenugreek

1 teaspoon ground cumin

1 teaspoon ground coriander

8–10 chicken thighs, or 4 chicken legs, skinned

450ml/¾ pint whole milk

4 sprigs of coriander, chopped

sea salt

To serve:

2 bananas, cut into 1cm/½ inch chunks and dressed with

lime juice

2 tablespoons flaked almonds, toasted in a dry pan until golden

Melt the butter in a large pan and add the chilli, garlic, onions and spices. Cook gently for 1 minute, then remove from the heat. Roll the chicken meat around in the spice mixture in the pan. Allow to stand for half an hour, then pour over the milk and bring to the boil. Turn down the heat and simmer for 20 minutes, then taste for salt and throw over the chopped coriander. Serve with the bananas and toasted almonds on the side.

pork cooked in milk, oregano and lemon

An interesting recipe with its roots in the Mediterranean. I like to think that it was discovered during a springtime glut of creamy milk, when lemons were on the trees, wild oregano on the hillside and the first fresh garlic had been lifted from the ground. I use steaks of boneless shoulder of pork, as they allow the sauce and its flavours to penetrate the meat. Remember to keep the pork rind to make crackling for salads (see page 197).

Serves 4

4 rindless pork shoulder steaks, weighing about 300g/10oz each

1 tablespoon olive oil

60g/2oz butter

2 garlic cloves, crushed

1 teaspoon dried oregano

about 1 litre/1¾ pints milk

4 parings of lemon zest

salt and freshly ground black pepper

Season the pork, then brown each piece quickly on both sides in the olive oil. Melt the butter in a casserole, add the garlic and oregano and cook for 2 minutes. Add the pork, turning it once to get a good coating of the fat. Cover with milk and bring to the boil. Push the lemon zest under the pork and simmer for 1–1½ hours, until the pork is very tender and the milk has cooked down to soft brown curds. Eat with new potatoes. Jerseys are best for their lemony flavour.

pan-cooked rice pudding with caramel, figs and pistachios

This rice pudding with its old-fashioned spices tastes best when it is not too sweet. It is a pudding to put you in mind of old manor houses, dairy cows in the pasture and a store cupboard filled with precious rice, dried fruit, sugar and spices.

Serves 4

60g/2oz pudding rice

600ml/1 pint whole milk

1 vanilla pod, split in half

a pinch of grated nutmeg

2 tablespoons double cream

120g/4oz golden caster sugar, plus extra for sweetening the rice

4 dried figs, soaked in warm Earl Grey tea until softened

2 tablespoons chopped unsalted pistachio nuts

Put the rice in a pan with the milk, vanilla pod and nutmeg. Place over a low heat and bring to the boil, then turn down and simmer slowly for at least 20 minutes, until the rice is cooked to the bite (this can take up to 50 minutes, depending on the rice). Remove from the heat and immediately add the cream to stop any further cooking. Add sugar to taste – it should be only faintly sweet. Transfer the rice mixture to a shallow dish. Squeeze the liquid from the dried figs, slice them and submerge them in the rice.

Put the 120g/4oz sugar in a small, heavy-based saucepan, cover with just enough water to soak it and bring slowly to the boil. Raise the heat and allow to boil fast, until it changes to the colour of maple syrup. Remove it from the heat immediately and pour the caramel over the rice. Throw over the chopped pistachios and leave to cool to room temperature, then serve.

✳ kitchen notes ✳

✳ After you have cooked the rice and sweetened it to taste, the mixture will keep for about 3 days in a container in the fridge. Making a double quantity will yield puddings for children, and for your own unexpected urge to eat them.

✳ Clean your caramel pan by filling it with water and bringing it back to the boil.

milk ice cream

On the Italian island of Giglio, there is a small *gelateria artisanale* down an alley near the port, where ice cream is made as fast as it is being sold. The various *gelati* are packed with fresh local fruit – peaches in July, plums in August, blackberries in September – and a day never passes when there is not also a vat of ice cream made simply with fresh milk, egg yolks and a pinch of sugar.

This is a silky ice – more of a milk sorbet than an ice cream. Two things are essential to its success: the best milk and eggs you can find. In order to hold on to the pure milk flavour, I do not use vanilla. Fruits, nuts and honey on the side show off the taste perfectly. Make it very fresh – on the day you eat it, if possible, just like the best *gelateria*.

Serves 4–6

6 egg yolks

1 tablespoon cornflour

600ml/1 pint non-homogenised whole milk (Guernsey or Jersey
is best)

1–2 teaspoons light brown raw muscovado sugar

Put the egg yolks in a stainless-steel pan – off the heat – and mix with the cornflour until smooth. Gradually whisk in the milk. Place over a low heat and stir until the mixture thickens, but do not let it boil. Remove from the heat, still stirring, then transfer immediately to a bowl to cool. Taste and add 1 teaspoon of sugar; taste again and add the second one if you wish. Refrigerate until cold, then put in an ice-cream maker and freeze in the usual way. Alternatively, pour into a container and freeze until soft ice crystals have formed. Remove from the freezer, stir thoroughly and freeze again until solid. Take out of the freezer 15 minutes before you want to eat it.

Serve each person a spoonful of ice cream zigzagged with runny honey and scattered with freshly chopped nuts – walnuts, pecans, pistachios or almonds – or with fresh or soaked dried fruit and a drop or two of rich, dark balsamic vinegar.

✳ kitchen note ✳

An ice made from milk has no more than a 2-week life in the freezer before it sours.

cooking with yoghurt

Always look for yoghurt that has been made from pure milk and not milk powder. Organic is a good standard, but as usual, read those labels.

yoghurt marinade for meat

The acidity in yoghurt tenderises the cheaper cuts of meat, which can then be skewered, Turkish soldier style, and grilled. Diced, boned shoulder of lamb, or rabbit or chicken, is ideal.

Makes enough for 1–2kg/2¼–4½lb meat

480g/1lb Greek yoghurt or whole-milk yoghurt

4 tablespoons olive or sunflower oil

3 garlic cloves, crushed to a paste with a little salt

1 tablespoon ground cumin

juice of 1 lemon

salt and freshly ground black pepper

Mix all the ingredients together, submerge the meat in them and leave for at least an hour. Lift out the meat and thread it on to skewers, then cook over hot coals outside or under a grill. Serve with bread, salad and the yoghurt sauce below.

✳ kitchen note ✳

You can use the same marinade for whole boned lamb shoulders and chops or jointed chicken to grill or barbecue.

yoghurt sauce for grills and pilaffs

240g/8oz plain yoghurt

2 tablespoons avocado oil (or olive oil)

1 teaspoon ground cumin or *ras el hanout* (a spice blend from

Morocco, available in Middle Eastern shops)

1 teaspoon black onion seeds (nigella)

I prefer not to mix this sauce, instead covering the bottom of a shallow bowl with the yoghurt and shaking the oil over it, followed by the spices.

cheese

Talk about cheese takes us back to the disputed territory of living food. The use of raw milk in making cheese has been under constant threat by the authorities responsible for food safety in Britain. These people do not believe in allowing consumers to take responsibility for what they eat. But the new rules they create are frequently based on questionable science. These authorities, who include the Department of Health, Defra and the Food Standards Agency, loathe raw milk and the bacteria that gives great cheese its multistorey flavours. Their erratic demands have tormented small food producers and pose a real threat to a burgeoning British industry of which they should be proud. I know of people who have stopped making cheese because they cannot face the red tape and the inconsistent demands made of them.

The most frustrating thing about the regulations stifling this industry is the fact that they are scarcely necessary given that the nature of the business means that the onus is on the producer to maintain the highest standards. Like many small-scale producers of good-quality, handmade food, artisan cheesemakers cannot afford to make mistakes. A whiff of dirty practice would destroy their business.

buying british cheeses

Be curious. Good cheese shops will allow you to taste a sliver of cheese before you buy. Don't be afraid to try more than one Cheddar; you will find that each is different, and you should keep testing until you find the one you want. I have noticed that a few supermarkets will now let you do this, if asked. So ask.

local cheese

If you know of a good cheese that is made near your home but is not sold in your local supermarket, why not ask them to supply it? Supermarkets are coming around to the idea that branches should stock local foods. This practice boosts the local economy, so it is good for everyone.

cheese shops

Specialist cheesemonger's are a joy to visit; the individuals who run them equal the farmhouse cheesemakers in their vast knowledge and enthusiasm. Contact the Specialist Cheesemakers' Association to find your nearest source of good cheese. Websites and home delivery services are also gradually becoming established. It is often possible to buy cheese direct from the farm, in perfect condition, via overnight delivery. This is the most reasonable way to buy cheese, although you may have to buy in larger quantities (see the Shopping Guide).

looking after cheese

Cheese is like a living creature: it must be nurtured and allowed to mature. How you look after it is almost as important as which type you buy. Keep it in conditions that are too cool or too dry and you will ruin even a great cheese, whether cut or whole. Artisan cheese is precious and expensive, so do not waste it. Even old cheese is useful in cooking, providing it has not been allowed to become overripe (if so it will smell of ammonia). Just a little used sparingly will make delicate sauces, soufflés and tarts. If I find mould has grown on the cheese itself rather than the rind, I dab it with kitchen roll dipped in a solution of equal parts white wine vinegar and water.

Unfortunately supermarkets are novices when it comes to handling cheese. Often you will see a cheese from a great dairy wrapped in sweaty cling film and refrigerated at a temperature so cold it cannot ripen. I always rewrap cheese in greaseproof paper when I get it home, because it both seals it and allows it to breathe. If you have a room with a constant, cool temperature, it's the best place to keep cheese, but the top of the fridge will do. Specialist cheese shops offer good advice on keeping different types of cheese.

british versus continental cheese

Artisan cheesemakers on mainland Europe have succeeded in holding on to their traditions rather more successfully than the British. I grew up believing – quite correctly for the time – that Brie de Meaux, Camembert, Roquefort and Emmental were the cheeses to eat or cook with. But a day spent with Mark Newman at Hamish Johnson's cheese shop in Northcote Road, Battersea, taught me that many of the new cheeses from Britain and Ireland (particularly County Cork and Limerick) can be substituted for the Continentals. With the help of an electric grill and plenty of bread, Mark, his assistants, and I came to some interesting conclusions.

stars among british and irish cheeses

✳ Bishop Kennedy – A British cow's milk cheese with rind that has been washed in liquor to enhance the aroma, which tastes almost exactly like the smelly but delicious German cheese, Munster, and melts like it too. Good for a fruity soufflé or gratin.

✳ Cerney – A good fresh British goat's cheese that can be used for cooking in soufflés and tarts.

✳ Chabis and Golden Cross – Both these British goat's cheeses make good replacements for light fresh goat's cheese in grilled goat's cheese salads.

✳ Coolea – An Irish cow's milk hard cheese that imitates Gouda. Coolea is sold in various stages of maturity. It has a classic nutty Gouda flavour and melts to a smooth cream. Use in cheese sauces and soufflés. Two other cow's milk cheeses, Remarkable Valley and Cilowen Organic, can stand in for raw Gouda, but do not melt as well.

✳ Durras – A new Irish washed-rind cow's milk cheese that has a subtle flavour when raw. It melts to a wonderful runniness that would be useful when making *fonduta*, the eggy Italian equivalent of fondue. Not only does it keep its flavour when melted, but it has a pleasing, slow build-up of flavours.

✳ Flower Marie – A fresh ewe's milk cheese with a delicate rind and flavour. Looking at it you would think it too dense to melt well, but it does, to a wonderful puffy light cream. I put this cheese on half potatoes that have been baked or boiled and put them in the oven until the cheese melts. It has the added bonus of returning to its raw state when cool, so is an ideal cheese for picnic pizza. When melted it's close to a Fontina or Taleggio, although it is modelled on the Corsican Fleur de Maquis.

✳ Gubbeen – A semi-soft, butter yellow cow's milk cheese from Ireland with a thin rind. This mild cheese is beautifully crafted, melting to a white cream with a gentle flavour. For cooking, use it in soufflés, fondue or *fonduta*.

✳ Lord of the Hundreds – A hard British ewe's milk cheese with a texture and flavour close to Manchego. Raw, it is slightly chalky with small bubbles, and is very good eaten with fruit cheeses. It melts to a pleasant white cream, keeping its tart flavour and if anything becoming slightly citrus. Melt between slices of bread or on gratins.

✳ Malvern – A young Pecorino taste-alike ewe's milk cheese with a pale curd. It is piquant with citrus tones when raw, an aroma it keeps when melted. But it has enough presence to make itself felt in sauces, risottos and lasagne.

✳ Saval – Taking half its name from the late campaigning cheesemaker, James Aldridge, Saval is a cow's milk cheese made in Wales. With a piquant smoky flavour, it melts to a thick cream and is wonderful in toasted cheese sandwiches and recipes, like risotto, that call for Pecorino.

✳ Somerset Rambler – Another ewe's milk cheese very similar to a young Pecorino. Dry and chalky enough to pare over a rocket salad or use in home-made pesto when raw, it becomes chewy and sweet when melted. Good for risotto.

✳ Stinking Bishop – A soft, washed cheese made to a similar recipe as the Swiss-French favourite, Vacherin. It has a powerful aroma, but if kept well has a silky texture and delicate flavour. When melted it puffs pleasantly and becomes a pale cream. Another good cheese for *fonduta* and soufflés.

✳ Wigmore – A ewe's milk, soft, bloomy rind cheese with a simple delicate flavour. It makes a good alternative to Taleggio and Fontina.

british blue cheese

The following blue cheeses compare well to European cousins for taste, although I have not attempted to melt them:

✳ Beenleigh Blue – A blue, British ewe's milk cheese. Sweet-sour, dry and lovely, it is so similar to a Picos d'Europa, the Spanish cheese you eat with *membrillo* or quince cheese, that it would be hard to tell them apart.

✳ Devon Blue – Made by the same dairy as Beenleigh, Devon Blue is the cow's milk version. It is sweet, fruity and powerful.

✳ Oxford Blue – A cow's milk cheese that I dare say I prefer to Stilton. Really well kept Oxford Blue can stand up to a Fourme d'Ambert or even Gorgonzola, although it lacks the latter's beautiful gelatinous quality.

unique british cheeses

Some British cheeses have no Continental equivalent. There is nothing to compare to a good Cheddar, Caerphilly, Cheshire, Stilton, Lancashire or Double Gloucester – look for the naturally made farmhouse versions, or those with a PDO mark (Protection of Designated Origin). These are completely different animals to the factory-made cheeses shrink-wrapped in blocks. But I wouldn't dismiss block cheese entirely. Although it may lack the many-layered flavours of handmade cheese, it's a good source of inexpensive protein, and a great alternative to meat or fish. Buying these cheeses supports large-scale milk production, of course, whereas hand-crafted cheese tends to boost small-scale dairies.

ways to eat cheese

There's something very right about a simple lunch of bread and cheese. Served alongside little bowls of cress, pickles and chutneys, or a slab of sticky boiled dark ginger cake with a pat of salty farmhouse butter, and this erstwhile former lunchtime cop-out turns into a feast.

Good artisan cheese can play a part in bigger feasts, too. One of my friends celebrated her wedding in Wales, in a place and among people she had known all her life. To mark this she put a huge half round of locally made Caerphilly on each table for the guests to eat with the cake. Not only was it one of the most stylish gestures I have seen, but the hungry wedding guests fell upon its creamy, crumbly interior like vultures. The party almost didn't end that night.

I also like to eat cheese the French way, after the main course, with a plain lettuce salad dressed in olive oil. It may seem a simple case of throwing a few items together, but finding good cheese and the things to eat with it requires know-how. For these reasons I haven't included dozens of cheese recipes in this book beyond a few essential favourites. Obviously some cheese is ideal for cooking, but you will get a lot of pleasure if you eat cheese in the raw, appreciate the flavours, and use anything leftover for cooking.

This seems the right moment to give away a family secret; the best ginger cake of them all and one that, if you make it now, will last weeks in a tin – improving all the time.

boiled dark ginger cake

Based on Constance Spry's great dark and sticky Belvoir ginger cake, this is served with the cheese course, and is excellent with Cheddar, Malvern or Somerset Rambler, or a moister pressed cheese such as Caerphilly or Wensleydale. Boiling the sugar, treacle and butter before baking is a revelation – it is almost impossible to make a dry cake using this method.

120g/4oz butter

120g/4oz soft brown sugar

120g/4oz sultanas (optional)

2 tablespoons water

300g/10oz black treacle

1½ teaspoons ground ginger

2 eggs

180g/6oz plain flour

½ teaspoon bicarbonate of soda

60g/2oz ground almonds

1 tablespoon blanched split almonds

Preheat the oven to 150°C/300°F/Gas Mark 2. Put the butter, sugar, sultanas, water and black treacle into a saucepan and bring to the boil. Boil for exactly 5 minutes, then set aside to cool until just hand hot. Beat in the ginger, then the eggs, one by one. Sift in the flour with the bicarbonate of soda and almonds and fold in well.

Turn the mixture into a greased 20cm/8 inch square cake tin and bake for about 1 hour, scattering the almonds on top after 40 minutes. Cool on a wire rack. This cake benefits from being made a day or two before it is needed.

✳ kitchen notes ✳

✳ To make a sticky fruit cake, leave out the ginger, replace the black treacle with golden syrup and add about 180g/6oz chopped dried fruit.

✳ For people who suffer from gluten intolerance, this cake works really well using 180g/6oz of a mixture of brown rice flour and tapioca flour instead of the plain flour.

recipes for fresh cheeses

When the rich springtime milk comes in, artisan cheesemakers make the first fresh cheeses with their loose, pale and faintly furred rinds. Now you have a seasonal ingredient that's second to none. Think of these as the fillet steak of cheeses. Eat them raw with young leaves or rolled in herbs. During the rest of the year, you can use the nearest equivalent. I particularly love those small pots of fresh goat's cheese you can buy in supermarkets. With the addition of herbs and pepper they take on a grandeur they never possessed in their little plastic pot, and cook in a useful way, too – softening when hot but returning to a creamy curd when cold.

raw fresh cheese

cheese salads

Make it up as you go along. A bowl of salad leaves, any type, to begin with, then 90g/3oz fresh cheese per person, crumbled loosely straight on top using your hands. Add toasted pumpkin seeds or pine nuts; crushed walnuts or sliced dried figs; perhaps sultanas or crisp bacon, with a few fine shreds of white onion or shallot. Herbs could be chervil, mint or parsley. Sometimes I roll small pieces of fresh cheese in the chopped herbs to throw over the salad or make a green herb dressing, working together olive oil with basil or parsley in a pestle and mortar or food processor. Black pepper is important – or perhaps pink. It is up to you how you throw together these informal salads – you cannot go wrong.

cottage cheese

I like cottage cheese – it was about the first so-called health food I ate and I have enjoyed its wet texture and gentle flavour ever since. It is possible to buy farmhouse cottage cheese made from whole milk, which is distinctly nicer than the mass-produced version. As a cooking cheese, it makes a viable alternative to ricotta, although you may want to put it in a cloth suspended in a sieve overnight to rid it of excess moisture.

blue cheese

Most blue cheeses come under the semi-soft label, but treat them as fresh cheese in salads.

blue cheese, pears and cobnuts

A salad that is associated with French food but even nicer when made with British ingredients – especially Kentish cobnuts which, when fresh in September, have milky-sweet kernels.

Serves 4

360g/12oz blue cheese, such as Beenleigh, Devon Blue or Colston Bassett Stilton, sliced

3 pears, cored and sliced

3 bunches of watercress

3 tablespoons Kentish cobnuts, lightly crushed (or pine nuts)

For the dressing:

1 heaped tablespoon wholegrain mustard

2 tablespoons red wine vinegar

2 tablespoons water

8 tablespoons olive oil

1 teaspoon sugar

a large pinch of salt

freshly ground black pepper

Put all the ingredients for the dressing in a jar and shake until emulsified. Loosely mix all the salad ingredients together and divide between 4 plates. Pour the dressing over them.

cooked fresh cheese

In the Middle East fresh cheeses are rolled in the thinnest pastry, either alone or with cooked greens like spinach, to make substantial little parcels. This won't be news to you. I'm talking about the ubiquitous filo parcel, which has now entered our cooking vernacular, along with pasta, pilaffs and curries. Restaurant reviewers are snobby about food in parcels, but in home cooking filo or 'brik' sheet pastry is without doubt a brilliant freezer store item, lasting much longer than standard pastry made with fat.

cheese pastries

These are big, fat parcels – avoid fiddling around with tiny triangles unless you have nimble fingers and time on your hands. Use whole-milk cottage cheese or Flower Marie. Alternatively you could use feta, ricotta or goat's cheese.

Serves 4

200g/7oz chard or spinach leaves, chopped

400g/14oz fresh cheese (see above)

4 sprigs of coriander leaves and their roots, chopped

120g/4oz unsalted butter, melted

8 sheets of filo pastry

paprika

salt and freshly ground black pepper

Cook the greens in a pan over a medium heat with a little water until tender. Drain, squeeze out the excess water and season with salt and pepper. Leave to cool. Mix loosely with the cheese and coriander and 4 teaspoons of the melted butter, then refrigerate.

Preheat the oven to 220°C/425°F/Gas Mark 7. Brush a filo pastry sheet with melted butter on both sides, repeat with a second and place one on top of the other. Spoon a quarter of the cheese mixture into a high pile in the centre of the pastry, then bring up the edges and scrunch them into a twist at the top. Place on a buttered baking sheet, brush with a little more butter and scatter a pinch of paprika on top. Repeat this process to make 3 more parcels. Bake for about 20 minutes, until crisp and golden brown. Eat the pastries hot or lukewarm, with a little more melted butter.

fresh ewe's milk cheese with tomato and chilli

When I think of a pan filled with tomato and peppers, cooked until sweet with oil and hot, molten ewe's milk cheese, I remember the tax inspector on the island of Syros, where the writer, Elizabeth David, lived in 1940. This was the place where she first lived as a Mediterranean housewife, taking the local food to her heart. Half a century later, in 1999, I co-produced a film about her life. We retraced her footsteps to the island, searching for people who would cook for the programme's presenter, Chris Patten, in the manner so perfectly described in her first book, *A Book of Mediterranean Food*. Everyone pointed us in the direction of a restaurant run at weekends by the local tax inspector. This dish was one among a dazzling tray of *meze* – and the undoubted star. I tried to imitate it as soon as I returned home, finding I could only get it right with semi-dried or sunblush tomatoes.

Serves 4

2 tablespoons olive oil

1 onion, finely chopped

1 red pepper, roughly chopped

2 large red chillies, deseeded and chopped

4 tomatoes, deseeded and roughly chopped

12 sunblush tomatoes, roughly chopped, plus 3 tablespoons of their oil

240g/8oz feta cheese, broken into 1cm/½ inch pieces

freshly ground black pepper

mint leaves, to garnish

Heat the oil in a frying pan, add the onion and red pepper and cook until soft but not coloured. Add the chillies, tomatoes, sunblush tomatoes and their oil and stew for about 15 minutes, until sweet to the taste. Add the cheese, allow the mixture to bubble, then remove from the heat. Season with black pepper – do not stir – and scatter mint leaves over the pan as you take it to the table. Eat with any type of toasted or grilled bread.

easy fresh cheesecake

This simple cheesecake is very good eaten with crème fraîche and an orange salad. This recipe makes a large cake, so there is spare for lunches, lunchboxes or weekday after-supper treats.

240g/8oz whole-milk cottage cheese or ricotta

5 eggs, separated

5 tablespoons golden caster sugar

90g/3oz plain flour

1 teaspoon vanilla extract

240g/8oz mascarpone or cream cheese

grated zest of ½ lemon

grated zest of ½ orange

icing sugar for dusting

Preheat the oven to 180°C/350°F/Gas Mark 4. Line a round, shallow 25cm/10 inch cake tin with baking parchment, taking it up the sides of the tin. If using cottage cheese, mash it with a fork and set aside.

Whisk the egg yolks with the sugar until pale and thick. Fold in the flour, then the vanilla, cottage cheese or ricotta, mascarpone or cream cheese, and the citrus zest. Do this gently, to retain as much air as possible in the egg yolks. In a separate bowl, whisk the egg whites to a stiff foam, then fold them into the cream cheese mixture. Pour into the tin and bake for about 30 minutes, until firm and slightly puffed, with tinges of brown on the surface. Serve at room temperature, dusted with icing sugar.

semi-soft and hard cheeses
cheese and toast

Or, in other words, putting together a forgotten piece of cheese and a dryish piece of bread, with perhaps a few other items – the most sophisticated gadget you need is a heavy-based frying pan. Use off-cuts of semi-soft bloomy-rind cheeses, which become rivers of silky, molten goo – the need to use a knife and fork to eat these snacks is a good sign.

toasted cheese and ham sandwiches

Place a slice of cheese and a slice of ham between 2 slices of bread, then butter the bread on the outside. Heat a heavy-based frying pan and fry the sandwich over a medium heat on both sides until the cheese melts.

toasted flat breads with cheese

Lay slices of cheese between sheets of flat bread with a layer of thick tomato sauce and herbs – or simply with ham. Brush on both sides with olive oil and toast under the grill or in a dry frying pan on both sides until the cheese has melted.

cheddar tart

Take this rich tart straight to the table while it is still puffed up from the heat of the oven. Keen's, Montgomery and Daylesford Cheddar are good but you could also explore others (see the Shopping Guide).

Serves 4

120g/4oz cooked ham, diced

90g/3oz farmhouse Cheddar cheese, grated

2 eggs

2 egg yolks

300ml/½ pint single cream

a pinch of grated nutmeg

freshly ground black pepper

For the pastry:

240g/8oz plain flour

a pinch of salt

90g/3oz chilled unsalted butter or lard, diced

1 egg yolk

2–3 tablespoons cold water

To make the pastry, put the flour and salt in a bowl and rub in the fat lightly but thoroughly with your fingertips so the mixture resembles breadcrumbs. Work in the egg yolk and enough cold water to form a dough (this can all be done in a food processor, if you prefer). Roll the pastry out on a lightly floured work surface and use to line a deep 20cm/8 inch tart tin. Prick it randomly with a fork and chill for 15 minutes.

Preheat the oven to 190°C/375°F/Gas Mark 5. Cover the pastry with greaseproof paper and fill with dry rice or beans (this will prevent the pastry bubbling up). Bake for about 15 minutes, until the pastry is dry. You may want to lift away the paper and rice or beans for the last 5 minutes of cooking so the base can dry out.

Scatter the ham over the pastry case, followed by the cheese. Mix together the eggs, yolks, cream, nutmeg and some pepper and pour this mixture over the ham and cheese. Bake the tart for 25–30 minutes, until risen and glossy brown.

dry or overripe cheese

Never throw away that small piece of cheese that is too scruffy to put on a cheeseboard. If it has been well kept and still has a good aroma, melt it in soufflés (see page 390) and tarts such as the one above.

cheddar crisps

Light as anything, easy-to-make wafers to eat with drinks or soup. They are so quick you can make lots in half an hour. They work best with dry cheese but do not use a fan oven to bake them in – they can turn to dust. These crisps keep well in an airtight plastic container.

Makes about 16

120g/4oz mature Cheddar cheese, grated
4 teaspoons plain flour

cayenne pepper and sliced pistachio nuts or flaked almonds (optional)

Preheat the oven to 190°C/375°F/Gas Mark 5 and line a baking sheet with baking parchment. Mix the Cheddar with the flour and place a heaped teaspoon of the mixture near the top corner of the baking sheet. Spread out to a biscuit-sized disc. Repeat until the baking sheet is covered, leaving about a finger of space between each one. Scatter a few grains of cayenne pepper and some nuts over each one – or leave them plain, if you wish. Bake for 5 minutes or until golden and bubbling. Remove from the oven and allow to cool a little. It is then easy to lift the crisps from the paper using a palette knife. Make more batches until you have used up all the cheese mixture.

hot soft cheese with mushrooms and truffle oil

This is true Saturday lunchtime food for lining tummies before long after-noon walks. It is similar to *fonduta*, the Italian version of fondue. Use ripe, sweet-tasting Brie-type cheese for this liquefied pot of cheese and eat it with a small spoon and some bread, cured meat and watercress on the side. You could also dip blanched vegetables in the cheese – purple sprout-ing broccoli in winter, asparagus during the spring/summer glut.

Serves 4

300g/10oz very ripe, soft bloomy-rind cheese, such as Flower Marie, Durras or Gubbeen

120g/4oz butter

4 egg yolks

300ml/½ pint whole milk

For the top:

2 tablespoons dried porcini mushrooms, soaked in hot water until soft, then drained and chopped

a little white truffle oil (see Kitchen Note below)

Heat 4 ramekin dishes in the oven. Remove and discard the rind from the cheese, then dice the cheese. Place a bowl over a saucepan of simmering water and melt the butter in it. Add the cheese and stir until it has melted. Mix in the egg yolks, one by one, then gradually add the milk, whisking continuously for about 10 minutes with a balloon whisk until the sauce is thick and shiny.

Serve in the ramekin dishes, with the chopped dried mushrooms on top and a few drops of white truffle oil. Eat immediately, with small spoons, bread to one side.

✳ kitchen note ✳

You can buy white truffle oil from Italian delicatessens. Buy only very small bottles, as it has a strong taste and perishes quickly.

veal

Due to its dairy diet, veal is very rich and filling. When cooked the sweet flavour of veal is very pronounced, quite different to beef, and it is not actually necessary to buy as much as you would beef – 150g/5oz per person is plenty. The meat varies in colour, from very pale pink to a deeper rose red, and tends to be loose grained. It should be well hung, just as for beef, to tenderise the meat.

spotting the imports

It is often impossible to tell whether the veal you eat in restaurants or see in butcher's or supermarkets is European or British. However, you can bet that if it is not labelled British that means it's come from elsewhere. No shops advertise the fact that they're selling veal from the Netherlands, Belgium, France or Italy, the countries most associated with cruel practice. British veal is only available in certain supermarkets. Indeed, amazingly there are some with 'free-range only' egg policies that seem happy to sell Dutch veal.

organic veal

Organic veal calves are reared alongside their mothers, on a mixed diet of milk and grass. Their meat tends to be redder. This is arguably the kindest way to rear a veal calf, but having visited non-organic farms, I have no problem with either standard.

rosé veal

You may come across rosé veal in butcher's. This meat, an alternative to milk-fed veal, is from calves reared to the age of eleven months in barns on a diet of mainly grain and straw. The flesh is darker and less tender, but the flavour is less buttery, rather like mild beef.

the veal to buy

When asking for veal, insist on proof that it was reared in Britain. You will find – thanks to the high rearing cost of British veal – that the prime cuts (loin, best end and rump, also called fillet) are expensive. Expect to pay about £20 per kilo, but it can be bought for less direct from a farm (see the Shopping Guide). There are plenty of other cuts to choose from, such as shoulder, breast, cushion, middle neck, and shin, also known as osso buco. They braise well, and I have also found that even these cuts, taken from British milk-fed veal, need only to be cut thin and hammered to produce very tender escalopes. These so-called cheap cuts are not cheap exactly, but once the bones have been simmered for a stock, there will be another delicate, extremely valuable cooking ingredient ready and waiting in the fridge or freezer.

cold loin of veal with watercress and anchovy sauce

Use some meat left over from a roast loin, shoulder or loin of veal to make a luxurious supper or lunch dish. To roast veal, rub with butter; season and roast as for beef. Use the skewer test on page 182 to test for doneness. Roast veal should be slightly pink in the centre.

Serves 2

8 very thin slices of cold veal

a bunch of watercress

4 tablespoons olive oil, plus a little extra for the watercress

1 egg yolk

1 anchovy, chopped

1 teaspoon capers, chopped

juice of ¼ lemon

1 hard-boiled egg yolk

Put the veal slices on a plate. Cut the stalks off the watercress, put the leafy ends beside the veal and shake over a little oil. Chop the stalks finely, discarding any dried ends, and put them in a small bowl. Add the egg yolk, anchovy and capers, then add the 4 tablespoons of oil drop by drop, stirring all the time. Stir in the lemon juice. Push the hard-boiled egg yolk through a sieve over the watercress. Eat the veal with a good spoonful of the sauce to one side.

escalopes

If you buy a piece of veal rump, make it into escalopes by cutting it into slices across the grain, 1cm/½ inch thick. Place them between 2 pieces of greaseproof paper and hammer with a meat mallet or wooden rolling pin until about 3mm/¼ inch thin. The meat can be stored in the freezer like this until you need it. Butchers will do the hammering for you but you do need to check that they cut the meat Continental style, across the grain.

breadcrumbed escalopes

Dipped in seasoned flour, egg, then breadcrumbs (see page 33), escalopes make a one-pot meal – all you need is something green to eat with them. Children like them, too. Fry in a little sunflower oil for 2 minutes on each side, being careful not to burn the crumbs. Squeeze a little lemon over the escalopes; it cuts any oiliness. Serve with egg noodles or potatoes.

veal escalopes with tarragon and cream

An easy, elegant way to eat veal – I like them in winter with smooth mashed or puréed potato. Escalopes cut from the rump of veal are the most expensive, but you could make this dish from other cuts of milk-fed veal, providing you pound them between 2 sheets of greaseproof paper to flatten them (see page 441).

Serves 2

2 veal escalopes weighing about 180g/6oz each, pounded until thin (see page 441)
1 tablespoon olive oil or butter
1 glass of white wine
leaves from 2 sprigs of tarragon
125ml/4fl oz crème fraîche or double cream
salt and freshly ground black pepper

Season the veal with salt and pepper. Heat the oil or butter in a frying pan and fry the veal for 1–2 minutes on each side. Transfer to 2 warmed plates, then add the wine to the pan, stirring over the heat as it boils and scraping any bits from the base of the pan. Add the tarragon and cream and simmer until it thickens. Pour the sauce over the veal and take to the table.

veal meatballs

Veal mince can be taken from the cheap cuts. Eat these simple meatballs with pasta dressed with a dash of sherry and cream. The uncooked meatballs freeze well, so it's worth making double the quantity and storing half of them in the freezer (or in the fridge for 3 days).

Serves 4

2 tablespoons olive oil

1 small glass of sherry or white wine

300ml/½ pint veal or chicken stock

125ml/4fl oz double cream

parsley leaves

For the meatballs:

480g/1lb minced veal

a few gratings of lemon zest

60g/2oz breadcrumbs

1 egg, beaten

½ tablespoon freshly grated Parmesan cheese, or similar British cheese

salt and freshly ground black pepper

Combine all the ingredients for the meatballs and roll them into spheres the size of golf balls. Heat the oil in a large casserole and gently fry the meatballs until golden all over. Add the sherry or wine and the stock, carefully scraping up any juices from the bottom of the pan without breaking up the meatballs. Simmer for 20–30 minutes, until the meatballs are cooked through. Quickly stir in the cream. Serve with spaghetti or egg noodles, scattering over the parsley as you take it to the table.

✳ kitchen note ✳

If you prefer, you can use 600ml/1 pint Tomato Sauce (see page 358) instead of the sherry, stock and cream.

veal kidneys

Veal kidneys are a bother to prepare; removing their ducts is a fiddle, so ask the butcher to do this for you. They should then be gently fried whole and sliced when pink in the middle. They are wonderful added to Black Pudding, Dry-cured Sausage and Bacon with Leaves (see page 222).

calf's liver

Calf's liver is my favourite liver to fry. Sweet flavoured and lemony, it lacks the rough edges of lamb's liver. There are two ways to eat it:

✳ Thinly sliced, then fried on both sides for 1 minute in butter; it is nicest when still a little pink in the centre.

✳ Rubbed with butter and a little chopped rosemary, black pepper and salt, then roasted whole. Cook as for a fillet of beef, using a skewer to check for doneness (see page 182). It should be served pink but not rare in the centre, sliced, with a big dish of mashed potato and various mustards.

shopping guide

1: bread and flour

buying flour in bulk

Sarre Windmill
Sarre, Kent
tel: 01843 847573
www.foodfirst.co.uk

Shipton Mill
Tetbury, Gloucestershire
tel: 01666 505050
www.shipton-mill.com
Home delivery and farm gate sales

N. R. Stoate & Sons
Shaftesbury, Dorset
tel: 01747 852475
Farm gate sales only

specialist breads

Graig Farm Organics
Llandrindod Wells, Powys
tel: 01597 851655
www.graigfarm.co.uk
Home delivery and selected retail outlets –
see website

Long Crichel Bakery
Wimborne, Dorset BH21 5JU
Shop or contact for stockists

Staff of Life Bakery
Kendal, Cumbria
tel: 01539 738606
Home delivery and shop

Poilane
46 Elizabeth Street, London SW1
tel: 020 7808 4910
Shop only but available via mail order
from Mortimer & Bennett (see above)

Village Bakery
near Penrith, Cumbria
tel: 01768 881811
www.village-bakery.com
Home delivery. Also available from
Waitrose, selected branches of Sainsbury's,
Tesco and other retail outlets – see website

2: store

avocado oil

E. H. Booth & Co. Ltd – The Grove avocado oil
For branches tel: 01772 251701
www.foodfirst.co.uk
The Grove avocado oil is also available from Tesco

Mortimer & Bennett – Pacifica Culinara oil
33 Turnham Green Terrace, London W4
tel: 020 8995 4145
www.mortimerandbennett.com
Home delivery and shop

british bacon, sausages and other dry-cured meat

Denhay Farms Ltd
Bridport, Dorset
tel: 01308 458963/422770
www.denhay.co.uk
Home delivery. Also available from selected branches of Safeway and some Asda stores in the south west

John Robinson and Sons
Stockbridge, Hampshire
tel: 01264 810609
No home delivery but worth the journey

Sillfield Farm
Kendal, Cumbria
tel: 015395 67609
www.sillfield.co.uk
Products available from Furness Fish, Poultry & Game Supplies
Ulverston, Cumbria
tel: 01229 585037
www.morecambebayshrimps.co.uk
Home delivery

canned wood-roasted peppers

Whole Spanish peppers with just a little bite – these are delicious served sliced on an antipasto plate, or mixed with pasta or rocket salad

Mortimer & Bennett – Navarrico
33 Turnham Green Terrace, London W4
tel: 020 8995 4145
www.mortimerandbennett.com
Home delivery and shop

Trencherman & Turner – Navarrico
Eastbourne, East Sussex
tel: 01323 737535
www.loadedtable.com
Home delivery and shop

english-grown herb plants and seeds

Jekka's Herb Farm
Alveston, Bristol
tel: 01454 418878
www.jekkasherbfarm.com
Home delivery

Suffolk Herbs
Kelvedon, Colchester, Essex
tel: 01376 572456
www.suffolkherbs.com
Home delivery

fresh english-grown chilli peppers

Peppers by Post
Dorchester, Dorset
tel: 01308 897892
www.peppersbypost.biz
Home delivery

frozen organic peas

Available from Sainsbury's and Waitrose

hot and cold smoked wild salmon

Frank Hederman – Belvelly Smokehouse
Cobh, County Cork
tel: 00353 21 4811089

Ummera Smoked Products Ltd
Timoleague, County Cork
tel: 00353 23 46644
www.ummera.com
Home delivery

olive oil in bulk

Elanthy extra virgin olive oil
Moreton in the Marsh, Gloucestershire
tel: 0800 169 6252
www.elanthy.com
Home delivery

The Oil Merchant
tel: 020 8740 1335
Home delivery

potatoes – unusual british old and new varieties

From Ocado/Waitrose and Sainsbury's

Carroll's Heritage Potatoes Ltd
Cornhill-on-Tweed, Northumberland
tel: 01890 883060
www.heritage-potatoes.co.uk
Home delivery

rice cooker

Nisbets Next Day Catering Equipment
1110 Aztec West, Bristol
tel: 0845 1405555
www.nisbets.co.uk
Home delivery and shop in Bristol

sustainably caught anchovies/sardines/tuna

Mortimer & Bennett – Ortiz and Ramon Bue
33 Turnham Green Terrace, London W4
tel: 020 8995 4145
www.mortimerandbennett.com
Home delivery and shop

Taste the Difference line-caught albacore in olive oil – from Sainsbury's

Trencherman & Turner – Ortiz and Ramon Bue
Eastbourne, East Sussex
tel: 01323 737535
www.loadedtable.com
Home delivery and shop

Waitrose – for Glenryck Maldives Eco-friendly tuna steaks in brine
Look out for Maldives as country of origin on cans of tuna from Tesco, Co-op, Morrisons, Sainsbury – and also on cans of Princes and Glenryck branded tuna.

3: stock

artisan meat retailers

See Poultry and Meat listings below for home delivery companies, butchers and farm shops

organic stock, fresh and frozen

Daylesford Organic Farm Shop
Nr Kingham, Gloucestershire
tel: 01608 731700
www.daylesfordorganic.com
Frozen stock, home delivery

Joubère – organic vegetable, chicken and beef stocks
Crawley, West Sussex
tel: 020 8992 6851
www.joubere.co.uk
Available from Fresh & Wild stores (see www.wholefoodsmarket.com for locations) and Waitrose

naturally fermented soy sauce

GoodnessDirect
Daventry, Northants
tel: 0871 871 6611
www.goodnessdirect.co.uk
Clearspring Organic Soy Sauce – home delivery

Kikkoman brand
www.kikkoman.com
Widely available from oriental supermarkets, independent specialist food shops and most supermarket chains

4: poultry

anodised roasting tins

Lakeland Limited
tel: 015394 88100
www.lakelandlimited.com
Home delivery

Nisbets Next Day Catering Equipment
1110 Aztec West, Bristol
tel: 0845 1405555
www.nisbets.co.uk
Home delivery and shop in Bristol

chickens

Creedy Carver Ltd
Crediton, Devon
tel: 01363 772682
www.creedycarver.co.uk
Home delivery

Ellel Free Range Poultry Co. – Poulet de Bresse chickens
Galgate, Lancashire
tel: 01524 751200
www.ellelfreerangepoultry.co.uk
Home delivery

The Farmyard Chicken Co. – Label Anglais brand
Harlow, Essex
tel: 01279 792460
www.labelanglais.co.uk
Home delivery

The Real Meat Company
Warminster, Wiltshire
tel: 0845 762 6017
www.realmeat.co.uk
Home delivery

Sheepdrove Organic Farm
Lambourn, Berkshire
tel: 01488 71659
www.sheepdroveshop.com
Home delivery and shop in Lower Redland Road, Bristol

msg-free hoi sin sauce

Lee Kum Kee Hoi Sin Sauce
From Wing Yip stores in London, Birmingham, Manchester
tel: 0870 608 8800
www.wingyipstore.co.uk

free-range ducks

Everleigh Pheasantry Ltd
Marlborough, Wiltshire
tel: 01264 850 344
www.pheasants.co.uk
Home delivery and shop

Pipers Farm
Cullompton, Devon
tel: 01392 881380
www.pipersfarm.com
Home delivery and shop in Exeter

free-range turkey – all year round/out of season

Richard Waller, Long Grove Wood Farm
Chesham, Buckinghamshire
Tel: 01494 772744
Farm gate sales and local shops

free-range turkey – seasonal

Ellel Free Range Poultry Co.
Galgate, Lancashire
tel: 01524 751200
www.ellelfreerangepoultry.co.uk

Helen Browning's Totally Organic
Swindon, Wiltshire
tel: 01793 790460
www.helenbrowningorganics.co.uk
Home delivery

House of Rhug
Corwen, Denbighshire
tel: 01490 413000
www.rhugorganic.com
Home delivery and shop

Kelly Turkeys
Danbury, Essex
tel: 01245 223581
www.kellyturkeys.com
Home delivery and selected shops
throughout the UK – see website

sausages for braising

Denhay Farms Ltd – dry-cured bacon and sausages
Bridport, Dorset
tel: 01308 458963/422770
www.denhay.co.uk
Home delivery. Also available from
selected branches of Safeway and some
Asda stores in the south west

5: beef, pork and lamb

Packages of meat can be stamped with
logos or marks as a statement of various
quality standards. There are five British
organic marks, with the Soil Association
acknowledged by organic experts as setting
the highest standards for animal welfare.
The Little Red Tractor (LRT) is the logo
for British Farm Standards (BFS). It does
not guarantee that the food marked with it
is British (although currently supermarket
chains will not buy imported meat stamped
with the BFS logo), nor does it assure the
highest standards. The criteria set by its
accreditation board have been criticised,
particularly by the farm animal welfare
organisation Compassion in World
Farming. BFS permits the usual ogres of
intensive farming: broiler houses, cramped
indoor rearing techniques and long-distance
transport.

butchers

The City Meat Co.
421 King's Rd, London SW10
tel: 020 7352 9894

A. Dove & Son Ltd
Northcote Road, London SW11
tel: 020 7223 5191

Pipers Farm
Cullompton, Devon
tel: 01392 881380
www.pipersfarm.com
Home delivery and shop in Exeter

John Robinson Family Butcher
High Street, Stockbridge, Hampshire
tel: 01264 810609

Home Farm Shop
Tarrant Gunville, Dorset
tel: 01258 830208
Home delivery within a 4-mile radius

charcoal

Dorset Charcoal Company Ltd – sustainable hardwood charcoal products
Hazelbury Bryan, Dorset
tel: 01258 818176
www.dorsetcharcoal.co.uk
See website for stockists in the south west
and for C. Lidgate in Holland Park

lamb boxes

Aran Lamb – certified organic Welsh mountain lamb
Bala, Gwynedd
tel: 01678 540603
www.aran-lamb.co.uk
Home delivery

blackface.co.uk – heather-bred Scottish blackface lamb
Irongray, Dumfries
tel: 01387 730326
www.blackface.co.uk
Home delivery

Farmer Sharp – fell-bred Herdwick lamb and mutton
Cumbria
tel: 01229 588299
www.farmersharp.co.uk
Stall only (at Borough Market, London
SE1), except by special arrangement

Hazel Brow Farm – Pennine-reared organic Swaledale lamb
Richmond, North Yorkshire
tel: 01748 886224
www.hazelbrow.co.uk
Home delivery

Traditional Devon Meats – Dartmoor whiteface lamb, known as 'angel meat'
Okehampton, Devon
tel: 01837 810416
www.traditionaldevonmeats.co.uk
Home delivery

Whitbysteads Hill Farm – pasture-fed Herdwick and Swaledale lamb
Penrith, Cumbria
tel: 01931 712051
www.whitbysteads.co.uk
Home delivery

meat – all types

Cranborne Farms Traditional Meats – rare-breed pork, beef and lamb
Cranborne, Dorset
tel: 01725 517168
www.cranborne.co.uk
Shop and home delivery

Daylesford Organic Farm Shop
Nr Kingham, Gloucestershire
tel: 01608 731700
www.daylesfordorganic.com
Home delivery

Donald Russell Direct – traditionally reared natural meats and fish
Inverurie, Aberdeen
tel: 01467 629666
www.donaldrusselldirect.com
Home delivery

Edwards of Conwy – North Wales saltmarsh lamb and Welsh black beef
Conwy, North Wales
tel: 01492 592443
www.edwardsofconwy.co.uk
Shop and home delivery

Graig Farm Organics – organic Welsh black and Hereford beef and Welsh lamb
Llandrindod Wells, Powys
tel: 01597 851655
www.graigfarm.co.uk
Home delivery and at selected retail outlets – see website

Northumbrian Quality Meats – locally produced organic and rare-breed meat
Hexham, Northumberland
tel: 01434 270184
northumbrian-organic-meat.co.uk
Home delivery and farmers' markets – see website

Orkney Organic Meat – organic Aberdeen Angus beef and Shetland/Cheviot-cross lamb
Holm, Orkney
tel: 01856 781345
www.orkneyorganicmeat.co.uk
Home delivery

Pipers Farm
Cullompton, Devon
tel: 01392 881380
www.pipersfarm.com
Home delivery

Sheepdrove Organic Farm – organic beef, lamb, pork and poultry
Lambourn, Berkshire
tel: 01488 71659
www.sheepdroveshop.com
Home delivery and shop in Lower Redland Road, Bristol

The Well Hung Meat Company – organic lamb, beef, pork and chicken
Buckfastleigh, Devon
tel: 0845 2303131
www.wellhungmeat.com
Home delivery

Wild venison – from Sainsbury's

6: wild meat and game

canned duck or goose fat

Mortimer & Bennett
33 Turnham Green Terrace, London W4
tel: 020 8995 4145
www.mortimerandbennett.com
Home delivery and shop

freshwater crayfish

Matthew Stevens & Son
St Ives, Cornwall
tel: 01736 799392
www.mstevensandson.co.uk

game birds, venison, rabbit, hare

Donald Russell Direct (see above)

Everleigh Pheasantry Ltd
Marlborough, Wiltshire
tel: 01264 850 344
www.pheasants.co.uk
Home delivery

Furness Fish, Poultry & Game Supplies
Ulverston, Cumbria
tel: 01229 585037
www.morecambebayshrimps.co.uk
Home delivery

Yorkshire Game
Richmond, North Yorkshire
tel: 01748 810212
www.yorkshiregame.co.uk
Home delivery

red deer shanks/osso buco

Donald Russell Direct
Inverurie, Aberdeen
tel: 01467 629666
www.donaldrusselldirect.com
Home delivery

7: fish and shellfish

fish merchants specialising in day-boat fished, sustainably harvested fish and shellfish

Andy Race Fishmerchants Ltd
Port of Mallaig, Highlands of Scotland
tel: 01687 462626
www.andyrace.co.uk
Home delivery

Matthew Stevens & Son
St Ives, Cornwall
tel: 01736 799392
www.mstevensandson.co.uk
Home delivery

Wing of St Mawes
St Columb, Cornwall
tel: 01726 861666
www.cornish-fish.co.uk
Home delivery

freshly picked unpasteurised crabmeat

Fishworks Direct
St Columb, Cornwall
tel: 0800 052 3717
www.fishworks.co.uk

Matthew Stevens & Son
St Ives, Cornwall
tel: 01736 799392
www.mstevensandson.co.uk
Home delivery

Blakes of Ventnor
The Esplanade, Ventnor, Isle of Wight
tel: 01983 852176
Shop

pilchards/sardines

Cornish Fish Direct
Newlyn, Cornwall
tel: 01736 332 112
www.cornishfish.co.uk
Home delivery

potted and cooked shrimps

Furness Fish, Poultry & Game Supplies
Ulverston, Cumbria
tel: 01229 585037
www.morecambebayshrimps.co.uk
Home delivery

Southport Potted Shrimps
Southport, Lancashire
tel: 01704 229266
www.pottedshrimps.co.uk
Home delivery

farmed salmon – conventional

The Sustainable Salmon Company at Loch Duart – salmon sold via Loch Fyne
Lairg, Sutherland
tel: 01499 600264
www.lochfyne.com
Home delivery

salmon – organic

Andy Race Fishmerchants Ltd – salmon from Orkney
Port of Mallaig, Highlands of Scotland
tel: 01687 462626
www.andyrace.co.uk
Home delivery

Club Chef Direct – organic Glenarm salmon from Northern Ireland
tel: 01275 472252
www.clubchefdirect.com
Home delivery

Organically farmed salmon is available from Tesco, Waitrose and Sainsbury's

salmon – wild

Wild Irish salmon from Cork has a short season in June and July and is a well-managed fishery; order it fresh from good fishmongers or buy smoked from:

Ummera Smoked Products
Timoleague, County Cork
tel: 00353 23 46644
www.ummera.com
Home delivery

Wild Alaskan salmon, certified as responsibly fished by the Marine Stewardship Council (MSC), can be bought fresh from Sainsbury's, Tesco and Waitrose, smoked from Marks & Spencer, and canned from Sainsbury's

smoked pollack

The Handmade Fish Company
Bigton, Shetland
tel: 01950 422214
www.handmadefish.co.uk
Home delivery

William Jolly
Kirkwall, Orkney
tel: 01856 873127
www.jollyfish.co.uk
Home delivery

sustainably caught, fresh tuna

From Marks & Spencer, Sainsbury's, Ocado/Waitrose

sustainably farmed shellfish

Loch Fyne Oysters Ltd
Cairndow, Argyll
tel: 01499 600264
www.lochfyne.com
Home delivery

sustainably farmed tiger prawns

Island Seafare
Port St Mary, Isle of Man
tel: 01624 834494
www.islandseafare.co.uk
Home delivery

8: gluts of fruit and vegetables

identifying puffballs and other fungi

Food for Free by Richard Mabey (Collins, 2001)

How to Identify Edible Mushrooms by Harding, Lyon, Gillmor and Hammond (Collins, 1996)

jersey royals

The Jersey Royal Potato Post
St Helier, Jersey
tel: 01534 861345
www.jerseyroyalpotatopost.com
Home delivery

multi-coloured sugar crystals

Belle de Sucre
Château de Cornou, Nargis, France
From Harrods Food Halls
tel: 020 7730 1234
www.harrods.com
Home delivery

nationwide and local vegetable box schemes

Abel & Cole
Milkwood Road, London SE24
tel: 020 7737 3648
www.abel-cole.co.uk
Home delivery to London and parts of the home counties, the south and west

Boxfresh Organics
Rodington, Shropshire
tel: 01952 770006
www.boxfreshorganics.co.uk
Home delivery to Shropshire and parts of the west Midlands

Fieldfare Organics
Wendover, Buckinghamshire
tel: 0845 601 3240
www.fieldfare-organics.com
Home delivery to London and the south east

Graig Farm Organics
Llandrindod Wells, Powys
tel: 01597 851655
www.graigfarm.co.uk
Home delivery nationwide

whole wheat (pasta wheat)

Ebly brand – from supermarkets and independent food shops

9: eggs

canned wood-roasted peppers

For Navarrico brand, see the Store listing on page 446

columbian blacktail eggs

From Ocado/Waitrose

cotswold legbar eggs

From Waitrose, Sainsbury's and Tesco

free-range/organic speciality eggs – duck, goose, quail and others

Farmers' markets will often sell speciality eggs; for the nearest, check
www.farmersmarkets.net or
www.lfm.org.uk
Local farm shops can be found through
www.bigbarn.co.uk

gulls' eggs – when in season (april to may)

Butcher & Edmonds
Leadenhall Market, London EC3
tel: 020 7329 7388

Everleigh Farm Shop
Marlborough, Wiltshire
tel: 01264 850 344
www.pheasants.co.uk
Home delivery and shop

H. S. Linwood
Leadenhall Market, London EC3
tel: 020 7929 0554

10: dairy

artisan-made british, irish and european cheeses

The Fine Cheese Company
29–31 Walcot Street, Bath
tel: 01225 448748
www.finecheese.co.uk
Home delivery

La Fromagerie
2–4 Moxon Street, London W1, and 30 Highbury Park, London N5
tel: 020 7935 0341 and 020 7359 7440
www.lafromagerie.co.uk
Home delivery

Hamish Johnston
48 Northcote Road, London SW11
tel: 020 7738 0741
www.hamishjohnston.com
Home delivery

Neal's Yard Dairy
6 Park Street, London SE1
tel: 020 7645 3554
www.nealsyarddairy.co.uk
Home delivery

butter and cream

Manor Farm Organic Cream
Godmanstone, Dorset
tel: 01300 341415 – call for nearest stockists
www.manor-farm-organic.co.uk

Pengoon Farm – clotted cream and Jersey butter
Helston, Cornwall
tel: 01326 561219
www.pengoon.co.uk
Home delivery

buttermilk

Cream of Cumbria
Howberry, Blackford, Carlisle
tel: 01228 675558

english milk-fed veal

Helen Browning's Totally Organic
Swindon, Wiltshire
tel: 01793 790460
www.helenbrowningorganics.co.uk
Home delivery

milk co-operatives

For suppliers of Yorkshire milk, Cadog (Wales) and Dairygate, email info@dfob.co.uk or call
tel: 0800 834 823

Milklink deliver West Country milk across the South of England
enquiries@milklink.com
tel: 01752 331800

non-homogenised milk

Duchy (most supermarkets); Manor Farm Organic (Waitrose and Fresh & Wild stores); Bowland Fresh (Booths); English Select Farm Milk (Marks & Spencer); White and Wild (major supermarkets); Rachel's Organic Dairy (major supermarkets); Horizon (independent health food shops)

organic milk or raw-milk producers

Suppliers can be found in *The Organic Directory 2005–2006* (Soil Association/ Green Books) and *The New Shopper's Guide to Organic Food* by Lynda Brown (Fourth Estate, 2003) See www.seedsofhealth.co.uk

pasteurised buffalo milk

Buffalo House
Leighton Buzzard, Bedfordshire
tel: 01525 220256
www.buffalogold.com
Home delivery. Also supplies British Buffalo Mozzarella

index

Figures in bold refer to recipes.